PRAISE FOR:

Veganomicon

"Exuberant and unapologetic . . . recipes don't skimp on fat or flavor, and the eclectic collection of dishes is a testament to the authors' sincere love of cooking and culinary exploration."—*Saveur*

"This is vegan cooking at its best."—*Vegetarian Times*

"Full of recipes for which even a carnivore would give up a night of meat."—*San Francisco Chronicle*

"Seriously good recipes with broad appeal."—*Washington Post*

Vegan Cookies Invade Your Cookie Jar

"[A] winning collection of vegan cookie recipes that should appeal to vegans and nonvegans alike. . . . Decadent recipes . . . show that you can be vegan and still indulge in delicious treats."—*Publishers Weekly*

"Moskowitz and Romero are icons in the vegan world. . . . All your favorite cookies are here, alongside many that are about to become your favorites."—*Bar Harbor Times*

"Outstanding."—*Providence Journal*

Vegan Cupcakes Take Over the World

"[Moskowitz and Romero] produce insanely fetching cupcakes." —*New York Times*

"Written chattily and supportively for even the most oven-phobic. . . . Each page of this cookbook contains an irresistible delight."—*Bust*

Viva Vegan!

Also by Terry Hope Romero and Isa Chandra Moskowitz

Veganomicon

Vegan Cookies Invade Your Cookie Jar

Vegan Cupcakes Take Over the World

200 Authentic and Fabulous
Recipes for Latin Food Lovers

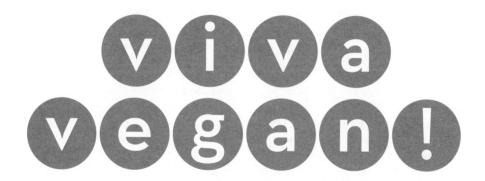

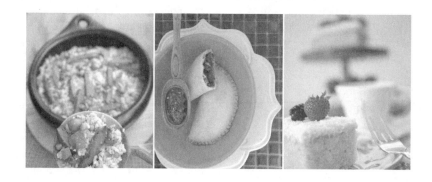

Terry Hope Romero

Da Capo

LIFE
LONG

A Member of the Perseus Books Group

Designed by Trish Wilkinson
Set in 11 point Goudy

Photographs by Angie Gaul
Café con Leche Flan photograph by Ana Cruz

Illustrations by John Stavropoulos and
Terry Hope Romero

Library of Congress
Cataloging-in-Publication Data

Romero, Terry Hope.
    Viva vegan! : 200 authentic and fabulous recipes for Latin food lovers / Terry Hope Romero. — 1st Da Capo Press ed.
        p.   cm.
    Includes index.
    ISBN 978-0-7382-1273-9 (alk. paper)
    1. Vegan cookery. 2. Cookery, Latin American. 3. Cookery (Hot peppers) I. Title.
TX837.R787 2010
641.5'636—dc22   2010000585

First Da Capo Press edition 2010

Published by Da Capo Press
A Member of the Perseus Books Group
www.dacapopress.com

Note: This book is intended only as an informative guide for those wishing to know more about health issues. In no way is this book intended to replace, countermand, or conflict with the advice given to you by your own physician. The ultimate decision concerning care should be made between you and your doctor. We strongly recommend you follow his or her advice. Information in this book is general and is offered with no guarantees on the part of the authors or Da Capo Press. The authors and publisher disclaim all liability in connection with the use of this book. The names and identifying details of people associated with events described in this book have been changed. Any similarity to actual persons is coincidental.

Da Capo Press books are available at special discounts for bulk purchases in the U.S. by corporations, institutions, and other organizations. For more information, please contact the Special Markets Department at the Perseus Books Group, 2300 Chestnut Street, Suite 200, Philadelphia, PA, 19103, or call (800) 810-4145, ext. 5000, or e-mail special.markets@perseusbooks.com.

10 9 8 7 6 5 4 3

For Nerio and Teresa.

CONTENTS

PART I
LATIN CUISINE AND VEGAN COOKING

Introduction   3

The Vegan Latin Pantry   7

Kitchen Tools (or How Do I Slice a Mango?)   23

PART II
THE RECIPES

1   A Few Essential Latino Vegan Recipes   31
     Annatto-Infused Oil (Aciete de Achiote)   31
     Basic Onion-Pepper Sofrito   32
     Steamed Red Seitan   34
     Steamed White Seitan   35
     Chorizo Seitan Sausages   36

2   Salsas and Condiementos   39
     Creamy Avocado-Tomato Salsa (Venezuelan Guasacaca)   39
     Green Tomatillo Sauce   40

Peanut Sauce (Salsa de Mani)   41

Chimichurri Sauce with Smoked Paprika   42

Pickled Red Onions   43

So Good, So Green Dipping Sauce (Green Ají Sauce)   43

Green Onion Salsa   44

Pine Nut Crema   45

Red Chile Sauce   45

Simple Latin Tomato Sauce   46

Classic Roasted Tomatillo Salsa   47

The Only Guacamole Recipe I Ever Make   48

Fresh Tomato Salsa with Roasted Chiles and Winter Salsa and
    Dried Chile Variation   50

Cashew Crema   51

Chocolate-Chile Mole Sauce (a Oaxacan Wannabe)   51

Spicy Salsa Golf   53

Habanero-Melon-Papaya Salsa   53

3 Bocadillos, Snacks, and Appetizers   55

Eggplant Torta Sandwich   55

Mashed Potato Pancakes with Peanut Sauce (Llapingachos)   57

Mixed Mushroom Ceviche   59

Tostones with Avocado and Palm Ceviche   61

Mini Potatoes Stuffed with Mushrooms and Olives (Papas Rellenas)   62

Mexican Side-Street Corn   63

Bite-Size Green Plantain Sandwiches (Patacones)   65

Cubano Vegano Sandwich   66

4 Ensaladas   69

Cilantro-Citrus Vinaigrette   69

Fresh Gazpacho Salsa Dressing   70

Creamy Ancho Chile Dressing   70

Classic Cabbage   71

Spinach-Avocado-Chile   72

Black Bean–Corn Salsa Salad 72

Fruity Chile Slaw 72

Spinach–Brazil Nut–Gazpacho Salad 72

Shredded Carrot-Jicama 72

Chipotle Caesar Mexicano 73

"Any Noche" Romaine and Fruit Salad with Candied Chile Peanuts 73

Chayote and Potato Salad with Capers and Peas 75

Tomato Salad with Sweet Crisp Onions (Ensalada Chilena) 76

Mango-Jicama Chopped Salad 77

Hearty Warm Yuca and Cabbage Salad 78

Salvadorian Marinated Slaw (Curdito) 79

Peruvian Red Chile–Corn Salad with Limas and Cherry Tomatoes 80

Quinoa Salad with Spinach, Olives, and Roasted Peanuts 82

5 Beans and Rice, Los Dos Amigos 83

Basic Beans from Scratch 83

Home-style Refried Beans 86

Red Beans with Dominican-style Sazón 87

Venezuelan-style Black Beans (Caraotas) 89

Colombian-style Red Beans 90

Drunken Beans with Seitan Chorizo 91

Costa Rican Refried Rice and Beans (Gallo Pinto) 92

Classic Stovetop Long-Grain White or Brown Rice 94

Cilantro-Lime Rice 95

Yellow Rice with Garlic 96

Arroz con Coco (Savory Coconut Rice) 97

Savory Orange Rice, Brazilian Style 98

6 Vegan Asado: Tofu, Tempeh, and Seitan 99

Chimichurri Baked Tofu 100

Tofu Chicharrones 101

Zesty Orange Mojo Baked Tofu 102

Latin Baked Tofu 103

Mojo Oven-Roasted Seitan   104

Peruvian Seitan and Potato Skewers (Seitan Anticuchos)   104

Latin Shredded Seitan   106

Seitan Saltado (Peruvian Seitan and Potato Stir-fry)   108

Tempeh Asado   110

Yellow Chile Grilled Tempeh (with Ají Amarillo)   111

Pan-fried Tempeh with Sofrito   112

7 Complete Your Plate: Vegetables, Plantains, and Grains   115

Fried Sweet Plantains   115

Sweet and Nutty Roasted Stuffed Plantains   117

Crispy Fried Green Plantains (Tostones)   118

Mofongo   120

Braised Brazilian Shredded Kale   121

Calabacitas (Mixed Squash Sauté)   122

Swiss Chard with Raisins and Capers   123

Pan-Grilled Vegetables in Chile-Lime Beer   124

Peruvian Potatoes with Spicy "Cheezy" Sauce   125

Crunchy Fried Yuca (Yuca Frita)   126

Yuca with Cuban Garlic-Lime-Mojo Sauce   127

Amaranth Polenta with Roasted Chiles   128

Quinoa–Oyster Mushroom Risotto (Quinotto)   130

8 One-Pot Stews, Casseroles, and Cazuelas   133

Potato-Chickpea Enchiladas with Green Tomatillo Sauce   133

Quick Red Posole with Beans   136

Green Posole Seitan Stew with Chard and White Beans   137

Creamy Potato Peanut Stew (Guatita)   138

Rice with Pigeon Peas (Arroz con Gandules)   140

Spicy Tortilla Casserole with Roasted Poblanos   142

Creamy Corn-Crusted Tempeh Pot Pie (Pastel de Choclo)   144

Arroz con Seitan   145

Portobello Feijoada (Brazilian Black Bean Stew with
Portobello Mushrooms)   147

9 Super Fantástico Latin Soups!   149

Creamy Potato Soup with Avocado (Locro)   149

Cuban Black Bean Soup   150

Hearty Pumpkin and Cranberry Bean Stew (Porotos Granados)   152

Sancocho (Vegetable, Roots, and Plantain Soup)   154

Sweet Potato–Chipotle Bisque   155

Quinoa-Corn "Chowder" with Limas and Ají   156

Tropical Pumpkin Soup   158

Potato-Kale Soup with Sizzling Chorizo   159

10 For the Love of Corn: Arepas, Pupusas, Tortillas, and More   161

Pupusas Stuffed with Black Beans and Plantains   162

Homemade Soft Corn Tortillas   165

Whole Wheat Flour Tortillas with Chia   166

Taquitos with Chorizo and Potatoes   168

Chorizo-Spinach Sopes   171

Black-Eyed–Butternut Tostadas   173

Chipotle, Seitan, and Potato Tacos   174

Arepas (Venezuelan- and Colombian-style "Tortillas")   177

Colombian Grilled Arepas with Corn and Vegan Cheese   179

Arepas Stuffed with Oyster Mushrooms and Pimiento Peppers   180

Arepas with Sexy Avocado-Tempeh Filling (Avocado Pepiada Arepa)   181

Savory Fresh Corn Pancakes (Cachapas)   182

11 You, Too, Can Tamale   185

Savory Vegan Masa Dough   188

Black Bean–Sweet Potato Tamales   189

Red Chile–Seitan Tamales   191

Chocolate Mole Veggie Tamales   193

Farmers' Market Tamales   194

Pineapple-Raisin Sweet Tamales   196

12 Empanadas!   199

Wheat Empanada Dough   199

CONTENTS

Creamy Corn-Filled Empanadas (Empanadas Humitas) — 201
Shredded Seitan and Mushroom Empanadas with Raisins and Olives — 202
Sweet and Spicy Seitan-Potato Empanadas (Bolivian Salteñas) — 204
Corn-Crusted Pumpkin-Potato Empanadas — 207
Beans, Rice, and Sweet Plantain Empanadas — 210

13 Drinks — 213

Creamy Horchata — 213
Real Brown Sugar Limeade (Agua de Papelón) — 214
Tropical Fruit Shake (Batido) — 215
Real Hot Chocolate and Variations — 216
Simple Syrup — 218
Sangria — 219
Mojito — 220
Michelada (Spicy, Salty, Ice-Cold Beer) — 220

14 Desserts and Sweets — 223

Churros — 223
Chocolate para Churros — 225
Sopaipillas with Orange Flower–Agave "Honey" — 226
Un-Dulce de Leche — 227
Crepes with Un-Dulce de Leche and Sweet Plantains — 228
Coconut Tres Leches Cake — 230
Fresh Mango and Guava Bread Pudín — 232
Simply Arroz con Leche — 234
Sweet Coconut Corn Pudding (Majarete) — 235
Dulce de Batata (Sweet Potato Sweet Mash) — 236
Chocolate Orange Spice Cake with Dulce de Batata — 238
Fresh Papaya-Lime Sorbet — 239
Sweet Corn Ice Cream — 240
Buttery Cookies with Thick Dulce de Leche Filling (Alfajores) — 241
Thick Dulce de Leche Filling — 242
Vanilla-Coconut Flan — 243
Café con Leche Flan — 245

Appendix A: Muchos Menus   *249*

Appendix B: Quick-Start Shopping List   *255*

Appendix C: Cooking Terms and Techniques   *261*

Appendix D: Metric Conversion Chart   *267*

Acknowledgments   *269*

Index   *271*

PART I

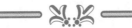

LATIN CUISINE
AND VEGAN COOKING

INTRODUCTION

When friends would ask me what new cookbook I was writing, my answer, "a vegan Latin cookbook," was often met with looks of "*como?*" How can that be? The meatiest cuisine on the planet (so say some) made meatless? Is she *loca*? Has she been living off of raw broccoli for too long? *Oye!* But Latin food and vegan cooking need not be mutually exclusive. In fact, they are a match of culinary perfection, just like beans and rice.

Imagine a world without tomatoes, potatoes, corn, beans, pumpkins, chili peppers, or even chocolate. Who would want to live there? Now imagine life without . . . cow tripe. You're probably thinking . . . *no problemo, senorita!* Well, that first set of ingredients gets me out of bed in the morning. These humble foods are not just culinary gifts but also part of the soul of Latin American cuisine. And even better . . . they're all naturally vegan.

Whether you're vegan, vegetarian, or just excited to give a few meatless meals some real estate on your dinner plate, this cookbook is for you. Interest in vegan cooking is exploding; the Latin community is expanding, and compassionate, healthy, affordable cuisine is more accessible than ever to anyone who loves tacos, tofu, or both.

The spirit and essential flavors of many of my favorite original Latin dishes are preserved in these pages. I aim to keep things authentic, but this is still not your *abuela's* cooking, even if she is vegan (and lucky for you if she is!). These recipes are meatless, dairy-free food fantasies made reality: seitan potato tacos, espresso-spiked vegan caramel flan, and melt-in-your-mouth *alfajore* (*dulce de leche* butter cookie sandwich), and none have ever known a cow. I've also created new recipes infused with Latin flavor, like gazpacho-inflected salad dressing, or a spicy dairy- and egg-free chocolate cake stuffed with a *dulce* made from sweet potatoes; my take on some "*Nuevo, nuevo Latino*" cuisine.

Is your neighborhood sadly lacking a Latin American grocery? I've got you covered. These recipes include the adjustments necessary to bridge the differences between a

North American or European supermarket and a Latin American *mercado*. I'll also encourage you to seek out uniquely Latin ingredients in one of the many Latino markets in most major American cities (hey, we're the largest and fastest growing minority!) or take shopping to the next level on *el Internet*.

WHY LATIN AND VEGAN?

My roots are Venezuelan, I was raised in New England, and then, soon after high school, I ran off to live in New York City (home to many Puerto Ricans, Cubans, and Dominicans). I had the break of a lifetime when I first moved here to work at one of the few Latino owned and operated vegan restaurants in NYC at the time. Bachué (named after an ancient Colombian goddess) was an ambitious mix of macrobiotic staples (brown rice, seaweed), flights of vegan fancy (savory vegan crepes), and an entirely Latino plate of "yellow" brown rice, beans, fried sweet plantains, and grilled seitan. I marveled over what I recognized from my childhood, now transformed and made even better by a Latina vegan fairy godmother (named Veganué?). All of the flavor, texture, and spirit of the real thing—and not an animal's life interrupted. This was what was missing from the vegan spectrum of eating. While my days at that café have long passed, I took with me all those lessons learned and a need to explore this crazy notion of vegan Latin cuisine.

ECONOMICAL AND MEAT FREE

Are you a budget-conscious foodista? Latin food, especially when meat- and dairy-free, is economical and a timely choice for today's challenging times. Many Latin staples are some of the cheapest yet most nutrient-dense foodstuffs you can find at most supermarkets: rice; dried or canned beans; root vegetables; aromatic fresh herbs like cilantro, garlic, and parsley; peppers and onions; creamy coconut milk. Dried Mexican chiles—an inexpensive, authentic ingredient—delivers vast yet nuanced flavor. I don't know about your grocery store, but those I frequent in NYC stock ultra-versatile green plantains that go for six, or sometimes even ten, for one dollar! With such savings it's easier to spend a little extra on good-quality olive oil, organic products, and dairy alternatives. All of these basic, inexpensive ingredients are then used for maximum effect—the greatest nutritional and delicious bang (for your hard-earned buck).

Continuing on with the theme of thrift, Latino food is all about embracing leftovers and repurposing previously cooked foods. Refried beans are likely the most beloved example. Leftover *tostones* (crunchy fried plantains) get a second, sublime life in *mofongo*. Last night's rice and beans are transformed into comforting *gallo pinto*, or quinoa and beans into crispy Peruvian-styled, free-form *tacu tacu*. Old tortillas regain their former glory fried into tostadas or baked into a casserole—some may say even better than they were before.

SEITAN TACO, WHERE HAVE YOU BEEN ALL MY LIFE?

So you're a vegan or vegetarian already and you've already mastered the dinner plate without the animal stuff on it. You get a golden tamale then! But perhaps you've longed for a taco that more resembles the delights found at a taco truck (usually off limits to those who don't eat animals) than it does fast food. Or you've longed for a world beyond standard vegetarian fare like bean burritos or soy cheese nachos. You'll find plenty to get started here. Many of my recipe testers have become devotees of Peruvian panca chili paste or homemade dairy-less *dulce de leche* sauce and have worked these into their regular vegan menu rotation.

FOR ALL YOU LATINAS OUT THERE: *NO TRIPE FOR ME, GRACIAS*

I also wrote *Viva Vegan!* with Latinas (and Latin food lovers) in mind. Perhaps you've picked up this book with an emerging desire to quit meat and dairy, or even just to eat less of it. You're nearest and dearest to *mi corazón* and I aim to get you off to a promising career as a vegan Latina (or Latino). The easy part is cracking open this book and cooking up a soothing bowl of vegetable-filled *posole* stew or a batch of *arroz con seitan*. The hard part (I know what you're thinking) is what to tell your mom when she presents you with a dozen pork tamales for Christmas, brimming with all those unmentionable animal bits you don't want to eat. Just remember, you're not alone. I'm a pragmatist and the easiest way to make things happen is to step into the kitchen and start cooking for yourself. Experience has taught me and countless others that the way to a complaining *familia* is through their stomachs. Learn to master delicious vegan adaptations of traditional dishes (or invent your own new takes on meaty favorites) and everyone will learn to come around to your way of thinking. Or, at the very least, ask you when you're making dinner again! Didn't grow up with all the Latin foods you wish you could have? Maybe your parents thought it was important you got to know chicken noodle soup instead of *sancocho*, tuna casserole instead of *pupusas*, baked beans instead of *arroz con gandules*, all in hopes that you'd fit in with the other kids at school. I'll say it just one more time . . . this book is for you, too! Think of it as a way to get to know your roots just a little more, one chomp of *yuca frita* at a time.

SPICY FOOD PHOBIC? DON'T DROP THIS BOOK!

A word on heat: Not all Latin American food is spicy or drenched in chilies. Throughout much of the Caribbean and many parts of South America, chilies (often called *ají*) are popular but used with care. In fact, you might even find that some of these foods in their native countries could use a little extra spice. In those cases I've included options to "pepper up" things in anticipation of the North Americans' love of chili-laced Mexican cuisine. But ultimately it's your kitchen and you can decide how hot you want your recipes to be.

FOOD FROM THE OTHER AMERICA(S)

Sometimes it's best to leave *mondongo* and *morcilla* to those who really want to eat it (if you don't know what those are, then well, I'm not going to tell you!). My goal is not to "veganize" every Latin recipe out there. Instead, I've taken all of the gorgeous diversity of herbs, spices, vegetables, legumes, and fruits, and intertwined it with these vegan recipes to convey the history, love, and *sabór* of the Latin palate.

Empanadas and tamales are as much an American staple as burgers and apple pie. Eating Latin American food is eating *American* food . . . we all live in the Americas (if you're on this side of the planet that is). That said, Latin American food has an entire place of its own in the culinary universe. If you're a Latina and know tortillas but not *arepas*, or are just someone hungry for an additional approach to eating meatless and dairy free, I hope this can be a map on your journey to exploring a few new cultures in the convenience of your own home kitchen.

Enough with the reading, let's get to cooking (and eating)!

THE VEGAN LATIN PANTRY

$\mathcal{N}$ow with the formalities out of the way, let's chat about all of the great ingredients that go into these recipes! Not meant to be an all-inclusive list, this is a rundown of things to have on hand. Some may be old hat to you if cilantro is a regular item in your veggie bin; others could be entirely new, such as *ají amarillo* paste or masa harina. Likewise, some of these ingredients are Latin-food-specific and found in friendly Latin American grocery stores; some are more vegan in nature and may require a trip to the health food store.

Read through this section, even if just a quick scan, to get an idea of what that next shopping trip should include or if you are already in the clear with certain ingredients. For a handy take-along guide for shopping in Latin markets or health food stores, step over to appendix B. And for suggestions on shopping online for hard-to-find ingredients, see (you guessed it) appendix B again.

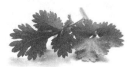

PANTRY AND GROCERY INGREDIENTS

I've broken down things that don't need refrigeration into three lists: basic items, Latin ingredients, and vegan stuff. Depending on where you live, this could mean three different shopping trips or just one stop and a thorough taking-stock of the kitchen cupboards.

The Basics

Both vegans and Latinos need cooking oils or flavorful broths for cooking. Because there is a lot of wiggle room regarding quality of that olive oil or brands of vegetable broth, I leave it up to your excellent personal taste to pick out what you enjoy. It's likely you may already possess some or all of these ingredients, but be sure to check exactly how much is there before starting a recipe.

Extra-virgin olive oil is the go-to olive oil especially in salads and uncooked items. More refined oils such as **virgin olive oil** and **olive oil blends** are less costly and easy to buy in bulk, but you might sacrifice a little flavor. Some like to reserve the more expensive extra-virgin oil where the flavor will more likely be savored, such as in salad dressings or drizzled on top of soup, and use cheaper oils for pan-frying.

Peanut oil, **canola oil**, **grapeseed oil**, and **coconut oil** are used to approximate other flavors in Latin American cooking. Peanut oil is superb for deep- and pan-frying and its aroma complements strong flavors such as hot chiles or tomatoes. Use canola for baking, frying, or where a light-tasting oil is needed. Grapeseed is very light and right for salads when the flavor of olive oil may overwhelm other ingredients. Coconut oil is used in some Latin dishes and is occasionally called for in these recipes. Look for organic, unhydrogenated natural coconut oil. Use refined coconut oil if you don't want a coconut flavor . . . unrefined coconut oil has a pronounced coconut aroma.

Shortening and **margarine** come into play when making tamales or baked goods. Both once had a bad rap sheet with nasty stuff like hydrogenated fats and chemicals, but some have since evolved to meet the needs of today's healthier chef who still appreciates a "buttery" cookie or rich, tender piecrust. These are useful ingredients in Latin cooking as they both step in for lard—the favored fat for tamales and flour tortillas—in very traditional recipes. Look for new brands of shortening and margarine that are labeled free of trans fats and non-

hydrogenated, and make sure that they're also vegan (some brands think it's cool to pump up margarine with whey or other milk solids). As of this writing Spectrum and Earth Balance are two common and excellent vegan brands; the latter is also available in a handy solid stick form.

Long-grain white rice is king in Latin American cooking and can be enjoyed with just about any Latin cuisine. Delicious and versatile organic long-grain white can be found lots of places; even the old-guard Latin grocery brand Goya is on the organic kick! I personally love to use nontraditional aromatic basmati hybrids (such as California basmati or Texmati) for my own home cooking, as the consistency is similar to white long-grain rice, plus they have a mouthwatering buttered-popcorn aroma, without the need of cows or corn. The only kinds of rice I suggest to refrain from using in these Latin recipes are Asian short-grain rice, risotto rice (unless called for), and sticky/sushi-type rice.

Long-grain brown rice can also be used in these dishes, keeping in mind that the total liquid content and cooking time will increase quite a bit (usually doubled).

Vegetable broth makes for moister and more flavorful casseroles, stir-fries and sauces. (Use it as broth in soups, too, of course.) Unless you really love making your own vegetable broth, use boxed broth or even broth reconstituted from vegetarian bouillon cubes. Try different brands to find one you like. Use low-sodium broth, if you prefer. There are also good "chicken"-flavored vegan cubes, and vegetable broth in a handy concentrated paste form (Better Than Boullion brand, for one) that's concentrated enough that it can easily be stored in the fridge but makes many quarts of broth whenever you need it. In general, avoid brands that have artificial additives or monosodium glutamate (MSG).

White wine and **red wine** are a flavorful cooking liquid that I love to use when deglazing (page 261) a sauté pan. The cheap stuff is perfect! Some wines might be filtered with animal-based ingredients, so just be sure to choose a certifiably vegan wine for your cooking needs. One handy site that can confirm the veganness of your wine is barnivore.com.

Red wine vinegar and **white wine vinegar** are widely used as seasonings in Latin cuisine. Just a tablespoon in a bean soup can help sharpen flavors and provide a perfect contrast to the spicy and earthy flavors present in lots of Latin foods. If you prefer something a little milder, **rice vinegar** can be substituted, or if you don't mind and have a big bottle of it already (since it has dozens of household uses), plain **white distilled vinegar** is a sharp and tangy addition to recipes. **Malt vinegar** is fine for use in soups or spicy marinades, as the malty flavors are compatible with salty or strong flavors. The only vinegar I don't recommend for Latin cooking is apple cider vinegar. Although it's the dar-

ling of health food cooking, I find that the strong cider aroma and flavor can overwhelm and just doesn't taste right with these foods.

Beer is remarkable not just for drinking—and in an ice-cold Michelada (page 220 anyone?)—but *fantastico* when used in marinades, as a substitute for vegetable broth in rice dishes, or even incorporated into hearty stews. I can't say enough about the flavor boost beer can bring to foods, especially spicy or garlicky dishes. Mexican beer is my go-to beer for cooking Latin stuff and most commonly available brands, such as Corona, Dos Equis, and Presidente, are vegan as of this writing.

Liquid smoke is my most favorite of sneaky flavoring ingredients. Entirely vegan and made by distilling wood smoke with water (sounds amazingly alchemical!), a shake or two into beans or marinades imparts a delicate smoky flavor that stands in nicely for bacon or ham. **Vegetarian Worcestershire sauce**, our vegan stand-in for its not-so-vegan counterpart, is used in many Latin countries, where it is called *salsa ingles*, as a common seasoning for beans, rice, and other savory dishes. Even **soy sauce** shows up in some cuisines (such as the Japanese and Chinese influences in Peruvian food) and, of course, since we're vegans we just can't get enough of the stuff, plus it helps flavor and balance such soy foods as tofu and tempeh. I like to use mild Chinese-style light soy sauce in Latin recipes (save the tamari and shoyu for Japanese cuisine, please).

Freshly ground black pepper is habit forming and not too expensive as far as habits go. For a few bucks, a decent pepper mill and a bag of mixed peppercorns bring endless moments of pepper-grinding joy.

Salt is also a personal preference item. I use two kinds of salt: coarse **kosher salt** is great for general all-purpose cooking, but I still use **granulated table salt** for baking. If you choose to use kosher salt, use just a teeny bit more than table salt, as it has more volume because of its flaky texture. **Sea salt** is a tasty all-purpose salt for all of you gourmet hippies out there.

The Vegan Pantry

It used to be that a drive to the health food store was necessary to get tofu or soy milk, but now it seems any generously stocked supermarket or corner grocery will have many of these items. *¡Viva la vegan revolución!*

Nondairy milk is a generic term for your choice of **soy milk**, **rice milk**, **almond milk**, **oat milk**, **hazelnut milk**, **hemp milk**, or other nut-based milk in these recipes. Excellent commercial brands now exist for all of these milks and it's worth trying a few to see which one you like. I'll list my preference for the type of milk in the recipe, but if you hate, say, almond milk, switch it to hemp or oat or whatever floats your boat. This flexibility of substitution, however, excludes coconut milk or soy creamer . . . which will be listed specifically and unequivocably if a recipe calls for it.

Here are my own personal preferences for using nondairy milks: I like to use **soy milk** mostly for baking and making flan, as it contains plenty of protein to help provide structure and body to the final product. I adore **almond milk** and use it when a baked good doesn't need much nondairy milk, say a tablespoon or two. And it makes a killer *horchata* and delightful *arroz con leche*. For a thick creamy *café con leche* or for use in vegan ice cream, I like **hemp milk, hazelnut** milk, or the new **coconut**-based drinking milk So Delicious Coconut Milk Beverage. And **rice milks** are a favorite for *merengadas* or for any sweet and delicate smoothie.

Heavy cream substitute is yet another generic term for the soy- or nut-based cream substitutes now available. Silk brand is the most commonly found **soy creamer** and the new MimicCreme, although not as widely available, is a wonderful heavy cream stand-in made from almonds and cashews. The unsweetened variety is excellent for use in soups. I generally use only plain soy creamer and unsweetened nut-based creamers.

Do not by any means use that powdered "nondairy creamer" designed for coffee; it's insanely artificial tasting and full of bad-for-you hydrogenated oils. Just say no!

Tofu usually comes up when the topic of vegan food arises. Properly prepared tofu is like the chameleon of foods and can be transformed into savory entrées, light desserts, and everything in between. Generally the water-packed, chilled "Chinese" firm style is used for baked tofu and savory dishes. "Japanese" silken tofu (either water-packed or boxed) is used for some desserts or where a smooth-textured, blended consistency is desired. Consult the recipe for which kind of tofu should be used.

Tempeh originally hails from Indonesia but has since spread like a mushroom all over the non-meat-eating community. The short story is that it's a fermented soybean cake, which sounds terrible but when properly made tastes awesome! It has a firm, distinctly non-tofu-like texture, and a rich, nuanced flavor. Tempeh should be lightly steamed first to help soften it up to absorb the flavor from marinating (the second step) just before frying (the last step that makes everything great, including tempeh).

Vital wheat gluten flour is special wheat flour whose starchy portion has been removed so only the protein gluten is left. Silky and a pale creamy color, it is used to make seitan (wheat meat) in these recipes. You'll most likely have to go to a health food store to find this item, or online to check out baking specialty stores. I recommend purchasing a lot of it, either in bulk or the largest packages you can, if you become really excited about making seitan.

Seitan is a wonderfully chewy "meat from wheat" crafted from seasoned vital wheat gluten, which can be purchased or made at home. Of the unmeat power trio (tofu, tempeh, and seitan), this one usually wins over omnivores first with its chewiness,

excellent grill-ability, and meaty appearance. Homemade seitan can be as involved a process as you like; the seitan recipes in this book (steamed rather than boiled or baked like most seitan) are fairly minimalist and don't require too much fiddling on your part. Seitan is great for individuals who can't handle soy (as long as it's not seasoned with soy sauce!); it pairs superbly with Latin cuisine; and when sliced and cooked just the right way, it even looks like meat.

Nutritional yeast is a special ingredient no vegan or health nut should be without, as it provides a cheeselike flavor to foods, along with a boost of vitamin B_{12}, protein, and other things to keep you alive. Look for golden yellow powdery flakes with a savory smell and melt-on-your-tongue texture, either sold in bulk or packed in jars. This book uses it primarily for flavoring seitan and in a few other cheeselike concoctions. Absolutely *do not* confuse with brewer's yeast, which smells like old socks and will not work in these recipes!

Textured vegetable protein (TVP) is made from soy and is available in dehydrated form (usually chunks or small bits). It always needs be rehydrated before eating and is best when tossed into a simmering sauce or soup. When flavored correctly it transforms in something hearty and chewy and provides a satisfying meatlike experience. TVP is an old-school vegetarian meat substitute that I only use occasionally in some soups and stews for a special hearty, chewy effect. You won't need to purchase much if you choose to use it with this book; one large bag of the large chunk style should suffice. You could also substitute Soy Curls—a dried, soy-based protein made with whole soybeans—for TVP in any recipe, too.

The Latin Pantry

Beans, rice, chile peppers . . . they're all right here, along with a few other things you may not be but should get more familiar with. These ingredients cover most everything you'll need to make the following recipes, but be sure to read through a recipe first to see if there are special things required.

Beans, cooked to perfection, are the heart and soul of so many of Latin recipes, not to mention one fine, filling, and wonderfully cheap source of protein, fiber, and nutrients. **Canned beans** are an ideal convenience food during those busy times and are useful when you require just a little bit of beans and not a whole pot. With a little advanced planning, you may find that **dried beans** need not be inconvenient at all and even lend themselves to freezing.

Purchased **frozen beans** are not as widely used, but frozen fava beans and frozen pigeon peas work well for these recipes. If you're lucky enough to find either, I promise you'll be delighted by the fresh, vegetable-like texture that big fava beans provide.

Frozen pigeon peas (*gandules*) are common wherever frozen Caribbean ingredients can be found and have superior flavor and texture to the canned variety. Frozen beans can be added directly straight from the freezer to rice prior to cooking and do not require thawing.

Coconut milk is practically a requirement for so many tropical dishes and desserts. Canned full-fat or reduced-fat coconut milk can be used interchangeably unless noted.

Coconut cream is the concentrated fat from coconut milk, often containing finely grated bits of coconut flesh. It's rich, creamy, and coconutty (perhaps as close to a decadent "dairy" thing as naturally vegan ingredients get) and can be obtained either by skimming it off the top of a can of full-fat coconut milk or by purchasing it separately in small cans or in solid blocks. Some solid brands of coconut cream are somewhat dehydrated and need to be chopped into chunks and soaked in water to be reconstituted into a creamy consistency once more. Check the ingredients label to be sure the brand you use is pure coconut and vegan.

Panela, a minimally refined natural brown cane sugar, is also known by many regional names such as *chancaca*, *papelón*, or *piloncillo* and can even be found in some Indian markets as *jaggery* or *gur*. It's a true brown sugar—it's not just white sugar with molasses added. *Panela* is not overly sweet and has strong molasses, caramel, and honey-like flavors. It

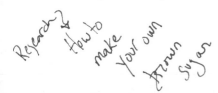

These Are a Few of My Favorite Beans

To love Latin cuisine is to get to know the bean better. Each region has its favorite "hero" bean, usually complemented by a few runners-up, but I think each bean is a superstar and should get equal plate time. Next time you take a visit to your local Latin market, pick up a bag of your favorite bean *and* a brand-new bean to try. Sometimes I even soak and cook two separate bean batches at a time if I'm anticipating a week or two of bean-centric eating. Anytime you find an intriguing bean, just swap it for a basic batch of cooked beans, pair it with rice, or use it in a soup. Beans encourage experimentation!

If you're at a grocer with a big Latin selection, you may find some of the more uncommon "ethnic" beans available in canned form, too. Usually they are not organic, but these are a good choice if you want to try out a new bean but don't want to commit to soaking and cooking a whole batch. If you can buy organic—pintos, black, and garbanzo are all fairly common organic choices now—do so, as they tend to taste better and some brands also use much less salt than nonorganic brands do.

All-Purpose Beans, Good for Any Cuisine or Meal

- Pinto (very Mexican/American Southwest)
- Garbanzo
- Black (essential for Cuban, Venezuelan, and Brazilian dishes)
- Red kidney
- White kidney (cannellini)
- Pink beans

Specialty Beans, for Variety and Extra Specialness

- Cargamanto, Roman, or cranberry bean (Colombian and Caribbean, with rice or refried)
- Bola roja, a large round red bean (Colombian, with rice)
- Dominican red, similar to red kidney (Dominican, rice 'n' beans)
- Canary, a creamy yellow bean (Peruvian, rice 'n' beans, soup)
- Salvadorian/Central American red, small red beans (*gallo pinto*, rice 'n' beans)
- Pigeon peas (Puerto Rican rice 'n' beans, *arroz con gandules*)
- Giant or small lima/butter beans (Peruvian, soups and salads)

gives everything it's made with a pretty caramel-amber color. Not granulated like more refined sugars, *panela* is sold in heavy, golden brown cakes or cones, and if relatively fresh, is easy to grate or chop. Once the package is opened, use *panela* as soon as possible,

as it will start slowly to dry out and become more difficult to grate. Dried-out *panela*, if not a little hard, is still perfectly fine for melting for use in syrups or drinks.

Dried and ground or precooked corn flours, commonly known as **masa harina** or

Research & How to make your own Brown Sugar

masarepa, are absolutely essential if you want to make homemade tortillas, tamales, arepas, and so many more uniquely Latin American "breads." Previous generations of Latinos made masa harinas by grinding prepared dried corn by hand on stone or wood. These days, if you have a lot of time on your hands, you could try that, too, but if you're wondering if it's hard, thankless work, then yes, *amiga*, it certainly is! Fortunately, packaged Mexican-style masa harina and Colombia/Venezuelan-style *masarepa* flour is widely available.

"Mexican"-style masa harina flour is made with corn first treated with lime water (a process called *nixtamalization* . . . try that one in your next Scrabble game), hulled, dried then ground into a fine flour. All of that work makes the nutrients in the corn more accessible and gives masa harina its characteristic delectable aroma and flavor. **Instant masa harina** is the most common and widely available variety—it's typically sold in 5-pound paper sacks and specifically labeled "for tortillas, tamales, *pupusas, sopes*. . . ." It has a pale creamy color and a fine texture. Fresh masa is highly revered by masa harina snobs, but like many things valued by snobs it may be difficult to obtain (at least outside of Central America). MASECA is probably the easiest brand to find in the United States; Bob's Red Mill also makes an excellent golden masa harina, too.

The other kind of precooked corn flour is *masarepa*, sometimes called by the brand name of Harina PAN or *harina para arepas*. Got all that? Don't worry, just look for "arepa" on the bag and you likely have the right thing. This special corn flour is used almost exclusively in Colombia and Venezuela and has a totally different character and taste from masa harina. Look for this in typically plastic, smaller 1- to 2½-pound bags. It comes in both white and yellow (no difference in flavor, though) and has a coarser texture that more closely resembles American-style cornmeal (but still it's not the same!). This corn flour is made from corn kernels that have been cooked, hulled, dried, and then ground into a rough flour without the lime water soak. *If in doubt*, always check the bag to see where it's imported from; it should be from either Colombia or Venezuela. *Mexican masa harina cannot be substituted for masarepa* (and vice versa). They taste completely different!

There really is no substitution for either of these masa harinas. What I refer to as "North American" cornmeal—the coarse stuff that's used for cornbread or polenta—is entirely different from Latin corn harina and won't work in these recipes. If you're in doubt as to what kind of corn product you have, simply stir some with a little warm water. Regular cornmeal will just become a runny mush, whereas either masa harina or *masarepa* will form a soft dough that you will be able to roll and flatten and make shapes with.

The good news is that both styles of corn harina are readily found in most New York

City (and large North American cities in general) supermarkets that carry basic Latin American products (if you see Goya stuff, you're probably in luck).

Dried chiles are essential to Mexican and Central American cuisine. This book calls for a flavorful selection not too overwhelming (to me at least) in the heat department. Good-quality dried chiles should appear shiny and not dusty. Depending on the variety, such as the fleshy ancho or morita chile peppers, the dried chile will

An Absolute Beginner's Guide to Dried Chiles

At some point in pursuing your daily requirement of chile peppers, you may find yourself standing before a bewildering selection of bagged dried chiles. What to do next? Just get excited and recognize that there are no mistakes to be made here, just willingness to get a little burned (but hopefully in a delicious way). Some exclusively Latin stores may not even label their bagged chiles . . . you just have to ask what is what!

Use rubber gloves when handling fresh or dried hot chiles. Or if you don't, just be sure not to rub your eyes (or other sensitive areas; just thought you should know) for a while after handling chile peppers.

There are a lot of hot chile pepper slingers out there who are more than willing to profess expertise on this subject. While I may not be a chileologist, the following are some of my favorites:

Ancho, guajillo, or **pasilla**. These earthy, raisiny/fruity chiles range from mild to medium heat and are extremely versatile when used in many sauces and salsas. They go great with Mexican food, of course, but also pair well with American foods whenever you want to add a special chile kick.

Chipotle (which is just a generic term for a dried smoked chile, but jalapeño chipotles rule the roost) chiles are another flexible pepper useful in sauces, stews, and salsas and excellent in marinades.

Dried **Peruvian mirasol peppers** are similar in heat to **jalapeños**, with a dark yellow color and warm tropical flavor. Large soft, dried **Peruvian panca peppers** are mild but loaded with delicious, earthy, sweet flavor.

There are numerous thin-skinned, shiny red chile peppers that look prettier than their raisinlike cousins and generally range from medium to hot to very hot. Large, tapered **costeños**, fiery thin **chile de arbol** dried chiles, and little hot **pequín** chiles are flavorful and can be stretched out over many uses. I generally like to use them blended with a milder, moister chile such as ancho, for a sauce or salsa that has a full range of flavors and more nuanced heat. As a general guide, I use the seeds from chiles for a hotter final product, but I also like to remove the seeds from soft chiles such as ancho, as they tend be too large and tough. Tiny chiles, such as pequín, usually don't need to have their seeds removed and can be ground up whole.

Different chiles hit our taste buds in different ways. Some hit you immediately with bright heat, whereas others linger toward the back of the palate and build up with every bite. I rarely buy just one bag of dried chiles . . . it's too much fun to blend and experiment with them, plus they last nearly forever stored in a cool, dark cabinet. (If you do intend to store them forever, keep your chiles in an airtight container or a tin.)

feel flexible, sort of like dried fruit or leather (or pleather, for vegan's sake!), and not completely tough or hard. Chiles with thin walls, such as costeño or arbol, will be somewhat brittle but should also be dust free to denote good quality and relative freshness (for a dried-out chile, that is).

Canned chiles, such as chipotle in adobo sauce, are an excellent Mexican product to have on hand, so stock up two or more cans.

About Ají, or Just When You Thought You Were onto Chiles

A*jí* (ah-HEE) is a general term for "chile pepper," used primarily in South America and the Latin Caribbean. Hundreds of varieties exist and each region has its favorites, from the *ají dulce* of Puerto Rico and Cuba to the *ají amarillo* and *ají panca* of Peru, Bolivia, and Ecuador. Unfortunately, most of these chiles are difficult to find fresh in the United States, but it's easier to find them as jarred pastes (or *crema*) that blend effortlessly into sauces and soups. Always refrigerate jars of *ají* paste after opening.

These *ajís* in this easy-to-use paste form have steadily become a regular in my cooking. They could become a whole new way for you to enjoy spicy Latin food (beyond more familiar Mexican cuisine), too! Look for these superconvenient *ají* pastes wherever South American groceries can be found, or order them online.

Ají amarillo is a yellow chile pepper found throughout Peruvian and Bolivian cuisine. It's shaped a little like a large jalapeño with a wide end at the stem and a rounded taper at the other end. With deep yellow-orange flesh, a heat level somewhat less than a jalapeño, and a sweet, fruity finish, I am certain it could take North American chile fans by storm if given a chance.

Ají panca is a large, tapered dark red chile with an irresistible deep earthy flavor with strong sweet notes of ripe fruit, smoke, and red and black berries. It is very mild, more so than red ancho chiles, but packs so much flavor. The paste made from this *ají* is my favorite in marinades, sauces, and dressings.

Ají rocoto is a general term for a group of large, rounded South American chiles that are fiery and flavorful. A jar of rocoto paste will last you, unless you are a true hot sauce freak. I've also found frozen rocoto, that make a nice addition finely minced and use sparingly, in fresh salsas or tossed into ceviches.

If you can't find premade pastes, you can improvise with dried *ají*. For about 1 tablespoon of amarillo paste, take one dried *ají amarillo*, remove the seeds and stem, tear into pieces, soak in 2 tablespoons of boiling water until soft, and then grind into a paste. Follow this same technique for the other chiles, adjusting the liquid to a little more if using very large dried chiles.

If you're lucky enough to find frozen whole *ají* (or fresh, lucky you!), slice and seed the chiles. Cover with boiling water and let sit for 5 minutes. Drain, reserve the soaking liquid, and peel the skins off, if desired (this is traditional but if I'm feeling lazy, I don't bother). Puree the chiles in a food processor, scrape the sides a few times, and pour in enough reserved soaking liquid to form a smooth paste. Or roast to remove the skins, for a different flavor. Use this fresh paste as soon as possible. Estimate about one whole amarillo-size *ají* for every tablespoon of sauce.

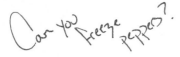

Can you freeze peppers?

These smoky chiles in tangy tomato sauce can't be beat and are majorly habit-forming in sauces, soups, or dips. Canned mild green chiles, on the other hand, don't taste nearly as good as fresh Anaheims and so I only use these in moments of desperation (or just use fresh Cubanelles instead). **Pickled jalapeños** (or **jalapeños en escabiche**) are better from a jar but, in a pinch, canned works. These are essential companions to tacos.

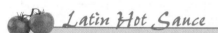

Latin Hot Sauce

Fans of Latin food, in particular Mexican cuisine, just have to have a bottle of hot sauce. The hot sauce one is raised with tends to be a lifelong relationship, so I'm not about to steer anyone away from their partner-in-hot sauce. But if you're shopping around, the following are good, authentic sauces to test out. Avoid using American-style hot sauces with Latin food; it just ain't right. A good hot sauce is an affordable luxury that makes just about anything taste better.

Tapatío (that handsome sombrero man) is always a safe and moderately spicy bet for beans, tacos, marinades, and even Micheladas (page 220). **Valentina** is another good choice, and **Cholula** is a saucy lady whose mellow ways are for hot sauce newbies. **El Yucateco** habanero hot sauces are a great way to enjoy this feisty pepper on just about anything.

Although Mexican sauces get lots of face time, try out other regional hot sauces. I like Ecuadorian hot sauces, typically thick and moderately spicy concoctions seasoned with tomatoes and garlic.

Dried corn husks can't be eaten but are necessary for making tamales. Corn husks are a very natural product and can vary in quality, so shop around! Inferior husks may be packaged sloppily; not properly cleaned, with globs of dried corn silk remaining or husks that are small and uneven. Quality corn husks will look clean, be split and spread open, and stacked in easy-to-use bundles. These bundled husks are often a larger size that helps greatly in making tamales . . . so if you encounter a bunch on your next shopping trip, stock up! Kept in a dry and cool place, tightly wrapped corn husks will keep indefinitely. Just make sure they don't get wet (or they can go moldy), and tamales can be yours today, tomorrow, or next year.

LATIN PRODUCE

This list includes essential vegetables and fruits that you can find in most any grocery stores (tomatoes, onions, and bell peppers, for instance) and specialty items that require a trip to the Latin market or a supermarket that services a Latin community.

Fresh Latin **chile peppers** can vary greatly by region, especially in North America. **Jalapeño** and **serrano** are safe bets and have become almost commonplace in most supermarkets. Those living in the American West and Southwest will probably be the lucky ducks and have some of the best selection of fresh chiles outside of Central and South America, so make me proud and try every kind of chile you chance upon. Fiery **habaneros** are popping up in supermarkets with greater frequency, and the mild and deliciously stuffable **poblano** and **Anaheim** appear increasingly at farmers' markets and sometimes Whole Foods.

Probably the most familiar to Norte Americans, Mexican chiles such as the jalapeño and the serrano have been workhorses in the quest to take over gringo palates. Anaheim chiles are the large bright green chiles with a mild kick that you'll often find in lots of Mexican-style dishes in restaurants and are great for grilling and stuffing. Poblanos are the blocky, large dark green (or bright red when ripe) chiles that usually star in chiles rellenos, but are great also roasted, sliced, and added to stews, soups, tamales, casseroles, and anything Mexican. Habaneros are now famous (and rightly so) for their fabulously high Scoville rating (Scovilles measure peppers' heat, with bell peppers at zero and habaneros at 100,000 *escovilles*!) but also for the tropical fruity flavor they impart to foods.

Cilantro was once unknown outside of Latin and Asian cuisines, but now can be found almost everywhere. If you don't like cilantro's aromatic and slightly "soapy" taste, you may substitute flat-leaf parsley for color, but the flavor will not be the same. Don't bother with dried cilantro; it's tasteless and therefore useless. Save your money and buy an extra bottle of good Greek oregano, Mexican oregano, or extra ground cumin!

Flat-leaf (Italian) parsley is used in parts of South America, especially where the cuisine has strong European or Italian influences. It's essential for chimichurri sauce and is also a visual substitute for cilantro, when serving dishes to people who don't like cilantro.

Plantains look like large green monster bananas but are far more versatile, ranging from starchy to sweet, for a wide range of texture and flavor. Buy green plantains if that's what your recipe calls for, or if you don't need ripe plantains for at least 3 days. Unlike the familiar banana, it may take up to a week or more for a green plantain to get truly ripe. Plantains can be found usually stocked with Latin American produce, often in big bins. If you're lucky, your grocery may have separate bins of both green and ripe plantains.

Yuca (also known as **cassava** or **manioc**) is a large, starchy tropical tuber eaten in many parts of the world and an important food source in many areas of tropical Latin America. It looks like a long, thick yam with white flesh and dark brown, barklike skin, often covered with wax to keep in moisture. Yuca has an ultrastarchy consistency with a somewhat creamy texture. The flesh has lots of fiber and its nutty, light sweetness is well suited for frying, mashing, or just boiling. Yuca must always be boiled before a second cooking, such as frying. Look for it in supermarkets where root vegetables or Latin produce is displayed. You can also find in the

If you're lucky and have access to a farmers' market that services a sizable Latin American community, then maybe, just maybe, you'll be able to source interesting fresh herbs that rarely are seen outside of home-cooked meals.

Culantro (also called **recao** or **Mexican/wild coriander**): Not to be confused with cilantro, tropical-growing culantro is far less widely known and also used in some Southeast Asian cuisines in addition to Central and South American cuisines. Look for a tender green herb with long, jagged-edged leaves 1 to 1½ inches wide. It has a flavor similar to cilantro yet is stronger and more pronounced.

Verdolaga, also known as **purslane**, is a favorite of mine. A common weed practically all over the world, it's popular in soups in Central America and is just too damned nutritious—besides having excellent crunch, with loads of nutrition (Omega-3s galore!)—to pummel with a weed whacker. Try some fresh in salads or in sandwiches or tacos.

Papalo is a leafy herb with rounded wide leaves with a sharp herbal scent a little bit like cilantro's. Enjoy it fresh as a leafy green tucked into tacos or salads, or layered in a *torta* sandwich.

Huazontle is sometimes referred to as **Mexican broccoli**. A large herb with a substantial flowering head, it's traditionally cooked in an omelet-like entrée and topped with a light tomato sauce. A vegany way to enjoy this is to lightly blanch the flower buds in salted boiling water, drain, chop, and add to the filling of chiles rellenos (page 142).

Occasionally you'll be able to find fresh **epazote**. It's quite different from the dried stuff and very pungent. Use in beans and as you would use dried epazote, substituting 1 scant tablespoon of chopped fresh herb for 1 teaspoon of the dried.

frozen aisle prepeeled, frozen chunks of yuca that are very convenient to use.

Besides yuca, there are other fun tropical tubers to try. A favorite of mine is **ñame**, which has yellow flesh and a sweet, ripe plantainlike aroma. **Batata** is similar to yellow-flesh sweet potatoes. **Yautia** is part of the vast yam family and has a subtle sweetness and starchy texture.

Yellow, white, and **red onions** are a staple and should always be on your shopping list!

Green, red, and **yellow bell peppers** play an important role in making the *sofrito*

recipes in this book. Sweet Italian long green "frying" peppers or pale green tapered Cubanelles are tasty and interesting substitutes for the standard sweet bell pepper; I like to use a few of each when making a big batch of *sofrito* or *sazón*. Large sweet Hungarian red peppers are also nice in place of red bell peppers.

Garlic and **green onions** are always VIP guests at this Latin cooking party. I invite you to add as much garlic as you require to any recipe, as it's often a personal thing, keeping in mind if you really go nuts with the garlic, you may have an interesting time getting some people to get personal with. Whatever, you know you're delicious.

Always have a bulb (or more) of garlic on hand. Choose bulbs that feel heavy for their size and are very firm. Garlic is old and dried out when the bulb feels light or the skin on the bulbs collapses or releases dust when squeezed.

Green onions add a sharp, fresh oniony flavor to soups, beans, and salsas.

Fresh lime juice is used over and over, so purchase two or more limes at a time, or invest in a bottle of concentrated lime juice if you don't want to mess around with squeezing. Lemons can be substituted for limes, if needed. Yummy little Key limes have that special tropical zing that reminds me of the *limóns* of tropical Latin America and taste extra special in Latin drinks, desserts, or vegetables.

Avocados are now enjoyed all over North America. My dad came to America in the late '60s and recalls when finding an avocado in suburban New England was as likely as tripping over a palm tree . . . luckily, those days are just a memory. Guacamole is a universally loved way to get a dose of this creamy green fruit, but any Latin meal can benefit from a few slices of perfectly ripe *aguacate*.

As with beans or plantains, proper use of an avocado requires a little bit of advance planning. Most avocados are sold unripe and require 1 to 3 days to get that perfect "sweet spot" but not so ripe as to become mushy, the flesh streaked with brown veins, or bitter. Unripe avocados will be rock hard and

Which Avocado?

The small, pebbly green-black-skinned **Haas avocado** rules the fruit stand in North America. And no wonder—it has a dense and buttery flesh that makes outstanding guac and jazzes up most any meal you can think of. Haas is the one truly all-year-round avocado.

Perhaps you're wondering if there are other challengers out there to Haas's tasty green reign. Actually, many varieties of avocados are cultivated in North America and Central America, but only a few make it to grocery stores countrywide and most of them are seasonal, providing just a brief but interesting window of avocado opportunity. One place to learn more about this is the California Avocado Board (www.avocado.org/about/varieties), quite helpful in figuring out if you're about to sacrifice to an arepa an avocado with a nonvegan-like name of Bacon or Lamb (Lamb Haas, that is).

A sometimes overlooked type of avocado is the large, smooth-skinned variety sometimes referred to as **Caribbean** or **Florida avocado**. Florida avocados are truly tropical fruits (the Haas-type avos are somewhat subtropical) and typically are very large, sometimes football shaped, or round with smooth, glossy yellow-green skin. The flesh has a flavor that's milder and less fatty than the Haas variety, hence the somewhat creepy marketing name "SlimCados." Enjoy them not as a diet food but, better, as an authentic taste of the islands!

difficult to pierce with a knife . . . don't rupture the skin of an unripe avocado or it won't ripen properly, and that's just sad. And remember, don't refrigerate avocados, especially unripe avos . . . let them hang out in a bowl to ripen on your kitchen counter until it's guacamole time.

DRIED HERBS AND SPICES

Epazote is a Central American herb typically associated with Mexican cooking. It has a unique aroma, with a flavor that reminds me of a combination of oregano and cilantro with hints of tarragon and anise. Dried epazote is a commonly found herb in Mexican markets and is often added to beans (see page 85), but growing epazote in your garden shouldn't be too hard, as epazote is considered a weed in parts of the country. A little goes a long way.

Cumin is an Old World spice that's essential to the New World Latin cuisines. For Latin foods, a big jar of ground cumin will go far in everything from salads to soups. Cumin imparts a well-rounded savory base particularly well suited for beans and protein-rich seitan dishes.

Oregano is widely used throughout Latin America, another European export spread far and wide by its popular use in Spanish cuisine. Grow your own or use high-quality Greek or Italian dried herbs for really aromatic results (much better than run-of-the-mill supermarket stuff).

Mexican oregano is actually an entirely different plant than standard oregano and is native to Central America. It's a relative of lemon verbena but has a pungent oregano-like flavor with citrusy notes. You can tell Mexican oregano apart from the gringo stuff, as the dried leaves are pointed with jagged edges, a lighter shade of green, and have tiny, pointed flower clusters.

Other dried herbs and spiced that make an appearance are **dried thyme, freshly ground black pepper, ground cinnamon, cloves,** and both **hot** and **sweet ground paprika. Smoked hot paprika** is one of my favorites to add to foods, such as Chorizo Seitan (page 36), for its warm smoky flavor and deep red color.

Annatto or **achiote seeds** are dark red, hard little seeds from a tropical shrub native to the Americas. Valued for its vibrant yellow-orange-reddish hue, annatto generously adds intense color to Latin American foods. You'll find this in most any grocery that carries Latin American herbs and spices, often sold in large containers in its whole seed form, from which you can make Annatto-Infused Oil (page 31) to use in recipes. If you can find preground annatto or achiote paste, you may also use this to color foods instead of preparing the oil.

FROZEN PRODUCE

Frozen Latin produce offers an exciting way to sample exotic fruits, vegetables, and chiles that would otherwise be impossible to obtain fresh but just are not the same when consumed dried. Yeah, of course a frozen chile isn't the same as a fresh blah blah blah, but at least you'll be able to get a truer sense of what it tastes like off the vine. And some things, such as frozen yuca chunks, are just plain convenient!

Speaking of, frozen South American chiles are some of my favorite fun frozen Latin ingredients. **Frozen ají amarillo** and huge fiery **rocoto** are convenient, never go bad, and just require a brief rinse in hot tap water to thaw slightly before using.

Frozen tropical fruit purees are incredibly flavorful and easily broken up into smaller pieces to be blended with rice milk, sugar, or anything else for fast tropical drinks. Buy one, two, or a little of everything and be ready for the next heat wave!

Frozen gandules and **fava** beans are my preferred choice for both of these beans. Frozen favas are fresh, large green-hued beans (looking a little like limas) and you may want to remove their outside peel after cooking, which is relatively easy as the beans will pop out of their peel with just a little gentle pressure.

Precut, peeled, and ready to cook **frozen yuca chunks** require only a big pot of boiling salted water on your end, for faster *yuca frita* or served with garlicky *mojo* sauce.

Frozen choclo corn is the next best thing to fresh giant white corn kernels from South America. A fun snack and an authentic partner to Peruvian-style ceviches.

KITCHEN TOOLS
(OR HOW DO I SLICE A MANGO?)

*I*t may surprise you to learn I don't own a stand mixer. My food processor is tiny and doubles as a blender (with the proper attachment), and I do almost all of my mixing with a rubber spatula. The point is, kitchen equipment is ultimately about personal preference and it should work for you, not the other way around.

But if you're wondering what to get if you're just starting out, or suspect that cutting melons with a butter knife is not the best method, then this is the place to start. Following are the basics that will serve you well, along with a few special Latin cooking tools that make certain jobs much easier and are also just really fun to have (especially if you become a hard-core tortilla or *tostone* fanatic).

BASIC EQUIPMENT
Some things will make your kitchen time go faster, smoother, and more efficiently.

Anything to get you eating sooner than later is a helpful part of your kitchen arsenal.

Chef's knife: An 8-inch knife can conquer most any chopping task at hand. The sharper the better, as dull knives are more likely to slide off foods and slide onto you, definitely not fun. You don't have to spend too much, either . . . a good quality thirty-dollar knife will do everything you ask of it and then some.

Thin, sharp, serrated knife: This type of knife is ideal for slicing soft foods with a thicker peel, including tomatoes and plantains, and is essential for slicing mangoes (see box, page 233).

Heavy-duty cutting board: I like bamboo, but use wood, heavy plastic, or whatever you're comfortable with. A heavy cutting board is better than the skimpy one (such as glass or thin plastic) as it will move around less and be able to withstand more. To keep any cutting board from rocking around on the countertop, place a thick kitchen towel under it; it will help absorb some of the shock and keep it grounded.

I like to have at least two cutting boards handy: a small board for quick jobs and a great big one for chopping up everything for a big *sancocho* soup, for example. I also have a tiny cutting board made out of eco-friendly "paperstone"—it's made from some super-high-tech method of recycling paper into a tough-as-nails surface—that holds up in the dishwasher nicely. It's the lowest-maintenance cutting board I've ever owned.

Heavy skillet, cast-iron and stainless steel or nonstick: Cast iron is very popular through most of Latin America and it's an ideal surface on which to cook items at very high heat, when grilling or pan-frying. I love my cast-iron skillets. Use the best quality you can afford; a properly cared for cast-iron pan will outlast you. A lovingly tended cast-iron *casuela* will often be passed down through a Latin family.

But if your skillet isn't cast iron, just make sure that at least it's heavy bottomed, so as to be able to conduct heat well. A 12-inch-wide, deep stainless-steel skillet with a lid is great for sautéing anything or braising vegetables. It may require more oil to keep stuff from sticking, unlike well-seasoned, properly maintained cast-iron (see tip box).

- I've been phasing out nonstick cookware from my kitchen but will admit that it has an advantage with easy cleanup. If you do use nonstick cookware, for safety concerns, I suggest using it only for quickly cooking foods at medium or low heat, such as sautéing a big pile of leafy greens. Nonstick is safer to use with a few basic rules:
- Buy a high-quality pan with a hard, glossy finish (avoid dull finishes found on cheap cookware). Some of the big box stores now offer "greener" nonstick cookware that claims to be free of some of the more dubious chemicals of older nonstick technology.
- Never ever use metal utensils, including forks, metal tongs, or spatulas, on nonstick surfaces. Have handy a set of silicone-tipped cookware and tongs or use smooth wooden spoons for stirring or lifting food.
- Always use medium or lower heat when cooking with nonstick. Never use high heat and always have something (onions, vegetables, etc.) in the pan when you heat it up, to help keep the total temperature in the pan lower and prevent scorching (or potentially creating unhealthy nonstick fumes).

Large lidded pot that can be fitted with a steamer basket: For making tamales, of course, unless you hate tamales, puppies, and happiness. Look for at least a 4-quart pot set that comes with a fitted steamer basket and a tight-fitting lid, sometimes

Caring for Cast Iron

Considering they're made out of iron, cast-iron pans deserve a little bit of babying when you're first breaking them in. Some brands out there sell preseasoned pans, which I highly recommend to start with. I never clean seasoned cast-iron with soap, instead I just scrub with a mixture of kosher salt and warm water until the sticky bits are gone, rinse with hot water, and heat on the stove to evaporate any moisture to prevent rusting. When the pan is cool, wipe down the cooking surface with a thin coat of vegetable oil and you're done. A really well-seasoned pan can usually just be wiped down (also when cool) with a paper towel after cooking nonjuicy foods such as tortillas or pancakes, no need to scrub or clean. A quick Internet search for "cast-iron seasoning care" or "seasoning cast-iron pans" can tell you all these things in greater detail than can fit into this little box.

with adjustable steam vents for controlling the rate at which the water evaporates from the pot.

Heavy, large, solid-bottomed pot with a lid for frying: Again, I feel cast iron is best for this. It should have sides at least 4 inches high; a Dutch oven–style pot is perfect for deep-frying. This is the pot ideal for making refried beans or *tostones*, for example. I have another cast-iron pot, this one enamel-glazed and with a lid, which I use for making rice and other grains or foods that are acidic, such as those with lots of tomatoes, tomatillos, or beer.

Cast-iron grill pan: Another kind of cast-iron skillet, typically square, whose bottom has raised ridges for effective grilling and for making those spiffy grill marks on food. Nice for tofu, tempeh, seitan kebabs, corn, grilled vegetables, and even arepas or sandwiches. Season and care for as you would other cast-iron cookware.

Tongs: I use tongs to grill stuff, toss salad, pick up hot tortillas, sauté vegetables, you name it. They're nice for turning vegetables roasting in the oven (they're even handy for grabbing stuff off really high shelves!). I have long-handled metal ones for grilling and silicone-tipped ones for use with any nonstick cookware.

Large, heavy, nonreactive pot—ideally stainless steel—for cooking beans and soups. Could even just be the pot and lid you steam tamales in. Who said I don't believe in multitasking?

Hopefully, you have other stuff, such as **baking sheets, baking pans, measuring cups and spoons, mixing bowls, a whisk, and a few rubber spatulas,** too. I'm also a fan of **Microplane graters,** for tackling citrus zest and turning garlic into a fine pulp that works readily into seitan dough.

HANDY EXTRA EQUIPMENT

I'll keep this short so you don't have to completely clutter up the kitchen just on my account. But there are a few tools I love and use all the time to get this fiesta going.

Immersion blender: Lots of smooth sauces, creamy soups, and special effects thanks to pureed silken tofu can happen faster, neater, and easier via a handheld immersion blender (as opposed to a food processor or blender). Look for model that comes equipped with a mini–food processor jar that's super useful for grinding up toasted spices and chiles for mole and chile sauces.

Corn zipper: If you're serious about your summer corn enjoyment, then you just might need this rather silly-sounding gadget, which wins the award for most unlikely combination of words . . . corn + zipper = a tool that neatly and quickly separates the kernel from its cob for perfectly shucked kernels.

Heat diffuser for gas burners: A ventilated metal plate with a handle, heat diffusers are your friend for more even heating and less burning for stovetop cooking. Just put your pots (especially big pots of thick stew) on a heat diffuser when cooking at very high heat or for a long time. Also useful for roasting little chiles that might slip through the grille of your gas burner (see page 264 about chile roasting).

SPECIAL LATIN COOKING EQUIPMENT

You could make every recipe in this book without any of these specialty items. But you and your kitchen will be all the more interesting with a lovely tortilla press or a pretty *comal* on your stove. Most Latin cooking equipment (at least the most basic models) is really cheap, so why the heck not have a *churrera* or a *tostonera*?

Tortilla press: I have an aluminum one scored from Chinatown, NYC, of all places. It even says "tortilla press" on it to dispel any doubts and has two round plates with a hinged handle that snap together to turn masa dough into ready-to-grill tortillas in mere seconds. Built-to-last cast iron versions are available, too.

Tortilla warmer: Probably the least important Latin gadget. If you've ever ordered fajitas in a Mexican restaurant at a mall, you've seen these round lidded boxes. Oddly enough, I do end up using my tortilla warmer for other things, such as letting freshly grilled chiles rest (to self-steam the skins for peeling) or hiding cookies from unsuspecting housemates (oh well, time to find another hiding place). Some warmers can be popped into the microwave or oven for a fast method for reheating a stack of cold tortillas.

Tostonera: Looks like a hinged wooden paddle, rectangular or round. It functions kind of like a tortilla press but for squashing fried plantains before the second frying. Not essential for making *tostones* but fun to use, plus it makes them more consistent in shape and size. *Tostoneras* can be made of supercheap and flimsy wood, but may also be found crafted from long-lasting bamboo or plastic, for many years of fried plantain joy.

Churrera: Churros are already special, so why not seal the deal with a special churro maker? Well, not as in a person who lives in your kitchen and makes churros (Mom deserves a break!). A *churrera* is a plastic press that makes pressing churro dough fast and easy. See Churros (page 223) for more *churrera* talk.

Kitchen twine, white cotton, is useful when making tamales and is sometimes located near the tamale-making section of your local supermarket. No such section (yet)? Many Latin stores keep it in the produce aisle or with the paper goods.

Parchment paper for tamales is pretty much just that. It is sold cut into large squares as "*papel para tamales*" and is water and grease resistant and useful if you're all out of corn husks. Usually cheap enough, it's worth buying for just tamale making, as parchment paper for baking can be more costly.

Comal, budare, or other wide pan for grilling tortillas, arepas, or for even making things like *cachapas*. *Comals* are Mexican/Central American and are often oval shaped or sometimes round with a long handle. *Budares*, found in Caribbean countries and parts of South America, are round with a small bumplike handle that has a little hole. Cheap ones are aluminum; better quality are made from cast iron. If you're thinking that you can just use your cast-iron skillet instead, you are 110 percent right. Somewhere I even have a vintage *budare* passed down from my aunt, which I should use to make arepas . . . and I will when I find it! (Just don't tell my aunt, okay?)

PART II

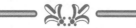

THE RECIPES

1

A FEW ESSENTIAL
LATINO VEGAN RECIPES

*E*veryone needs a few basic recipes to use in everything from simple snacks or entire meals. This chapter is a little collection of essential recipes—*sofrito*, annatto oil, and seitan (easy, steamed "meat from wheat")—that contribute to so many satisfying "meaty" Latin vegan dishes in this book. There's even a seitan chorizo-style sausage—(okay, perhaps it's a little beyond basic but nevertheless, a flavorful element to sink your teeth into). Diced and fried, it makes a tasty addition to just about any savory meal in this book.

You can, of course, substitute premade seitan for homemade, but I encourage you to give homemade a try just once; it requires just a few minutes of mixing and half an hour of steaming on the stove.

All of these basic recipes can be made days, weeks, or, in the case of the annatto oil, months in advance.

• • •

ANNATTO-INFUSED OIL (ACIETE DE ACHIOTE)

- Makes 1/2 cup oil
- Time: Less than 10 minutes
- Gluten Free, Soy Free

Annatto seeds, known as achiote, are as all-American a seasoning as you may ever hope to find. Annatto trees are native to the tropical Americas and the seeds are a natural powerhouse of bright orange color. Achiote-infused oil is used in Latin American cooking to add a vibrant splash of red-orange to rice, soups, breads, tamales, and beyond. My *papá* makes an occasional batch to tint empanada dough. The flavor of annatto is very subtle, perhaps a little nutty, so you don't have to worry about it clashing with other elements in your recipes.

Making this oil takes only a few minutes and it lasts forever stashed away in the spice cabinet. If you prefer ground achiote seeds, as a general rule, use 1 tablespoon of oil for every 1/2 teaspoon of ground achiote seeds.

Tip: For neater pouring, place a funnel into the mouth of the jar or bottle, then top with the strainer and pour the oil through!

> 2 tablespoons annatto (achiote) seeds
> 1/2 cup mild vegetable oil, such as canola or grapeseed or light olive oil

1. Combine the annatto seeds and vegetable oil in a small saucepan. Bring the oil to a simmer over medium-low heat, then lower the heat to low. Simmer for 2 to 3 minutes, until oil turns a very dark orange. Remove from the heat and let cool completely. Using a fine-mesh metal strainer, strain the oil into a small, clean glass jar and cap tightly. Discard the seeds. Annatto oil can be stored at room temperature and lasts almost forever.

About Achiote

You just might be able to find achiote in paste form on your Latin grocer's shelves. It's convenient and works easily into sauces and moist foods. Don't cook the paste into oil; it is ready to use as is. Substitute 1 to 2 teaspoons of paste for every tablespoon of oil. Just be sure to give the ingredients list a quick glance to make sure it's not harboring any hidden animal products. You may also find ground achiote powder; use 1 teaspoon per tablespoon of oil.

BASIC ONION-PEPPER SOFRITO

- Makes about 1 1/2 cups *sofrito*
- Time: About 45 minutes
- Gluten Free, Soy Free

Sofrito is the soul of so many Latin dishes it behooves you to learn how to make a good one. Simmering onions, peppers, and garlic in oil (plenty of it!) for a long time transforms them into a richly sweet and piquant base. *Sofrito* isn't consumed on its own but is used to create a flavorful foundation for countless dishes. It can be made well in advance, keeps for weeks in the refrigerator (just pour a thin layer of olive oil on the top to help keep it fresh), and is a fast and easy way to add flavor to beans and soups.

> 1/2 cup olive oil
> 6 cloves garlic, peeled and chopped coarsely
> 2 pounds green bell peppers, seeded and chopped finely
> 2 pounds yellow onions, diced
> A generous pinch of salt
> Freshly ground black pepper

1. Pour the olive oil into a cast-iron pot or large, heavy skillet and add the garlic, bell peppers, onions, salt, and ground pepper. Over medium-high heat, fry for 10 minutes, stirring occasionally. Lower the heat to low and fry for another 25 to 30 minutes, stirring occasionally,

until the vegetables are very soft and mushy, have released plenty of liquid, and are reduced to about one-third of their original volume.

2. Remove from heat. Use immediately or cool to room temperature, then store refrigerated in a tightly covered container. Be sure to scrape as much liquid and oil as possible from the bottom of the pot as this contains plenty of delicious *sofrito* flavor.

3. Store unused *sofrito* in a tightly covered glass container in the refrigerator. To extend the life of your *sofrito*, spread a thin layer of olive oil on top. *Sofrito* can last up to 2 weeks if kept chilled this way.

Uses: *Sofrito* is used whenever a recipe requires sautéing onion and garlic together in oil before adding the major players (such as more vegetables, proteins, and so on). *Sofrito* is used in these recipes as a base for many soups, rice dishes, and even tofu.

Variations

Sofrito con Tomate: Seed and finely dice 1 pound of ripe red tomatoes. Add with the other vegetables. You may need to cook for another 5 to 10 minutes to reduce the *sofrito* more if the tomatoes are especially juicy.

Sofrito con Cilantro and Achiote: Substitute Annatto-Infused Oil (page 31) for the olive oil. Stir in 1 cup of firmly packed, finely chopped fresh cilantro (or culantro, see page 19) into the *sofrito* during the last 10 minutes of cooking. A handful of chopped parsley makes a nice addition to this, too.

Sofrito con Ají: Add 1 to 3 seeded and finely chopped hot chiles with the rest of the vegetables.

Try adding 1 to 2 teaspoons of the following spices to your simmering *sofrito*: ground cumin, ground coriander, or sweet or hot ground paprika.

Sofrito for the People

Sofrito can be a time-consuming thing to make. I know that standing over a hot stove frying up peppers and onions doesn't feel like the first thing you want to do when you get home from the office. If you want to experience some genuine Latin cooking without cooking all that much, there is something be said about grabbing a jar of premade *sofrito*, and lots of people do. But it will never taste as sweet or nuanced as your own homemade *sofrito*.

If you're home on a rainy day, I recommend putting a big pot of *sofrito* on the stove to cook (and steam some seitan, too!) while you catch up with your *telenovelas* or call your parents to hear them complain about how you don't call enough. Tightly covered, firmly packed *sofrito* keeps for weeks in the fridge and can also be frozen.

STEAMED RED SEITAN

- Makes four seitan "loaves," each loaf serving 2, generously incorporated into entrées and other dishes
- Time: Less than 45 minutes

Latin food is meaty food, as any quick glance at a Latin American menu will tell you. That's where a few "loaves" of easy homemade seitan come to the rescue as an exceptional meat substitute. I love the look and texture of seitan in many traditional Latin dishes. Unlike the latter, you can almost pull a fast one over omnivores by serving up seitan entrées (unlike trying to convince your *abuela* that she's eating *mondongo* when it's just a lump of tofu).

Seitan's chewy, firm texture seamlessly works with many traditional cooking techniques (shredding, grilling, and marinating) and can hold its own paired with hot chiles and bold salsas. In fact, you may even encounter seitan—or in Español, *seitán*—if you travel in Latin America. Always keep a few seitan loaves wrapped up and waiting in your fridge for a variety of "meaty" meals.

This tomato-flavored seitan is designed for use in "beefy"-style dishes. For more "chickeny" or "pork" dishes, use Steamed White Seitan (page 35). This seitan is my go-to seitan when wheat meat is required for more complex dishes, as it's easy to steam this while attending to more time-consuming recipes.

Make-ahead Tip: For best texture and flavor, prepare this seitan a day or two in advance. An overnight chill helps firm up the texture and lets the flavor fully develop. Seitan should not be eaten straight up; rather, serve it fried, roasted, marinated, or grilled for maximum enjoyment.

1½ cups cold vegetable broth
4 cloves garlic, peeled and pressed or grated with a Microplane grater
3 tablespoons mild soy sauce
4 tablespoons tomato paste
2 tablespoons olive oil
1½ cups vital wheat gluten flour
¼ cup chickpea (garbanzo) flour
¼ cup nutritional yeast
1 teaspoon dried oregano
½ teaspoon ground cumin

1. In a measuring cup, whisk together the broth, garlic, soy sauce, tomato paste, and olive oil. In a large bowl, combine the wheat gluten, chickpea flour, nutritional yeast, oregano, and cumin, and form a well in the center. Pour the liquid ingredients into the well and stir with a rubber spatula until the dough leaves the sides of the bowl. Knead the dough for 2 to 3 minutes to develop the gluten. Let the dough rest for 10 minutes; knead again for 30 seconds. Place the dough on a cutting board and with a sharp knife, cut the dough into four equal pieces and lightly knead each piece a few times. Shape each into a roughly oblong loaf shape.

2. Tear off four 12-inch-square sheets of aluminum foil. Place a piece of dough in the center of a piece of foil. Fold the short sides of foil over the loaf, then fold over the ends. The foil should be secure but there should be some loose space around the dough to allow it to expand during steaming. Repeat with the other three pieces of dough. Place the wrapped dough in a steamer basket and steam for 30 minutes. Allow the dough to cool to the touch before chilling in the fridge for an hour or overnight.

3. Store the seitan in the fridge, tightly sealed in a plastic bag or airtight container, for up to 2 weeks. Seitan can also be frozen (wrap tightly), then thawed in the fridge for later use.

STEAMED WHITE SEITAN

- Makes four seitan "loaves," each loaf serving 2, generously incorporated into entrées and other dishes
- Time: Less than 45 minutes
- Soy Free (be sure to use soy-free vegetable broth)

Steam up a batch of this soy-free seitan for "chicken"- and "pork"-style dishes in this book, or anytime for seitan that's fast and relatively mess free. This seitan is very chewy (more so than the Red Seitan) and is well suited for cooking with moist foods (stews, rice dishes) or slicing very thin, marinating, and grilling or roasting (heav-

enly in a Cubano Vegano Sandwich [page 66]). This seitan (and the red recipe, too) are also firm enough to grate for surprisingly realistic-looking ground "meat." This recipe makes four compact loves for use in two recipes.

Tip: Make sure to look for soy-free vegetable broth if you're looking to completely eliminate soy. Vegetarian "chicken"-flavored broth is a sneakily easy way to season this seitan!

1 1/2 cups cold vegetable broth or "chicken"-flavored vegetable broth
4 cloves garlic, grated
2 tablespoons olive oil
1 1/2 cups vital wheat gluten flour
1/4 cup chickpea (garbanzo) flour
1/4 cup nutritional yeast
1 teaspoon dried thyme
1/2 teaspoon ground sweet paprika
1/2 teaspoon ground cumin
1 teaspoon salt, or more to taste

1. In a measuring cup, whisk together the broth, garlic, and olive oil. In a large bowl, combine the wheat gluten, chickpea flour, nutritional yeast, thyme, paprika, cumin, and salt, and form a well in the center. Pour the liquid ingredients into the well and stir with a rubber spatula until the dough leaves the sides of the bowl. Knead the dough for 2 to 3 minutes to develop the gluten. Let the dough rest for 10 minutes; knead again for 30 seconds. Place the dough on a cutting board and with a sharp knife, cut the dough into four equal pieces and lightly knead each piece a few times. Shape each into a loaf shape.

2. Tear off four 12-inch-square sheets of aluminum foil. Place a piece of dough in the center of a piece of foil. Fold the short sides of foil over the loaf, then fold over the ends. The foil should be secure but there should be a little give around the dough to allow it to expand during steaming. Repeat with the other three pieces of dough. Place the wrapped dough in a steamer basket and steam for 30 minutes. Allow the dough to cool to the touch before chilling in the fridge for an hour or overnight.

3. Store the seitan in the fridge, tightly sealed in a plastic bag or airtight container, for up to 2 weeks.

CHORIZO SEITAN SAUSAGES

- **Makes six 6- to 7-inch sausages**
- **Prep Time: 15 minutes**
- **Cook Time: 35 minutes**
- **Cooling Time: 40 minutes**

These past few years, steamed or baked seitan sausages became something of a vegan Internet meme. Suddenly vegan home cooks everywhere were doing something most of their omnivorous contemporaries only dream of . . . making sausage in their own kitchen! And being vegan makes it easy, far less messy, and requires only a fraction of the time.

In the spirit of that home industry, here is our friend seitan, tarted up with plenty of paprika (the essential flavor and coloring spice of chorizo), more spices, and vinegar, shaped into links, and baked for a sliceable texture. This recipe makes a tangy, moderately spicy chorizo that has a slow afterburn from the cayenne for a pan–Latin American (not just Mexican) cuisine application. Depending on your preference, you can add Mexican or Peruvian hot chiles, more or less spices, or more or less vinegar, to customize it to your liking.

If you store it in the refrigerator, it's easy to toss the chorizo into soups, stews, and beans, fry it again with potatoes or vegetables, or tuck it into tacos or *pupusas*. A little chorizo sausage goes a long way, especially if you make it very spicy, so freeze any portion that might go unused longer than a week. For best results, chill seitan chorizo, then slice and fry before adding to your favorite recipes.

1½ cups vegetable broth

4 tablespoons tomato paste

3 tablespoons Annatto-Infused Oil (page 31) or olive oil

3 tablespoons red wine vinegar

6 cloves garlic, grated

1⅔ cups vital wheat gluten

¼ cup chickpea (garbanzo) flour

3 tablespoons nutritional yeast

4 teaspoons ground smoked sweet or smoked hot paprika

4 teaspoons ground dried chile powder (a standard store-bought blend is fine)

3 teaspoons dried oregano or Mexican oregano

2 teaspoons ground cumin

1 1/2 teaspoons ground cayenne, or more to taste

1 teaspoon ground coriander

1 1/2 teaspoons salt

1/2 teaspoon ground black pepper

1. Tear off six pieces of foil about 8 inches wide each. Preheat the oven to 350°F. In a measuring cup, whisk together the broth, tomato paste, oil, vinegar, and garlic. In a large bowl, combine the wheat gluten, chickpea flour, nutritional yeast, paprika, chile powder, oregano (rub between palms first to eliminate any chunky leaves or stems), cumin, cayenne, coriander, salt, and pepper and form a well in the center. Pour the liquid ingredients into the well and stir with a rubber spatula until the dough leaves the sides of the bowl. Knead the dough for 3 minutes to develop the gluten. Let the dough rest for 10 minutes; knead again for 2 minutes.

2. Divide the dough into six equal pieces. Place a piece on the foil and shape it into a log about 6 inches long by 1 1/2 inches wide. Bring the wide ends of the foil together, fold over the dough, and firmly wrap it around the dough to form a sausagelike shape. Wrap it so that it's fairly secure but leave it a little bit loose so that the sausage can expand during baking and not burst through the foil (it can happen if you wrap your seitan too tightly, so leave some slack!). Twist the foil at each end of the sausage (so it looks like a candy wrapper). Repeat for the other five pieces of dough.

3. Place the foil-covered chorizo directly on the middle baking rack in the oven and bake for 35 minutes. Cool the chorizo for 40 minutes before using, to allow the texture to firm and the flavors to meld. For best flavor and texture, chill overnight before slicing. Store seitan chorizo in the fridge, tightly sealed in a plastic bag or airtight container, for up to 2 weeks or freeze.

Variations

Chipotle Chorizo: Replace half or all of the tomato paste with chipotles in adobo sauce. Remove the seeds and puree the chipotles with their sauce, then measure out in tablespoons to add as desired.

Hot Ají Chorizo: Add 1 to 2 tablespoons amarillo, panca, or—for really hot chorizo—*rocoto ají* paste, along with the wet ingredients.

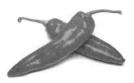

Un Pocito Ways to Serve Up Chorizo

The best and most direct way to enjoy this chorizo is to slice and fry it in a little oil to crisp the edges. This is easy to do by slicing prepared "veganrizo" into thin rounds or diagonal slices and lightly sautéing it for 4 to 6 minutes over medium heat in a few tablespoons of the oil. For that proper neon orange, oily glow that resembles the grease that accompanies the traditional sausage, use Annatto-Infused Oil (page 31).

Use fried chorizo immediately with the following:

- Stirred into beans (as with Drunken Beans with Seitan Chorizo, page 91, or Portobello Feijoada, page 147)
- Tucked into tacos (see "Taco Toppings!," page 176)
- Served as "croutons" on top of a thick soup (see Potato-Kale Soup, page 159)
- Kneaded into arepa dough (see Arepas, page 177)
- Stirred into either side dish rice or main entrée rice dishes right before serving (such as Rice with Pigeon Peas, page 140)
- Embraced in enchiladas, sprinkled on salads, quombined (okay, not a word but . . .) with quinoa, tossed into tortillas, or enfolded in empanada filling!

Seitan chorizo is great grilled, too! Slice the sausages down the center, brush or spray generously with olive or any vegetable oil, and grill for 2 to 4 minute per side, until hot. Serve paired with any beans and rice plate. Or savor it in a simple but outstanding Argentinean-style chorizo sandwich, the *choripán*.

2

SALSAS AND CONDIEMENTOS

Salsa isn't just the tomato stuff in a jar you pick up at the store when you're grabbing a bag of tortilla chips. Not only does *salsa* mean "sauce" in Spanish, it covers a huge array of warm cooked sauces, spicy chile sauces, creamy sauces with nuts, or "dairy" sauces made better with dairy substitutes or cool purees of vegetables, fruits, or herbs. Fans of Mexican-style salsas will see familiar ingredients—tomatoes, cilantro, avocados—done up in both familiar and new ways, depending on what cultural lens they're looking through. And that's a good thing! Stepping out of the tomato salsa safety zone can take you to new and exciting experiences, such as zesty green *ají* sauce or a savory peanut sauce with a totally Latin twist.

When I say salsa is exciting, I mean it . . . a great sauce can really make a meal— or make an already great meal even better. Latin sauces have the advantage of using full-flavored herbs and fresh vegetables and fruits and chile peppers, all ingredients that often require only minimal effort on your part. So while your tortillas or arepas are baking or the beans are bubbling, make a salsa (or two). As they say, you'll be really cooking with gas (but really with an even better natural resource, salsa!).

CREAMY AVOCADO-TOMATO SALSA (VENEZUELAN GUASACACA)

- Makes about 1¹⁄₂ cups salsa
- Time: Less than 10 minutes
- Gluten Free, Soy Free

You think you know avocados by way of guacamole, but avos are enjoyed, too, in a saucy form. This juicy salsa (called *guasacaca*) hails from Venezuela, where it's used as a condiment with lots of stuff. It's not so much a guacamole but more a cool, tangy sauce with a hint of extra richness from the olive oil. I love it with empanadas, but it's also stellar tucked into an arepa or heaped alongside beans and rice. In Venezuela, it's typically served with grilled foods, so do it right and serve with grilled tofu or tempeh.

Tip: In Venezuela you don't see hot chiles (called *ají*) used here, but I suspect that if you're used to other chile-fired Latin cuisines, you may want to sneak a little heat into this salsa. I like a few dashes of bottled red hot sauce.

> 2 cloves garlic, minced
> 1 ripe avocado, peeled, seeded, and
>   diced finely
> 1 large ripe tomato (about 1/2 pound),
>   seeded and diced finely
> 1/2 cup finely minced white onion
> 3 tablespoons lime juice or white wine
>   vinegar
> 2 tablespoons good-quality olive oil
> 3 tablespoons finely chopped fresh
>   cilantro
> 1/2 teaspoon salt, or to taste
> Lime juice or vinegar (optional)
> 2 tablespoons of finely chopped parsley
>   (optional)
> A few dashes of your favorite red hot
>   sauce (optional)

1. Place all the ingredients in a mixing bowl. Using a potato masher or a large fork, gently mash the ingredients just enough to create a creamy texture but still leave some chunks of avocado. Taste and adjust the flavor with more salt, lime juice or vinegar, parsley, and/or hot sauce, if desired. Serve immediately.

GREEN TOMATILLO SAUCE

- Makes 4 cups sauce
- Time: About 40 minutes
- Gluten Free, Soy Free

Tomatillos, the green, jacket-wearing cousins of tomatoes, are what make this classic green sauce a refreshing alternative to tomato-based chile sauces for enchiladas and tamales, just for starters. When I get the craving for tangy tomatillos served with fresh vegetables or warm-weather dishes, nothing but this sauce will do. (A touch of sweetener—either from sugar or agave nectar—rounds out the sharpness of the sauce, but leave it out if you like.) Try serving with Farmers' Market Tamales (page 194) or as an essential part of Potato-Chickpea Enchiladas with (you guessed it) Tomatillo Sauce (page 133).

Tip: Tomatillos, once their papery husks have been removed, may have a slightly tacky, soapy film on their skins. I like to wash them by placing them in a salad spinner, fill with enough warm water to cover, slosh them around and lift the spinning basket out of the washing water. Try with a few changes of water until the water seems less soapy and the tomatillo skins feel smoother.

1 pound tomatillos, husks removed, washed

2 cloves garlic, chopped

2 jalapeño, serrano, or other green chiles, washed, sliced in half, and seeded if desired (for hotter sauce, leave the seeds)

1 medium-size onion, chopped

1/2 cup fresh cilantro leaves, lightly packed

1 teaspoon dried oregano or Mexican oregano

2 tablespoons peanut or olive oil

1 1/2 cups well-seasoned vegetable broth

2 teaspoons sugar, or 1 teaspoon agave syrup (optional)

1/2 teaspoon salt, or to taste

1. Fill a large pot with enough water to allow the tomatillos to float, cover, and bring the water to a rolling boil over high heat. Add the tomatillos and cook for 10 minutes, stirring them occasionally, or until the skins start to split and the tomatillos' bright green color turns a dull olive green. Use a slotted spoon to transfer the cooked tomatillos to a bowl to cool for 20 minutes. Cooked tomatillos may collapse and release some juices while they cool.

2. In a blender jar, pulse the cooled tomatillos with their juices, garlic, chiles, onion, and cilantro to form a thick sauce. In a large saucepan over medium heat, heat the peanut oil, add tomatillo mixture, and bring to a boil, stirring occasionally. Slowly stir in the vegetable broth and bring to a boil again, then lower heat to a simmer. Cook for about 10 minutes, stirring occasionally; the sauce should thicken enough to thinly coat the back of a spoon lightly. Season with sugar and salt to taste.

PEANUT SAUCE (SALSA DE MANI)

- Makes a little over 1 cup sauce
- Time: Less than 15 minutes
- Gluten Free, Soy Free

Who doesn't love a good peanut sauce? Even if you're not entirely sure you do, give this sauce a try! Peanuts (natives of South America) are as American as it gets. Latin American–style peanut sauces tend toward mild and creamy and go perfectly with just about anything from yuca to rice to steamed vegetables. I like to offset the richness of the sauce by serving it with steamed kale or broccoli.

This sauce was born to be with Ecuadorian *llapingachos* (page 57), tender mashed potato pancakes. This recipe makes just enough sauce to top the pancakes, but try doubling it to have some extra peanut sauce whenever the craving strikes.

1 tablespoon peanut or canola oil

1 small onion, minced

1 large tomato, seeded and chopped finely
1/4 teaspoon ground cumin
1/2 cup warm vegetable broth
1/3 cup smooth natural peanut butter
1/4 cup almond milk or favorite
    nondairy milk
Salt and freshly ground pepper

1. In a saucepan over medium heat, combine the peanut oil and minced onion. Fry the onion until very soft, about 5 minutes. Stir in the tomato and cumin and cook for 2 minutes. In a measuring cup, stir together the warm vegetable broth and peanut butter until the mixture is emulsified, then pour into the pan. Stir and add the nondairy milk, lower the heat to low, and cook for about 2 minutes, stirring constantly.

2. Remove from the heat and serve warm. If desired, puree the sauce for a smoother consistency, or serve as is.

CHIMICHURRI SAUCE WITH SMOKED PAPRIKA

- Makes about 1 1/2 cups sauce
- Time: Less than 10 minutes
- Soy Free

A fresh, lively Argentinean sauce that's just too good to be secreted away by steak eaters any longer. Think of it as a spicy pesto—*chimichurri* begs to be tucked into sandwiches, served with any appetizer as a

pâté, paired with empanadas, and dabbed onto grilled tempeh or seitan. Try Chimichurri Baked Tofu (page 100) for an easy protein entrée.

Chimichurri has many variations in Argentina. The smoked paprika, in this case, adds a rich depth. Sometimes *chimichurri* is chopped by hand, but it's easier by far and perhaps even tastier just to throw everything into a food processor for a creamy paste. This sauce gains more flavor by getting a chance to mellow, so make a day in advance or at least an hour before serving.

4 cloves garlic, chopped
2 large shallots, chopped
1 large bunch fresh flat-leaf (Italian)
    parsley, thick stems removed
1/3 cup olive oil
3 tablespoons red wine vinegar
1 teaspoon smoked sweet paprika
1 1/2 teaspoons dried oregano
1 teaspoon dried basil
1/2 teaspoon red pepper flakes, or more
    to taste
1/2 teaspoon sea salt

1. Place the garlic, shallots and parsley into a food processor and pulse until finely chopped. Stream in the olive oil, red wine vinegar, paprika, oregano, basil, red pepper flakes, and sea salt, and pulse until creamy. Taste the sauce and adjust with more salt or red wine vinegar, if desired. Store in a tightly covered container and keep chilled until ready to use.

PICKLED RED ONIONS

- Makes about 3 cups onions
- Time: Less than 15 minutes, not including marinating time
- Soy Free

This may not be a sauce, but I bet you'll be reaching for these refreshing onions as much as your favorite salsa. Variations of pickled onions are found throughout Latin America, and although these aren't exactly pickled (more like strategically marinated), you won't hold it against them after tasting their tangy sweet flavor and soft yet crunchy texture. Their bright rosy color instantly beautifies any potato dish, tofu, taco, *lla-pingachos* (page 57), Creamy Potato Peanut Stew (page 138), or rice and beans platter. This recipe makes a lot, perfect for also spontaneously beautifying your favorite sandwich or even atop veggie hot dogs.

1¹/2 pounds red onions, sliced in half lengthwise and then very thinly
1/3 cup lime juice
2 tablespoons red wine vinegar or lemon juice
2¹/2 teaspoons kosher salt
A pinch of sugar

1. In a large pot, bring 2 quarts of water to a rolling boil. Place a metal colander in the sink. Add the onions to the rapidly boiling water. Stir for about 30 seconds, then drain into the colan-der and rinse thoroughly with cold water to stop the onions from cooking. Shake the colan-der well to release excess water. In a 2-quart plastic or glass container, combine the drained onions, lime juice, vinegar, salt, and sugar. Toss to mix everything, tightly cover the container, and chill for at least 2 hours to allow the flavors to blend. The onions will taste best if allowed to marinate overnight.

2. To serve, grab a few generous tablespoons of onions and shake off any excess juice. Pile generously on the serving plate. The cool, crunchy onions go especially well with hot, spicy, moist foods. Kept tightly covered in the refrigerator, these onions will last for at least 2 weeks but have a habit of disappearing long before that.

SO GOOD, SO GREEN DIPPING SAUCE (GREEN AJÍ SAUCE)

- Makes about 2 cups sauce
- Time: Less than 10 minutes, not including chilling time

Green and mean, this fresh sassy sauce is a mainstay of Peruvian cuisine with any meal and hot snack foods. Generally known as *salsa ají*, it's simultaneously cool, spicy, creamy, and herby. It's ideal served up with root vegetables, or on most any baked or fried potato dish, and also great with fried or roasted protein foods, drizzled in a creamy winter squash soup, or as a dip for french fries, sweet potatoes, or yuca. Who would think all that from a salsa made with lettuce?

There are many of variations of this sauce, using regional green herbs or relying on dairy or eggy mayonnaise for the requisite creaminess. But we don't need any of that for a great green sauce at home with traditional but easy-to-find fresh ingredients such as cilantro, onions, or green onions.

Tip: Use any fresh green chiles you can find; serranos are a good choice. If you're not used to cooking with green chiles blend a little piece at a time into the sauce to see what level of heat you're comfortable with.

1 to 3 fresh green chiles, such as jalapeño or serrano, seeds removed for less heat, if desired

2 cloves garlic, chopped coarsely

1/3 cup vegan mayonnaise

2 tablespoons olive oil

3 tablespoons lime juice

1/4 pound romaine lettuce (about 1/4 of a large head), thick base removed, leaves chopped coarsely

1 cup fresh cilantro leaves, lightly packed

3 whole green onions, trimmed and chopped

3/4 teaspoon salt, or more to taste

2 to 4 tablespoons water

1. In a food processor or blender, blend all of the ingredients except the water until smooth and creamy, stopping occasionally to scrape the sides of the processor bowl with a rubber spatula. Add a tablespoon of water at a time to thin the sauce to your desired consistency, if at all necessary. Taste the sauce and season with more lime juice or salt, if you like. Chill the sauce in a tightly covered container for 30 minutes or overnight before using. Keep chilled when not using.

GREEN ONION SALSA

- Makes about 3/4 cup
- Time: Less than 10 minutes
- Soy Free

A fresh, tangy *salsita* typically associated with empanadas in Colombia but just as well used with beans, tofu, or seitan for a blast of zippy green onion flavor. It tastes best if given an hour or more to mellow and let the flavors blend.

1 large bunch green onions (about 4 ounces), trimmed and chopped

2 cloves garlic, chopped

1/2 cup fresh cilantro leaves, packed

1/4 cup white or rice vinegar

1/4 cup lime juice

1 teaspoon salt, or to taste

1. Pulse all the ingredients together in a food processor to form a slightly chunky salsa. Chill or let sit at room temperature for at least 30

minutes prior to serving, to allow the flavors to blend. This salsa looks best served the day it's made and will darken somewhat the next day but still taste great.

PINE NUT CREMA

....

- Makes about 1 1/2 cups *crema*
- Time: Less than 10 minutes, not including baking time
- Gluten Free

....

This pine nut–based *crema* is the sauce you will go to again and again when a rich and cheeselike baked topping is what you crave. It's ideal on top of casseroles such as enchiladas, especially Potato-Chickpea Enchiladas with Green Tomatillo Sauce (page 40). The longer this sauce bakes, the better it gets, with a firm top "crust" and a creamy dairylike center. For an appealing browned crust, try broiling just before serving.

12 ounces soft silken tofu

1/2 cup pine nuts

2 tablespoons lime juice

1 tablespoon olive or peanut oil

2 teaspoons cornstarch

1 clove garlic, grated

1 teaspoon salt

1. In a blender jar, pulse together the tofu, pine nuts, lime juice, olive oil, cornstarch, garlic, and salt until smooth and creamy, scraping

down the mixture several times with a rubber spatula. Taste and adjust the flavor with more salt and lime juice if desired.

2. To use the *crema*, spread evenly on top of casseroles prior to baking. Pine Nut Crema sets up best when allowed to bake, uncovered, for at least 30 minutes at 350ºF. The longer it bakes, the more golden and slightly browned its surface will become. Baked *crema* will continue to firm as it cools. If desired, broil on high for an additional 4 to 6 minutes, until it develops golden brown spots.

RED CHILE SAUCE

....

- Makes about 3 1/2 cups sauce
- Time: About 25 minutes
- Gluten Free, Soy Free

....

If you've ever looked at a big bag of dried chile peppers and wondered what in blazes to *do* with it, then this sauce is for you. This is a smooth sauce with heat that ranges from gently piquant to blistering, depending on what chiles are used. My all-time favorite Mexican chile, the sweet, smoky, and mildly spicy ancho, gets top billing here. Or get crazy and use a blend of ancho plus others, such as pasilla, costeño, any kind of chipotle, or guajillo chiles, for a hot and nuanced sauce. There no end to the chiles you can try in this basic sauce that goes with well with beans, rice, enchiladas, or on top of tamales.

Tip: For more information on choosing and handling dried chiles, see the tip box on page 15 in the Pantry section.

3 to 4 ounces dried ancho chiles,
    or a mix of any dried red Mexican chile
    (such as pasilla, guajillo, costeño,
    chile de arbol)
2 tablespoons peanut or corn oil
2 cloves garlic, chopped
1 small yellow onion, diced
1 teaspoon dried oregano, Mexican
    oregano, or epazote
1/2 teaspoon ground cumin
1 (15-ounce) can diced tomatoes
2 cups vegetable broth
1/2 teaspoon salt, or to taste

1. In a large saucepan, bring 1 quart of water to a boil. Have ready a medium-size glass or metal heat-resistant bowl.

2. Heat a cast-iron skillet over medium heat. While the skillet is heating, slice open the dried chiles, remove the stems and seeds, and open the chiles so that they can be easily flattened when pressed with a spatula. (Wear gloves when handling hot chiles, or embrace a little pain.) Place the chiles in the heated skillet and use a metal spatula to press and flip them frequently to toast, about 1 minute. Watch the chiles carefully to prevent them from burning. Remove the skillet from the heat and transfer the chiles to the heat-resistant bowl. Pour the boiling water over the chiles and set aside for 10 minutes, to allow the chiles to soften. Drain the water from the chiles (this removes any overly bitter flavors from some dried chiles).

3. In a large saucepan, combine the oil, diced onion, and chopped garlic. Heat the pan over medium heat, stirring garlic frequently for about 1 minute until sizzling and fragrant. Stir in the oregano and cumin, then pour in the softened chiles, tomato sauce, and vegetable broth, and simmer for 1 minute. Either use an immersion blender or pour into a blender jar, and puree the mixture to create a smooth sauce. (Return to the saucepan if the blender jar is used.) Bring the pureed mixture to a simmer over medium heat and, stirring frequently, cook for about 10 minutes. Season to taste with salt and serve.

SIMPLE LATIN TOMATO SAUCE

- Makes about 2 1/2 cups sauce
- Time: About 20 minutes
- Gluten Free, Soy Free

This is a very simple tomato sauce, perfect to serve alongside *pupusas*, tamales, *sopes*, or grilled seitan with rice and beans. Unlike Italian-style sauces, Latin-style tomato sauces are cooked just enough to keep the texture light and flavors fresh tasting. Typically, these sauces are pureed until smooth, but you can leave this one chunky if you prefer. Try experimenting with different kinds of canned tomatoes for different textures. This recipe does not make a ton of sauce; rather, a nice amount to serve as a condiment—but go ahead and double or triple it if you're in need of tomato sauce for a crowd.

1 tablespoon olive or vegetable oil
3 cloves garlic, minced
1/4 pound yellow onion, diced small
1 1/2 teaspoons dried oregano
1/2 teaspoon ground cumin
1/4 cup vegetable broth, white wine, or
    water
1 (15-ounce) can tomato sauce, crushed
    tomatoes, or diced tomatoes
1 tablespoon lime juice
1/2 teaspoon salt
Freshly ground pepper

1. In a medium-size saucepan, combine the olive oil and garlic and heat over medium heat until the garlic starts to sizzle, about 30 seconds. Add the onion and fry for about 5 minutes, stirring occasionally, until the onion starts to turn golden and transparent. Stir in the oregano and cumin and fry for another 30 seconds. Add the vegetable broth to deglaze the pan; simmer for 1 minute. Add the tomato sauce and simmer for 10 minutes. Season with salt, pepper, and lime juice and remove from the heat. If desired, puree the sauce with an immersion blender until smooth, or leave as is.

Variation

Zesty Chipotle Sauce: This is easy and so good on tamales or with Amaranth Polenta with Roasted Chiles (page 128), with delicious chipotle flavor and a touch of chile heat. Simply stir in one 7-ounce can of prepared Mexican chipotle sauce (not whole chipotles in adobo, but the pureed, flavored tomato sauce), along with the diced tomatoes.

CLASSIC ROASTED TOMATILLO SALSA

- Makes about 3 1/2 cups salsa
- Time: About 20 minutes
- Gluten Free, Soy Free

So easy and so outrageously fresh you may never want to be seen with a jar of store-bought tomatillo salsa again. This smoky green salsa keeps well in the fridge for a week or more and is perfect for tortilla chips or tacos or dolloped on a sandwich. If ever you needed an excuse for a never-ending supply of fresh tomatillos, here it is!

Tip: Only canned tomatillos? Broil the other vegetables, then blend with the canned tomatillos with their juices as directed.

1 pound fresh tomatillos
3 to 4 serrano chiles, stemmed and seeded
    (use jalapeños if you can't find serranos)
4 cloves garlic

1 small white onion, chopped coarsely

2 green onions, separated into their white
and green parts

1 cup fresh cilantro leaves, lightly packed

1/2 teaspoon salt, or more to taste

2 tablespoons water, or more as needed

1. Remove the papery husks from the tomatillos, place in a large bowl, and cover with warm water. Slosh the tomatillos around for a few minutes to remove their sticky, waxy coating. Drain and pat dry.

2. Preheat the broiler to high. In a cast-iron skillet or a broiler-safe pan, place the serranos, garlic, onion, and white ends of the green onions and broil for 2 to 4 minutes, until the chiles are charred and blistered; some chiles may even split open. Remove the pan from the oven and scrape the serrano mixture into a mixing bowl to cool. Place the tomatillos in the hot pan and broil for 6 to 8 minutes, turning occasionally with tongs, until the tomatillos have softened, turned a dull green with charred spots. I usually remove the smaller tomatillos first and let the larger ones roast the full 8 minutes. Turn off the broiler and remove the pan from the oven. Transfer the roasted tomatillos to a bowl or plate to cool.

3. In a food processor, pulse the roasted serrano mixture for a few seconds. Add the green parts of the green onions and the cilantro and pulse again to chop finely, scraping down the sides of the processor bowl several times. Add the cooled tomatillos, salt, and water and pulse to a pureed or slightly chunky consistency, whichever you desire. If you like a thinner, pourable-style salsa, pulse in an additional 2 tablespoons of water or more, as desired. Taste and adjust with more salt, if desired. Best if served at room temperature.

Variation

Roasted Tomato Salsa: This one is easy. Just replace the tomatillos with ripe red plum tomatoes. Roast them whole in the oven until the skins are blistered and a little charred. Proceed as directed. Or use a combination of tomatoes and tomatillos for a beautiful roasted salsa.

THE ONLY GUACAMOLE RECIPE I EVER MAKE

- Serves 4 as a side
- Time: Less than 10 minutes
- Gluten Free, Soy Free

Guacamole, probably just after salsa, is a Latin food that's become second nature to most North Americans (it's almost shocking to meet somebody who's never eaten it!) and is a regular guest at parties and in burritos everywhere. But no mention of a guacamole recipe in a vegan Latin cookbook would be scandalous, so here it is. Speaking of scandal, I avoid putting too many things in my guac; I like it simple and straightforward.

The most important guac tip? Use only perfectly ripe avocados; the flesh should not have brown spots and should be soft and yielding without being mushy, and the skin should be dark but not pitted. I like it without tomatoes, but if you must, incorporate very finely diced ripe red ones after mixing all the other ingredients together. The legendary method for keeping it fresh is to place the whole avocado pit into the finished guacamole to help prevent its turning brown, but it's likely that that lime juice will do the real work.

Tip: Selecting good avocados is the hardest part of making good guacamole. Most avos are sold unripe and will ripen within 2 to 4 days of purchase, so timing is everything. A perfectly ripe avocado should feel firm but not rock hard; gently press the skin—it will yield slightly and a knife piercing the skin will slide easily into the fruit. Avocados that are too ripe feel mushy and have dark pits or patches on the skin; overly ripe avocados taste bitter or otherwise "off." Use a perfectly ripe avocado either that same day or early on the next day . . . ripe avocados may seem to get riper by the minute, especially in warm weather.

2 ripe avocados (any variety)
2 to 3 tablespoons freshly squeezed lime juice (about the juice from 1 large lime)

1 small yellow onion, peeled and minced
1 small green hot chile—serranos are ideal—minced finely (optional)
1/2 teaspoon salt, or to taste
2 tablespoons chopped fresh cilantro (optional)

1. Slice and peel the avocados and place in a mixing bowl. Sprinkle with the lime juice, minced onion, chile, salt, and cilantro, if using. Use a fork to mash everything together into a creamy, chunky paste. Taste and adjust the seasoning with more lime juice and salt, if desired. Serve immediately.

Variation

For a smoother guacamole, try grinding together the onion, chile, and cilantro with a mortar and pestle until smooth and then mash the mixture into the remaining ingredients. This is basically how a stone Mexican mole bowl (*molcajete*) works, grinding ingredients into pastes for smoother salsas. The onion and chile flavors will be distributed more evenly throughout your guacamole and you might just like it so much, you'll always make it that way from now on!

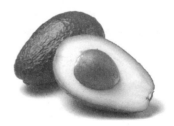

FRESH TOMATO SALSA WITH ROASTED CHILES

....

- Makes about 3 cups salsa
- Gluten Free, Soy Free

....

If you've heard of a burrito, you probably also know some kind of fresh tomato salsa, usually referred to as *pico de gallo*. This is what comes to mind when most people think of that certain five-letter word that's served up with tortilla chips: a chunky mixture of fresh tomatoes and herbs with a touch of chile and lime.

Of course, ripe red summer tomatoes make the best salsa, but up north we only have a few months of these heavenly tomatoes and that's when canned diced tomatoes come to the rescue. This is a perfectly delicious and affordable option during those long no-tasty-tomato months of the late fall, winter, and spring (see how desperate things can get?).

2 to 4 jalapeño or serrano chiles

2 pounds ripe red tomatoes, preferably plum, seeded and chopped finely

1 large white onion, diced finely

3 tablespoons lime juice

1/2 cup finely chopped fresh cilantro

1/2 teaspoon salt or more to taste

1. Roast the chiles as described on page 46, peel, and remove stems. If desired, remove seeds for a milder heat (or leave in if using serranos, as these seeds are smaller and softer than those of jalapeños). Mince the chiles as finely as possible and place in a mixing bowl.

2. Add the tomatoes and onion to the chiles and stir in the lime juice and salt. Chill the salsa for 30 minutes or let sit at room temperature, for the flavors to blend and the tomatoes to tenderize and release more of their juices.

Variations

Winter Salsa: It's February, it's snowing outside, and you need fresh tomato salsa. Don't even think of using those plastic pink wrapped things called "tomatoes." And perhaps you don't want to pay ten dollars a pound for tomatoes shipped from halfway across the world. Instead, reach for a 32-ounce can of diced organic tomatoes and stir into the chiles and other ingredients. If you prefer a less watery salsa, try draining off a little bit (but not too much) of the liquid first.

Dried Chile Salsa: Replace the fresh green chiles with dried bright red chiles. Chile de arbol or costeño are my favorites for tomato salsa. Leave the pods whole (with seeds) and gently toast (see Red Chile Sauce, page 45) until fragrant. Remove the stems and grind in a spice grinder, then stir into the salsa. Let this salsa sit for at least an hour before serving, to allow the dried chiles to soak in the tomato juices.

CASHEW CREMA

....

- Makes about 1 2/3 cups *crema*
- Time: Less than 10 minutes, not including cashew soaking time
- Soy Free and Gluten Free

....

Light, tangy, and a wee bit salty, this raw nut cream recalls the light, smooth *cremas* used to garnish soups, stews, tacos, or whatever cultured cream is used on in Latin American food. Although it's not to be confused with sour cream, it's equally rich and should be used within a week of blending. This recipe is a little thick but you can thin it with more water if you want a *crema* with a dressinglike consistency.

  1 cup raw cashew pieces

  1/2 cup water

  2 tablespoons lemon or lime juice

  1 teaspoon agave nectar

  1/2 rounded teaspoon salt, or more to taste

1. Place the cashews in a small glass or plastic bowl and cover with at least 2 inches of cold water. Let soak for at least 4 hours or overnight; the cashews will become very soft and expand a little in size. Drain, then pulse in

a food processor with the remaining ingredients, stopping occasionally to scrape the sides of the bowl with a rubber spatula. Blend until smooth and creamy, about 2 minutes in total. Taste and adjust with more salt or lemon juice, if desired. Store in a tightly covered container in the refrigerator.

CHOCOLATE-CHILE MOLE SAUCE (A OAXACAN WANNABE)

....

- Makes about 4 1/2 cups sauce
- Time: About 1 hour
- Soy Free, Gluten Free

....

I'm a little obsessed with those famously complex Oaxacan chocolate moles. Here's my most recent attempt: a dark sauce with hints of ripe sweet fruit, nuts, and spices that's probably not the most authentic but is plenty complex, with a velvety richness all its own. The bittersweet flavors contrast expertly with sweet vegetables such as *calabacitas* or with fresh corn tortillas, or use as a luxurious dip for fried sweet plantains. You can also drape this sauce on Tempeh Asado (page 110), get fancy and serve it on top of enchiladas, or craft up a batch of special mole-filled tamales.

Tip: Oaxacan chocolate-based moles are said to have at least three different kinds of dried chiles in them. I recommend that you at least have two, one of them being ancho or pasilla and the other being mulato (the other mole chile), or play with guajillo or morita chiles. This sauce is supposed to be nuanced, so have fun experimenting with a host of chiles.

3 ounces mixed Mexican dried chiles, such as ancho, pasilla, guajillo, or mulato

1/4 cup sliced almonds

3 tablespoons chopped pecans

2 tablespoons sesame seeds

1/2 teaspoon whole aniseeds

1/4 teaspoon ground cloves

1/2 teaspoon ground cinnamon

1/2 teaspoon ground cumin

1 generous teaspoon Mexican oregano

1/4 cup crushed tortilla chips

3 tablespoons peanut oil

4 cloves garlic, chopped

1 small yellow onion, peeled and diced

1/4 cup dark raisins

1 small ripe (soft, yellow with black) plantain, peeled and diced

11/2 cup diced tomatoes with juices

3 cups warm vegetable broth

4 ounces Latin drinking chocolate, preferably Mexican, such as Ibarra, or semisweet chocolate, chopped

3/4 teaspoon salt, or to taste

1. In a large saucepan, bring 1 quart of water to a boil. Have ready a medium-size glass or metal heat-resistant bowl. Heat a cast-iron skillet over medium heat. Slice open the dried chiles, re-move the stems and seeds, and open the chiles so that they can be easily flattened when pressed with a spatula. (See the chile user's tip box, page 15, for stuff about using gloves for chile protection.) Place the chiles in the heated skillet, and with a wide metal spatula press and flip them frequently to toast, about 1 minute. Watch carefully to prevent the chiles from burn-ing. Remove the skillet from heat and transfer the chiles to a heat-resistant bowl. Pour the boil-ing water over the chiles and set aside for 10 minutes, allowing the chiles to soften. Drain the water from the chiles and set them aside.

2. Reheat the cast-iron skillet over medium heat and place the sliced almonds, chopped pecans, sesame seeds, and aniseeds in the pan. Toast, stirring frequently, for 2 to 4 min-utes, until the almonds are pale golden and the anise is fragrant. Immediately remove from the heat, scrape the seeds into a food processor or spice mill, and add the cloves, cinnamon, cumin, oregano, and tortilla chips. Pulse to a fine grind.

3. In a large saucepan, combine the oil and garlic. Heat the pan over medium heat, stirring frequently, until the garlic is sizzling and fra-grant, about 30 seconds. Add the onion and cook until translucent and soft, 6 to 8 minutes. Stir in the raisins and plantain and fry for 3 minutes, until the plantain is mushy, then sprin-kle with the ground spice mixture. Cook, stir-ring, for 1 minute. Now stir in the softened drained chiles, tomatoes, and vegetable broth.

Either use an immersion blender or pour the mixture into a blender jar and puree to create a smooth sauce. (Return the mixture to the saucepan if the blender jar is used.) Bring the pureed mixture to a simmer over medium heat, stirring frequently, about 10 minutes. Stir in the chocolate and keep stirring until completely melted and incorporated into the sauce (the sauce will darken to a deep reddish brown), 4 to 6 minutes. Season with salt and serve. For a thinner sauce, stir in a little extra vegetable broth until your desired consistency is reached.

SPICY SALSA GOLF

- Makes 1/2 cup salsa
- Time: Less than 5 minutes

This sauce has nothing to do with hitting tiny balls with sticks or driving in little carts. Why the name for a simple but catchy blend of ketchup and mayo, who can say, but it's a strangely popular sauce that seems to find its way alongside lots of fried street and finger foods in many South American and Caribbean countries. I like to add a dash of hot sauce just so I don't have to think about the fact I'm eating ketchup and mayonnaise, but instead a creamy and piquant sauce that goes nicely with fried foods such as *tostones* (page 118) or finger foods such as Mini Potatoes Stuffed with Mushrooms and Olives (page 62).

1/3 cup vegan mayonnaise
2 tablespoons all-natural ketchup
2 to 3 dashes of red hot sauce

1. Whisk together all the ingredients in a small bowl until smooth. Serve immediately.

HABANERO-MELON-PAPAYA SALSA

- Makes about 4 cups salsa
- Time: Less than 10 minutes
- Gluten Free, Soy Free

This exquisite blend of cool fruit and searing roasted habanero chile is incredibly easy to eat for a refreshing side or even a light salad in warm weather. Use this recipe as a template to craft up other fruit salsas all summer long, using two or more fruits; I like to use a bulky tropical fruit (pineapple, papaya) with juicy locally grown fruit (peach, apricot, plums, and any melon, of course) for a sort of cross-cultural effect. Or use whatever really, it just tastes good. Serve with tortilla chips and thin slices of jicama as a snack or alongside any entrée.

Tip: See page 46 for tips on roasting chile peppers. As it's unlikely you'll need more than one habanero for this recipe, roasting on the stovetop on top of a heat diffuser is your best bet for small chiles like these. If you're not accustomed to habanero heat, go slow, adding a quarter or a third of the chopped chile to the salsa at first, then adding more as needed. If you've found that you've accidentally made your salsa a little too hot to handle, just stir in more chopped fruit.

1 habanero chile, roasted
3 green onions, trimmed and sliced thinly
3 tablespoons lime juice
1/2 teaspoon salt, or to taste
1 1/2 pounds ripe papaya, preferably
   Mexican/Latin American papaya
   (see papaya tip, page 215)
1 pound melon, such as cantaloupe,
   watermelon, crenshaw, honeydew

1. Remove the stem and seeds from the roasted habanero and mince the chile very finely, almost to a pulp if possible. (You may want to use gloves in this case, tough guy.) Place your desired amount of minced chile, green onions, lime juice, and salt in a large mixing bowl. Slice papaya in half, remove and discard seeds, and use a Y-shaped vegetable peeler to remove the papaya peel. Slice the papaya into bite-size pieces and add to the bowl. Slice the melon, remove and discard the seeds, and dice into 1/4-inch pieces. Stir the fruit to coat completely with the ingredients in the bowl and serve the salsa immediately. Fruit salsas are best eaten the day they are made.

3

BOCADILLOS, SNACKS, AND APPETIZERS

*B*ocadillo basically means "sandwich" in Spanish, but the word is so expressive it does double duty as a name for this chapter. *Boca* means "mouth," what you like to cram tasty things into, and *dillo* (dee-yo) is a general-use suffix meaning "cute" or "little." So here's an all-purpose chapter for small portions of tasty food that stand on their own. Sandwiches figure into the Latin *'dillo* factor in a big way, ranging from Mexican *tortas* piled high, tacos, arepas, or even a clever miniature version of the *patacones*, a sandwich built upon fried plantains.

You may also like to think of these little meals as appetizers (or tapas). Speaking of tapas, I say why not skip the idea of an entrée for dinner entirely and construct a meal of two to three different *bocadillos*. Then you don't have to worry about filling up before the entrée arrives, because the best part is already here.

• • •

EGGPLANT TORTA SANDWICH

- Makes 4 large sandwiches
- Time: About 50 minutes, including making the filling and roasting the eggplant

Think of this as eggplant hero goes south, really south, in the form of Mexico's beloved sandwich, the *torta*. *Tortas* are popular wherever a Mexican community calls home. This type of sandwich can be stuffed with all kinds of fillings, usually of the meaty persuasion, but is always overflowing and intriguingly decadent. Baking (or grilling) the eggplant instead of pan-frying keeps it a little lighter and allows for adding richer ingredients, such as spicy chipotle mayo and avocado.

Tip: Grilling the eggplant is an excellent option for a more smoky flavor that sings with the chipotle mayo. Either grill on a cast-iron grill pan or, if you're one of the lucky ones with an outdoor grill, double or triple the eggplant for use in sandwiches, tacos, and arepas. I prefer to salt eggplant to eliminate any bitterness, but if your eggplants are very fresh and not too big, skip this step.

Marinated Eggplant

- 1 pound eggplant, preferably small young eggplants
- 2 tablespoons freshly squeezed lime juice
- 4 tablespoons olive oil
- 3 tablespoons tomato paste
- 2 cloves garlic, smashed
- 1 teaspoon dried oregano, preferably Mexican
- 1/2 teaspoon ground cumin

Sandwich

- 2/3 cup vegan mayonnaise
- 2 chipotles in adobo sauce, seeds removed
- 1 cup Home-style Refried Beans (page 86), black or pinto
- 2 ripe red tomatoes, seeded and sliced into 1/4-inch slices
- 1 ripe avocado, peeled, seeded, and sliced into 1/4-inch slices
- 1/2 pound shredded romaine or iceberg lettuce
- 4 pickled jalapeño peppers, sliced very thinly
- 1/2 recipe Pickled Red Onions (page 43) or 1 red onion, sliced into thin rings
- 4 crusty French or rustic-style sandwich rolls

1. Preheat the oven to 375ºF. Prepare the eggplant first: Slice it lengthwise, about 1/4 inch thick, place in a colander above a sink, and lightly salt with kosher salt, if desired. Let the eggplant soften and drain for 30 minutes. While the eggplant drains, prepare the marinade by whisking together the lime juice, olive oil, tomato paste, garlic, oregano, and cumin. Add the drained eggplant, coat the slices with marinade, and let stand for 10 minutes, turning the slices occasionally.

When ready to roast the eggplant, lightly oil a rimmed baking sheet and spread with a layer of eggplant, trying not to overlap the slices too much. Brush each side generously with the marinade and roast for 10 to 12 minutes, flipping each slice and roasting for another 10 minutes until the eggplant is tender. Remove from the oven and wrap in foil to keep the eggplant warm.

2. Prepare the sandwich ingredients: To make chipotle mayonnaise, pulse the vegan mayonnaise and chipotle peppers in a food processor until smooth. Warm the refried beans either in a microwave or on a stovetop, adding a little water if necessary to create a spreadable consistency. Have ready the tomatoes, avocado, lettuce, and either Pickled Red Onions or thinly sliced red onion rings.

3. Slice each sandwich roll in half horizontally and, if desired, remove some of the bread inside each roll to allow more room for the filling. Toast or grill each roll half until hot. Assemble a sandwich by spreading the inside of a roll with chipotle mayonnaise, then topping that with refried beans. Stack on the bottom half a generous layer each of eggplant, tomato, avocado, shredded lettuce, jalapeño (if using), and some onions, and top with the upper half of the roll. Firmly press down on the sandwich, or to heat it panini style, grill it on both sides on a hot cast-iron skillet, pressing each side until the bread is browned and the edges crisp.

4. Slice each sandwich in half and serve immediately with a fresh lime wedge and slices of crisp radish.

Variations

Calabacita Torta: Replace the eggplant with young tender green or yellow summer squash.

Also see Taco Toppings! (page 176) for more ideas on what to put in *tortas*. Anything you would put on a taco can make a great *torta* filling, too, except for maybe supersaucy items.

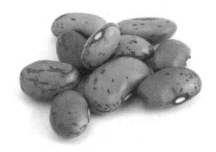

MASHED POTATO PANCAKES WITH PEANUT SAUCE (LLAPINGACHOS)

....

- Makes about eight 3-inch pancakes
- Time: About 45 minutes
- Soy Free

....

Tasty little mashed potato cakes pan-fried to perfection are an Ecuadorean favorite enjoyed as breakfast or hearty snack. *Llapingachos* can be served alone or with a traditional Peanut Sauce (page 41), but seem equally at home with So Good, So Green Dipping Sauce (page 43) and Pickled Red Onions (page 43). *Llapingachos* are hearty little *bocadillos* on their own but, for a full meal, serve with multiple sauces, a cabbage salad, and Latin Baked Tofu (page 103).

Typically *llapingachos* contain egg to help bind them, but in this case we're relying on the gluten in wheat flour do to the job. That being said, these are somewhat delicate and require a gentle hand, so a wide, firm spatula will be your friend when flipping and shaping these babies. Keeping the pancakes small—just under 3 inches wide—also improves the chances of your *llapingachos* staying together when being flipped.

Tip: Sometimes *llapingachos* are stuffed with a white cheese. Have some meltable vegan mozzarella-style cheese on hand? Then try placing a few thin slivers into the centers (depending on the ingredients, the cheese may not be soy free).

1 1/2 **pounds red- or yellow-skinned waxy potatoes**
1 **small yellow onion, minced**
1 **clove garlic, crushed**
1/2 **cup all-purpose flour, plus additional flour for coating**
1/4 **teaspoon baking soda**
2 **tablespoons nutritional yeast (optional, but adds a touch of cheeselike flavor)**
1 **tablespoon lime juice**
1/2 **teaspoon kosher salt, or to taste**
Freshly ground pepper
Peanut or vegetable oil for shallow frying

1. Wash the potatoes, peel if desired (I leave red-skinned potato jackets on, for color), and dice them into large chunks. Place in a large pot, cover with cold water, cover the pot, and bring to a boil over high heat. Lower the heat to medium and cook the potatoes for 20 to 25 minutes, or until tender.

Drain the water and pour the potatoes in a large mixing bowl. Add the minced onion and garlic and mash to form a chunky paste. Let the mashed potatoes cool to the touch and add the flour, baking soda, nutritional yeast (if using), lime juice, salt, and freshly ground pepper.

2. Pour the additional flour (use a little less than 1/4 cup) into a shallow bowl. Using your hands, knead the flour and other ingredients into the mashed potato mixture. Knead for about 3 minutes to stimulate the gluten in the flour, then separate the potato dough into eight equal pieces and roll into balls. Shape the *llapingachos* by lightly dusting your hands with flour and gently patting a ball of mashed potatoes into a small cake about 3/4 to 1 inch thick and about 3 inches in diameter. Dredge all the sides of the potato cake in flour. Repeat with the remaining dough and dredge each in flour.

3. Heat about 1/2 inch of peanut oil in a heavy cast-iron skillet over medium heat. The oil is ready when a pinch of potato sizzles when dropped in the oil. Carefully slide two or three cakes into the hot oil and cook for 2 1/2 to 3 minutes per side, occasionally pushing the cakes toward the sides of the skillet to help evenly cook their edges. Carefully flip the cakes once—they may be delicate during cooking—and cook for another 2 1/2 to 3 minutes. Well-cooked *llapingachos* should be golden on both sides. Slide the cooked cakes onto crumpled brown paper or paper towels to drain and cool for 1 to 2 minutes. Serve hot with Peanut Sauce (page 41), Pickled Red Onions (page 43), or any other salsa you like.

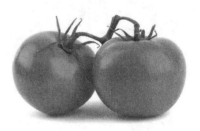

MIXED MUSHROOM CEVICHE

- Serves 3 to 4 as an appetizer or 2 as an entrée
- Time: About 30 minutes, not including marinating time
- Gluten Free, Soy Free

Ceviche, a method of "cooking" raw seafood in citrus juices, popular in many coastal parts of Latin America, is perhaps most commonly associated with Peru. But ceviche doesn't always have to equal seafood; mushroom ceviches like this are not uncommon and raw mushrooms are rendered juicy and tender after a few hours in a spicy and refreshing marinade.

Mushroom ceviche can be served as either a zesty appetizer or light entrée in warm weather. I like the flavor and visual variety of using a mixture of mushrooms but I do insist that you use light-colored mushrooms in this dish (save the portobellos for *feijoada*) as they look the most appealing after marinating. The huge king trumpet mushroom (mysteriously also known as an elf mushroom) costs more but is my favorite in this dish for juicy, long strips that are fun to eat. Oyster mushrooms live up to their name and provide a seafoodlike texture, and button mushrooms are reliable additions to any ceviche. Store raw, unsliced mushrooms in a closed paper bag in the fridge until ready to use.

Peruvian ceviches are often served with boiled sweet potatoes and seasoned corn kernels. The contrast of cool mushrooms, tender warm sweet potatoes, and chewy corn makes for an oil-free meal that is super low–calorie, refreshing yet substantial, too.

Tip: Regular fresh white corn is just fine if you have a well-stocked Latin grocery nearby; take a peek in their frozen section for *choclo* corn. These big fat white kernels of South American corn are the traditional sidekick of ceviche and really taste different from our sweet corn. Enjoy it boiled for 10 to 12 minutes, or until the kernels are no longer starchy but instead chewy and succulent. For a real Peruvian treat, cook the corn with a pinch of aniseeds and a tablespoon or more of sugar. I know it may sound strange but the chewy nuggets of sweet corn with a hint of licorice flavor is a quietly addictive snack even without the ceviche.

Ceviche

1/2 generous pound mixture of light-colored mushrooms such as oyster, white cremini, enoki, white button, or king trumpet mushroom

1 small red onion, cut in half, then sliced into thin shreds

1/4 cup freshly squeezed lime

1 to 2 small fresh hot chiles, seeded and finely minced, or 2 teaspoons *ají amarillo* paste (or both!)

3 tablespoons finely minced fresh cilantro

1 teaspoon salt
A pinch of sugar
Freshly ground pepper

Corn and Sweet Potato Garnish
1 1/2 cups white corn kernels, preferably
    fresh, or use frozen
1 pound orange-fleshed sweet potato
2 tablespoons lime juice
1/2 teaspoon salt
Lettuce leaves or tomato wedges,
    for garnish

1. With a clean kitchen towel, gently brush the mushrooms free of any debris and dirt. Use a sharp knife to remove and discard any tough stems. Slice very large mushrooms into strips no thicker than 1/2 inch. Leave very small mushrooms intact and slice medium-size mushrooms in half. The idea is to have a variety of shapes and sizes easy to eat in one or two bites.

2. Place the mushrooms in a large glass bowl and sprinkle the shredded onion on top. In a measuring cup, whisk together the lime juice, minced hot chiles, and/or *ají amarillo* paste, cilantro, salt, and freshly ground pepper. Pour over the mushrooms and onions and gently toss with tongs. Cover the container tightly and chill for 3 to 4 hours, occasionally stirring or gently shaking the container to redistribute the juices. The mushrooms are ready to eat when they are soft and juicy to the bite and have reduced in bulk by nearly half. Season with more salt and pepper, if desired, before serving.

3. About 45 minutes before serving time, peel the sweet potato, place in a large saucepan, and cover with cold water. Bring the water to a boil, lower the heat to a simmer, and cook the potato until tender and easily pierced with a fork, 35 to 40 minutes. During the final 10 minutes of cooking the potato, boil the corn kernels in a separate pan, cooking until the corn is tender but not mushy, 3 to 5 minutes, and drain. Drain the potato, slice into 1/2-inch-thick rounds, and sprinkle with half the lime juice and salt to taste. Sprinkle the corn with the remaining lime juice and season with salt.

Serve the ceviche in either an oval serving dish or shallow bowls. Arrange lettuce leaves and warm sweet potato slices on one end of the dish and mound the warm corn kernels on the other end. In the center, mound the chilled mushroom ceviche. Serve immediately. As you eat, nibble on alternate bites of mushrooms, sweet potato, and corn.

Variation

Use frozen (or fresh if you can find it) rocoto pepper in place of fresh hot chiles. Rocotos can be large, so finely chop 1 to 2 tablespoons and add as directed.

TOSTONES WITH AVOCADO AND PALM CEVICHE

- Serves 4 as a side or appetizer
- Time: About 30 minutes, not including marinating time
- Gluten Free, Soy Free

This is not a true ceviche, in the sense that nothing gets "cooked" by the citrus juice. But this zippy salad of creamy hearts of palm and avocado is a vegan riff on the traditional seafood ceviche filling for *tostones rellenos*, the fun Cuban snack of fried *tostones* formed into a cup, which is convenient for holding tasty fillings. A special variation of a *tostonera* is needed to make the *tostone* cups, but this filling is just as delectable scooped up with traditional flat *tostones*.

Tip: Look for organic, sustainably grown hearts of palm in glass jars or cans. If you can score actual fresh hearts of palm marinate them in the lime juice dressing for 20 minutes first and then stir in the avocado before serving with the *tostones*.

1 (14-ounce) jar or can of hearts of palm, drained and rinsed

1 large ripe red tomato (1/2 pound), seeded and diced finely

1 small red onion, peeled and diced finely

2 tablespoons lime juice

1 tablespoon white wine vinegar or more lime juice

1 tablespoon olive oil

2 tablespoons finely chopped fresh cilantro

1 teaspoon dried oregano

1/2 teaspoon salt

1 large ripe avocado

4 green unripe large plantains prepared as *tostones* (page 118)

1. Slice each palm heart down the center vertically, then slice into 1/2-inch pieces and place in a mixing bowl. Add the tomato and onion. Pour the lime juice, white wine vinegar, olive oil, chopped cilantro, oregano, and salt on top and mix well. Chill for 30 minutes to blend the flavor.

2. While the "ceviche" is chilling, prepare your *tostones*. Just before serving, peel and remove the seed from the avocado. Finely dice and thoroughly fold into the ceviche, making sure it's covered with the dressing. Mound the ceviche into serving cups and serve immediately with the hot *tostones*, or fill the *tostone* cups if you happen to have a special *tostonera* for making the cups.

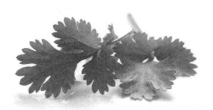

MINI POTATOES STUFFED WITH MUSHROOMS AND OLIVES (PAPAS RELLENAS)

- Makes 20 to 22 appetizer-size stuffed potatoes
- Time: About 1 hour, including boiling and baking, not including assembly
- Gluten Free, Soy Free

Papas Rellenas—deep-fried mashed potato balls filled with ground meat—are a popular street food all over Latin America. I've taken this snack through the great veganator-machine (a.k.a. my kitchen). Besides the obvious meatlessness, this recipe uses small new potatoes left whole, which have been precooked, hollowed out and stuffed with a savory concoction of ground mushrooms spiked with olives, raisins, and smoky paprika. A final baking frees you from messing around with deep-frying, too.

These can be time consuming to put together but make an impressive appetizer indeed. Of course, you could also make a meal instead and stuff the filling into large entrée-size potatoes. Either way, they're great on their own or served with a classic "street food"-style sauce—try So Good, So Green Dipping Sauce (page 43) or Spicy Salsa Golf (page 53).

Tip: Hollowing out little potatoes can be tedious, so consider making these a day in advance of filling. Or, if making larger potatoes, bake for double the amount of time and slice into bite-size pieces to use as appetizers.

2 pounds small new potatoes, each about 2 inches long or slightly smaller

Filling

1 pound cremini mushrooms
2 tablespoons olive oil
2 cloves garlic
1 small yellow onion, diced
1/4 cup walnuts, ground in a food processor into fine crumbs
1 teaspoon dried oregano
1/2 teaspoon ground cumin
1/2 teaspoon smoked sweet or hot paprika
1/2 teaspoon salt
1/2 cup dark raisins
1/2 cup black or green olives, chopped
2 tablespoons dry bread crumbs
A few twists freshly ground black pepper

1. Boil the potatoes until tender but not mushy, 14 to 16 minutes. Drain, rinse with cold water, and set aside until cool enough to handle. While the potatoes are cooking and cooling, prepare the filling.

2. Use a paper towel or a clean dishcloth to remove any dirt or debris from the mushrooms and trim and discard any tough stems. Use a food processor to finely chop the mushrooms; you may find it easier to cut them in half or quarters for easy chopping in the food processor. The

chopped mushrooms will look dark and moist; to avoid pureed mushrooms, do not overchop.

3. In a large skillet over medium heat, fry the garlic in the peanut oil until it starts to sizzle, about 30 seconds. Add the onion and fry until translucent and soft, 6 to 8 minutes. Stir in the mushrooms, ground walnuts, oregano, cumin, paprika, salt, and pepper, and fry the mixture. Stir constantly until the mushrooms have reduced in bulk and are dark and soft, 10 to 12 minutes. Stir in the raisins, chopped olives, bread crumbs, and freshly ground black pepper to taste. Continue to stir-fry the mixture until most of the mushroom liquid has evaporated but the mixture is still moist. Taste the filling and adjust the salt and pepper, if desired. Remove the pan from the heat and let the filling cool enough to be handled.

4. Preheat the oven to 375ºF and lightly oil a large metal baking tray. Carefully slice off the top third of each potato lengthwise; you may want to first see which side each potato can rest on without rolling around (much) and slice it from the opposite side to fill. Use a 1/2-teaspoon measuring spoon or a melon baller to remove as much of the potato interior as possible; leave a thin 3/8 inch or so of potato near the skin. Save the scooped potato for mashed potatoes or use in *llapingachos* (page 57).

5. Using the measuring spoon or your fingers, scoop as much of the filling as possible into the potato shells, mounding the filling on top and using your palm to shape it. Place the stuffed potatoes on the prepared baking tray and, if desired, spray or brush with a little extra olive oil. Bake for 15 to 20 minutes, until the potato is tender and the filling is hot. Serve immediately.

MEXICAN SIDE-STREET CORN

- **Makes 4 ears of corn**
- **Time: About 35 minutes, mostly inactive while roasting the corn**

It's as if you can't even step into the streets these days without somebody forcing on you *elotes*, perfectly cooked corn on the cob covered in savory Mexican spices. Well, I wish. If this isn't happening to you on a regular basis, then it's time to take matters into your own hands and make this zesty Mexican street food at home.

This corn is a great messy snack but makes an exciting casual side, too. I love Cashew Crema (page 51) here but vegan mayonnaise is a handy shortcut. Then you can hit the streets for your own roasted corn revolution.

4 whole ears corn, preferably completely covered with their husk
1/2 cup Cashew Crema (page 51), or
1/3 cup vegan mayonnaise
Coarse salt, such as kosher or sea salt
Your favorite ground dried Mexican chile, such as ancho or chipotle, or any chile powder blend

Finely crumbled dried Mexican oregano
2 limes, cut in half
Peanut or vegetable oil, if pan-grilling
   corn

1. For oven-roasted corn: This method is best done with fresh summer corn from the farmers' market. Your corn should have plenty of green fresh husk tightly wrapped around it. Preheat the oven to 350ºF and place the whole ears of corn, husks and all, onto a center rack and roast for 30 minutes. Remove from the oven and using oven mitts, peel back the hot husks and the corn silk. Add the toppings (see step 2) and eat immediately.

For stovetop-grilled corn: Also great for fresh farm-stand corn, this method works for corn with the husks removed or even thawed frozen corn on the cob. Preheat a cast-iron grill pan (the kind with raised grill lines on the bottom) or a regular cast-iron pan over medium-high heat. Remove any husk and silk, lightly oil the corn, and place on the hot pan. Grill the corn for 12 to 14 minutes, using tongs to rotate it occasionally. When the corn is golden or even a little charred, if you desire, remove from the pan, add the toppings, and serve.

For an outside grill: Once a year I get outside near a grill and when I do, I grill corn on the cob like this. Peel back the husks but leave them attached to the stem. Remove the silk, push the husks back around the corn, and soak the entire ears in cold water for 30 minutes. Throw on a hot grill and grill, turning occasionally, for 12 to 14 minutes, or until the kernels are tender.

2. To top the cooked corn, whisk the vegan mayonnaise (if using) until smooth. If the mayo is very thick, try adding a few tablespoons of lime juice to thin it out enough to easily spread. Divide the mayonnaise or Cashew Crema among the ears of corn and slather it on top. (If you're not the slathering type, put the mayo in an old condiment squeeze bottle and squeeze as desired on top of the corn.) Then sprinkle the corn with a little salt, a generous amount of chile powder, and a pinch of Mexican oregano. Take a lime half and squeeze as much juice as possible all over that corn. Eat right away!

Variations

Make this even more vegan by sprinkling the corn with nutritional yeast flakes (for a hint of cheeselike flavor) before finishing with the lime juice.

Viejo Bay: Omit the salt and oregano. Sprinkle Old Bay Seasoning as desired in addition to the chile powder and proceed as directed.

Tip: Just Roasted Corn

Roasting corn on the cob using any of these methods makes kernels deliciously ready to be used in burritos, tacos, or salads. Use a corn zipper (see Kitchen Tools, page 26) or a thin, sharp knife to remove the kernels from cooled cobs.

BITE-SIZE GREEN PLANTAIN SANDWICHES (PATACONES)

- Makes 10 to 12 appetizer-size "sandwiches"
- Time: About 30 minutes, not including making the seitan or salsa

Patacones, a specialty sandwich in the Maracaibo area of eastern Venezuela, is a miracle made of a whole fried green plantain *tostone* used as bread to "sandwich" fillings usually seen in arepas and are a popular street food or late-night snack. I prefer this scaled-down appetizer version for making at home and serving to friends.

This filling can be embellished with vegan cheese, beans, or other veggies, but considering the small scale of *tostones*, this amount fits just fine. The plantains here are cut thinner and gently rolled for a flatter *tostone* to properly sandwich everything together. Simplify and make the shredded seitan and the *golf* sauce a day or so before you fry the plantains.

4 green plantains
Vegetable oil, for deep-frying
1 recipe Latin Shredded Seitan, prepared in the "Venezuelan" style (page 106)
1 recipe Spicy Salsa Golf (page 53)
2 cups finely shredded romaine or other crisp lettuce

1 ripe avocado, peeled, seeded, and sliced very thinly
1 large ripe red tomato, seeded, sliced in half, then sliced very thinly

1. Peel and prepare green plantains for frying like *tostones* (page 118), *except* slice them thinly (about 1/2 inch) and make sure to slice them on a 45-degree angle to make long slices, about 2 inches in length. Before the second frying step, place a warm *tostone* between two sheets of brown or waxed paper and use a rolling pin to gently and evenly press the plantains flatter. Take care not to pulverize the slices, though, then fry again as directed and drain.

2. Keep the Latin Shredded Seitan warm (or reheat) either in a saucepan on the stovetop or in a microwave. If necessary lightly sprinkle avocado with lime juice to keep from browning. Have the lettuce and tomato handy and prepare the Salsa Golf now, if necessary.

3. To assemble a "sandwich," place a warm *tostone* on a cutting board and top with a small dollop of Salsa Golf. Add a little lettuce, a tomato slice, a generous tablespoon of seitan, and slice of avocado. Spread a little extra Salsa Golf on another *tostone* and press it on top of the whole pile. Serve immediately. For a cheeky presentation, you can spear each little "sandwich" with a cocktail toothpick to keep it all together while your guests grab at them, as things can get messy in the crazy world of *patacones*.

Variations

Replace the shredded seitan with a smear of thick black-bean Home-style Refried Beans (page 86)

If you want to use vegan cheese, arrange a layer of *tostones* on a baking sheet and top each one with a mound of finely shredded, meltable, mozzarella-style vegan cheese. Place under a preheated broiler and broil until the cheese melts, 4 to 5 minutes. Remove from the broiler, immediately top with whatever else you want, and finally top with another *tostone*. Serve right away.

CUBANO VEGANO SANDWICH

Makes 4 sandwiches
Time: 20 minutes, not including preparing seitan

I am pleased to present this unapologetically vegan version of the widely admired pulled-pork Cuban sandwich. Behold the perfect storm of tangy roasted seitan, vegan cheese, and sweet pickles embraced by buttery toasted bread. Don't even think of adding lettuce or mayo to this sandwich; this should be an undeniably "meaty" indulgence. Keep roasted seitan ready in the fridge and you'll have Cuban sandwiches in less than 10 minutes on a busy weeknight.

Press this veggie Cubano on a hot griddle to achieve its signature dense texture and crispy finish. A panini sandwich press is great, but an old fashioned hand-held grill press or even a brick wrapped in aluminum foil also work beautifully. A tour of your local construction site should yield something useful.

Note: It's said what really makes the Cuban sandwich special is the bread; Cuban bread looks similar to wide French bread but with a not-too-hard crust and a springy interior. Unfortunately for us, it is often made with lard and almost impossible to find outside of Cuban communities. For your sandwich-making adventure look for long sandwich rolls or French bread that has a moderately firm, thin crust and tender crumb and is wide enough (no less than 3½ inches thick) to properly contain the fillings.

1 recipe Mojo Oven-Roasted Seitan (page 104)

Sandwich

4 6- or 8-inch long sandwich rolls or 1 long, wide French bread loaf cut into 4 pieces
Nonhydrogenated vegan margarine
Prepared yellow mustard
1½ cups sweet pickle slices, drained (bread and butter pickles work great)
1 5-ounce package vegan ham slices
5 or 6 ounces white meltable vegan cheese, sliced very thin (⅛ inch)

1. Prepare Mojo Oven-Roasted Seitan, remove from oven, and let cool enough to handle. If you're not using it right away, cover it with foil and keep it warm in the oven. If you're using prepared seitan that's cold, heat it first in a microwave for 30 to 40 seconds. It will help melt the vegan cheese during the grilling.

2. Assemble the sandwich. Slice each roll in half and spread interior with margarine. Spread generously with mustard on one side, layer with pickles, then ham slices, sliced roasted seitan (sprinkle with any extra marinade), lastly slices of vegan cheese. Top with other half of bread. Spread with plenty of margarine on both outer sides of sandwich, top and bottom.

3. Preheat a wide cast-iron griddle over medium-low heat. You don't want it so hot that it burns the bread, but still hot enough to heat the insides of the sandwich and melt the vegan cheese. Place the sandwich on the griddle and, using your sandwich press (or foil-covered brick), press down very firmly, squashing the sandwich as much as possible. If using a brick, leave it on top of the sandwich and let it grill for 3 to 3$^{1}/2$ minutes, watching to make sure the sandwich doesn't burn. Remove the brick and use a wide spatula to carefully flip the sandwich. Press it again, applying as much pressure as possible. Grill for another 3 minutes or so until the vegan cheese looks softened and the bread is golden and crisp.

4. Move the sandwich onto a cutting board and use a sharp, serrated bread knife to diagonally slice it into two triangles. Serve immediately.

● ● ●

4

ENSALADAS

*B*asic elements of Latin cuisine, salads can be as simple as a mound of shredded cabbage, some tomato, threads of onion, or chunks of ripe avocado. And if the cook feels like elaborating, a splash of vinegar or lime juice, oil, and salt.

Some of the traditional salads here fit that bill perfectly—cabbage *curdito* and the simple Chilean salad of shredded onions and tomato—and are incredibly tasty just as they are. Some are lavish fiesta-ready creations, such as a contemporary version of a fruity Mexican holiday favorite and a potato salad with subtle chayote "pear" squash and capers.

And to also satisfy those North American cravings for big entrée salads, there are meal-worthy concoctions chock-full of vegetables, grains, and beans, too. And a few zesty salad dressings to liven up your regular fixings make any salad a potential Latin meal.

• • •

THREE LATIN SALAD DRESSINGS

These three easy dressings transport standard American salad ingredients with a boost of Latin *sabór*. Keep these fresh dressings in a tightly-capped glass or plastic jar in the fridge and use within a week for freshest flavor.

Cilantro-Citrus Vinaigrette

- **Makes about 3/4 cup dressing**
- **Time: Less than 10 minutes**
- **Soy Free**

An herby all-purpose vinaigrette fine for both large salads and tossing with fresh greens for a light side salad.

> 1/2 cup olive oil or grapeseed oil
> 2 tablespoons lime or orange juice, or a
>   combination of both
> 1 tablespoon red wine vinegar

2 tablespoons fresh cilantro leaves,
    lightly packed
2 cloves garlic, chopped coarsely
1 teaspoon mustard powder or prepared
    Dijon mustard
1/2 teaspoon salt
Freshly ground pepper

1 green chile pepper, seeded and chopped
3 tablespoons olive oil
2 tablespoons red wine vinegar
1 teaspoon dried oregano
1/2 teaspoon salt
A pinch of sugar (optional)
Freshly ground pepper

1. Combine all the ingredients in a blender or food processor and pulse until smooth. Use immediately or store tightly covered in the fridge for up to a week.

1. Combine all the ingredients in a blender or food processor and pulse until smooth. Use immediately or store tightly covered in the fridge for up to a week.

Fresh Gazpacho Salsa Dressing

- Makes about 1 cup dressing
- Time: Less than 10 minutes
- Soy Free

Gazpacho, that famous cold fresh tomato soup, is the inspiration for this tangy, sweet, and spicy dressing. I love how this tomato-y dressing hugs the leaves of fluffy green lettuces such as Bibb or red romaine and the thin rings of red onion. For a pleasing smoky touch, try roasting the peppers first (page 46) or roasting the tomatoes, using the oven method used for Classic Roasted Tomatillo Salsa (page 47).

1/2 pound ripe red tomatoes
1/2 cup diced sweet white onion
1/2 green, red, or yellow bell pepper,
    seeded and diced
3 cloves garlic, chopped coarsely

Creamy Ancho Chile Dressing

- Makes slightly less than 1 cup of dressing
- Time: Less than 10 minutes

Enjoy more spicy, creamy, tangy goodness with your salad! Not just for salads anymore, use this dressing as a dip for french fries or as an alternative topping for Mexican Side-Street Corn (page 63). The chipotle variation is even faster and easier, but don't let it distract you from making the tasty ancho original at least once.

2 ounces dried ancho chiles
    (3 to 4 large dried chiles)
3/4 cup vegan mayonnaise
2 tablespoons lime juice
1 tablespoon vegan ketchup

1. Slice open the dried chiles and remove and discard the stems and seeds. In a pre-

heated cast-iron pan over medium heat, toast the chiles, using a metal spatula to press them down onto the pan. Toast for about 1 minute each side until the chiles darken slightly and the skin appears somewhat brittle.

2. Place the chiles in a heatproof bowl, cover with enough boiling water to cover, and soak for 5 minutes. Discard the soaking water and, in a food processor, puree together the soaked chiles, mayonnaise, lime juice, and ketchup until very smooth. Taste the dressing and adjust the seasoning with more lime juice, if desired. For a thinner dressing, blend in a tablespoon of soy milk at a time until the desired consistency is reached.

Variation

Chipotle in Adobe: Omit the dried ancho chiles and vegan ketchup. Replace with 1 to 2 chipotles in adobo, removing the seeds from chipotles before blending. Add 1 to 2 tablespoons of the adobo sauce, as desired, and blend with the dressing.

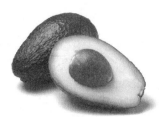

ENSALADA EQUATIONS: SIMPLE LATIN AMERICAN SIDE SALADS AND ENTRÉE SALAD IDEAS

Here's a lineup of tossed salad ideas that go together *rápido* while you're making the rest of your dinner or even just microwaving tamales straight out of the freezer. Most any of these salads can be transformed into a light but substantial meal with the addition of any baked tofu or grilled tempeh (see pages 100–108). There's enough to serve four or five as an appetizer or three or four as a large entrée. Use the ingredients as a guide, or go ahead and add less cabbage or more tomato or anything, really. Hey, it's your salad and I'm not going to tell you how to live it!

The instructions are the same for all of these salads: Place the ingredients in a large bowl, pour on as much or as little dressing as desired, and toss with tongs to completely coat everything with the dressing. Serve immediately!

CLASSIC CABBAGE

My favorite fast salad and typical of the shredded fresh cabbage salads found in many parts of Central and South America.

Cilantro-Citrus Vinaigrette (page 69) or vinegar + olive oil + dried oregano + salt and pepper + 4 cups finely shredded cabbage

2 large carrots, shredded

1 large tomato, seeded and diced

SPINACH-AVOCADO-CHILE

Top with sizzling Tempeh Asado (page 110) for a kick-butt hearty entrée salad.

Creamy Ancho Chile Dressing
(page 70) +

5 cups spinach leaves, well rinsed and
spun dry

1 small red onion, peeled and sliced
into thin rings

1 to 2 large tomatoes, seeded
and diced

2 ripe avocados, peeled, seeded, and
diced

BLACK BEAN–CORN
SALSA SALAD

Yet another way to dig into everyone's favorite pals, black beans and corn.

Fresh Gazpacho Salsa Dressing (page 70) +

6 cups Bibb or butter lettuce, torn into
bite-size pieces

2 cups roasted corn kernels
(see page 64)

2 cups or 1 (14-ounce) can cooked black
beans, rinsed and drained

1 ripe avocado, peeled, seeded,
and diced

FRUITY CHILE SLAW

Cool, fruity, and so pretty with red cabbage, pastel orange dressing, and red onions.

Creamy Ancho Chile Dressing (page 70) +

6 cups shredded red cabbage

2 large oranges, sliced into thin segments
and seeded

1 small red onion, sliced in half and then
into thin strips

1/2 cup toasted sliced almonds

SPINACH–BRAZIL NUT–
GAZPACHO SALAD

Your everyday spinach salad on a sassy tropical vacation.

Fresh Gazpacho Salsa Dressing (page 70) +

4 cups spinach, washed well and torn into
bite-size pieces

1 (14-ounce) can hearts of palm, drained,
rinsed, and sliced

2 cups or 1 (14-ounce) can cooked black
beans, rinsed

1/2 cup toasted chopped Brazil nuts

1/2 large sweet white onion, sliced into
thin strips

SHREDDED CARROT-JICAMA

A sweet and tangy slaw that's delighted to be in the presence of your favorite tacos or sandwich.

Cilantro-Citrus Vinaigrette (page 69) +

3 cups shredded carrot

1 large jicama, peeled and shredded

2 apples, shredded and immediately
  tossed with 1 tablespoon of lime or
  lemon juice

CHIPOTLE CAESAR MEXICANO

Snappy Caesar salad gets a Mexican
makeover.

Chipotle variation of Creamy Ancho Chile
  Dressing (page 70) +

5 to 6 cups romaine lettuce, torn into
  bite-size pieces

2 cups freshly made fried tortilla strips
  (see page 174)

2 cups seeded and diced ripe red tomato

"ANY NOCHE" ROMAINE AND FRUIT SALAD WITH CANDIED CHILE PEANUTS

- Generously serves 6 or more
- Time: About 1 hour, not including
  cooking the beets
- Gluten Free, Soy Free

This massive salad is inspired by the handsome sweet and savory fruity Mexican salads traditionally served on Christmas Eve,
Noche Buena. Such an exciting medley of
fruits, beets, greens, and even peanuts is
too much fun to save for only one holiday
night a year, so I've adapted this salad for
any season.

Pomegranate seeds traditionally garnish
this salad during the winter holidays, but
for a warm-weather variation, strawberries
make a pretty red substitute. This colorful
salad is right at home at parties or for feed-
ing many hungry friends during a leisurely
summer lunch or brunch.

Make-ahead Tip: Cook and peel the beets
up to three days in advance and store covered in the refrigerator. Make the candied
chile peanuts up to two weeks in advance
and store in a tightly covered container in
a cool, dark place.

Candied Chile-Peanut Topping

1 cup peanut halves

3 tablespoons light brown sugar

2 tablespoons water

1/4 teaspoon salt

1/4 teaspoon ground chile powder or
  cayenne, or more as desired

Salad

1/2 pound beets, green tops removed and
  ends trimmed

1/2 cup freshly squeezed orange juice

1/2 pound red apples, cored but
  unpeeled

1/2 pound jicama, peeled

1/2 pound fresh pineapple chunks, cut into
  bite-size pieces

2 large oranges, peeled, seeded, and
   sliced into sections
1 large head romaine lettuce,
   washed, dried, and ripped into
   bite-size pieces
1 small red onion, sliced in half, then into
   very thin rings
1/2 pound strawberries, stems removed,
   sliced

Vinaigrette
   1/3 cup light-flavored oil, such as
      grapeseed or sunflower
   1/4 cup lime juice
   1 tablespoon agave syrup
   1/2 teaspoon salt
   A big pinch of ground white pepper

1. Make the candied peanuts first. Spray a large piece of foil with nonstick cooking spray. In a nonstick skillet over medium heat, combine the peanuts, brown sugar, and water. With a heatproof silicone spatula, stir occasionally as the sugar melts into the water to form a bubbling syrup. Continue to stir for about 1 minute, then sprinkle in the salt and chile powder. Stir and cook the peanuts until syrup has thickened and coated them with a golden brown caramel, 6 to 8 minutes, watching carefully so they don't burn. Quickly spread the peanuts onto the prepared foil, breaking up any large chunks, and let cool completely before using. When ready to use, coarsely chop the peanuts into small pieces.

2. For the salad: Place beets in a small saucepan, cover with cold water, and bring to a boil over high heat. Lower the heat to a simmer and cook the beets for 25 to 35 minutes, or until easily pierced with a fork. Drain the beets, rinse with cold water, and let cool enough to be handled. Remove and discard the skins from the beets; slice in half and then into 1/4-inch-thick slices. Chill until ready to serve.

3. Pour the orange juice into a mixing bowl. Slice the apple into quarters, then into 1/4-inch-thick slices, and toss with the orange juice. Slice the jicama into 1/4-inch-thick matchsticks or bite-size pieces and toss with the apples. Stir in the pineapple chunks and orange sections.

4. In a measuring cup, whisk together all the vinaigrette ingredients until emulsified. In a very large salad bowl, toss together the lettuce, onion slices, and half of the dressing, stirring to coat the lettuce thoroughly with the dressing.

5. Arrange the juice-soaked fruit and the beets in an attractive pattern on top of the salad. Arrange the strawberries on top and drizzle the remaining dressing over everything. Sprinkle with the candied peanuts or serve them on the side. This salad is best eaten within a few hours of assembling.

Variation
Fall-to-Winter version: Omit the strawberries and replace with 1½ cups of pomegranate

arils (the deep red seeds and surrounding pulp); about one large, heavy pomegranate should have enough. Pomegranate is a traditional ingredient in this salad for Christmas Eve celebrations.

CHAYOTE AND POTATO SALAD WITH CAPERS AND PEAS

- Serves 5 to 6 as a starter course or side salad
- Time: About 45 minutes
- Soy Free

Pear-shaped, bright green, and puckered on one end like your granny's face after she's removed her dentures, chayotes are a fixture in Latin American tropical and Caribbean cuisine. And so are potato salads, so here's a happy meeting of the two! This recipe makes a ton of potato salad to serve with grilled foods or feed your next picnic.

This tropical squash is popular in soups and stews and also tossed into salad. Chayote squash has mild flavor and a subtle grassy aroma, with a crunchy texture. Boil this squash only long enough to remove any bitter undertones and its slightly sticky texture, but not too much, to retain its crispness.

Tip: Chayotes are also known as mirlitons (its Creole name, I do believe) or christophenes or cho-cho in the Caribbean. Next to plantains and yuca, they're a common item wherever Latin produce is sold.

2 chayote squash
1½ pounds white potatoes, scrubbed
2 carrots (about ¼ pound), peeled and diced into ½-inch cubes
1 cup fresh or frozen peas
¼ cup finely chopped parsley
2 tablespoons finely chopped fresh cilantro
3 green onions, minced finely
¼ cup capers, drained
⅓ cup red wine vinegar
¼ cup olive oil
1 teaspoon dried oregano
½ teaspoon dried thyme
½ teaspoon prepared Dijon mustard
1 teaspoon salt
Freshly ground black pepper

1. Bring 2 quarts of water to a boil in a large pot. Wash each chayote and cut into quarters, and remove and discard the soft white seed inside (it's edible but not that tasty). Dice the chayote into ½-inch cubes. Peel the potatoes and dice into ½-inch cubes; place in a large bowl filled with enough cold water to cover, to keep them from turning brown.

2. Add the diced chayote and carrots to the boiling water and cook for 7 to 8 minutes, until the chayote is slightly translucent on the edges and slightly tender but still firm to the bite. (Do not overcook chayote or it will become mushy.)

Drain in a metal colander set over the sink and rinse with plenty of cold water to stop the vegetables from cooking. Drain the potatoes, place in the pot, and add enough cold water to cover by about 2 inches. Bring to a boil, lower the heat to a simmer, and cook until the potatoes are tender, 14 to 18 minutes. Stir the peas into the boiling potato water within the last 2 to 3 minutes of cooking. Drain and rinse the potatoes and peas with cold water.

3. Place the drained vegetables in a very large mixing bowl. Sprinkle with the parsley, cilantro, green onions, and capers. In a measuring cup, use a wire whisk or fork to mix together the vinegar, olive oil, oregano, thyme, mustard, and salt until smooth. Pour over the vegetables, season with a few twists of freshly ground pepper, and use tongs to thoroughly mix the salad, making sure to completely coat the vegetables with dressing.

4. This salad is best served immediately slightly warm or at room temperature and is tastiest when eaten within a day of preparing.

TOMATO SALAD WITH SWEET CRISP ONIONS (ENSALADA CHILENA)

- Serves 4 as a side salad
- Time: Less than 30 minutes
- Soy Free

Chile has a national salad! It may be tempting to underestimate the deliciousness of just thinly sliced tomatoes and shredded sweet onions. But try it and eat your words (with a side of salad, of course). And you know the drill: a salad this basic requires the best possible produce, making this an ideal go-to when tomatoes are at their peak in mid- to late-summer. Don't fear the bounty of raw onions, as they are tamed by a soak in ice water and achieve a delicate juicy texture. This salad just screams for Vidalia onions, but large white Spanish onions work just as nicely.

1 very large Vidalia onion or other white
    sweet onion (about 3/4 pound)
1 pound ripe red tomatoes
2 tablespoons olive oil
4 teaspoons white wine vinegar
1/2 teaspoon dried basil, crushed finely
1/4 teaspoon salt
Freshly ground black pepper

1. Fill a large mixing bowl with about 2 cups of cold water and add a generous pinch of salt and a handful of ice cubes. You're preparing an ice water bath to soak the onions, to remove any bitterness and give them a crisp texture.

2. Peel the onions, slice in half, and with either a chef's knife, mandoline, or food processor, slice as thinly as possible. The slices should be nearly transparent, just under 1/8 inch thick. I prefer to use a knife, as it gives me the most control. If you use a food processor, take your time and make sure you don't end up accidentally pureeing your onions. Alternatively, if you have a trustworthy mandoline slicer, this would be a great time to use it. As you slice your onions, dump them into the bowl of ice water, stirring to cover completely with water. With your fingers, separate the sliced onions into individual shreds. Let the onions soak for 10 minutes.

3. Slice the tomatoes into quarters and remove and discard the pulpy seeds. Slice each quarter into thin slices, about 1/4 inch thick or slightly less, and place in a large bowl.

4. In a mixing cup, whisk together the olive oil, white vinegar, dried basil, salt, white pepper, and a few twists of black pepper with a fork or wire whisk, to create the vinaigrette dressing. When the onions are done soaking, drain them in a colander and vigorously shake to remove as much excess water as possible. Remove any ice cubes if they haven't already melted. Pour the onions on top of the tomatoes and drizzle the vinaigrette on top. Gently toss to coat vegetables with dressing and arrange as a pile on individual serving plates. Serve immediately.

Variation

Add 2 tablespoons of finely minced fresh cilantro, parsley, or basil to the dressing before pouring over the tomatoes and onions.

MANGO-JICAMA CHOPPED SALAD

- **Serves 4**
- **Time: Less than 20 minutes**
- **Gluten Free, Soy Free**

Jicama and mangoes just may become your next obsession after a bite of this crunchy cool tangy fruity salad. Enough adjectives for you? This salad completes just about any warm-weather meal—or alongside spicy Mexican or Central American eats. This tastes best given 30 minutes to marinate but should be eaten the day it's made.

1/2 pound jicama, diced into 1/4-inch cubes
2 mangoes, peeled and diced
    (see page 233 for mango-peeling tips)
1/4 cup chopped fresh cilantro
2 green onions, chopped finely
1 tablespoon chopped fresh mint
1/4 cup lime juice
1/4 teaspoon salt

1. In a large bowl, combine all the ingredients, tossing to coat everything with the lime juice, herbs, and salt. Serve immediately or store in a tightly covered container, kept chilled.

Variation

Mangoes, chile powder, and lime are a hit combo in Mexico and will be with you, too! Omit the mint. Combine 1/4 teaspoon of coarse salt with 1½ teaspoons of ground blended chile powder or, for authentic Mexican zing, use a single chile powder such as chile de arbol or pequín. Assemble the salad as directed, except omit the ¼ teaspoon of salt. Sprinkle the top of salad with the salted chile powder mixture and serve immediately.

HEARTY WARM YUCA AND CABBAGE SALAD

....

- Serves 2 to 3 as a main course, or 4 as an appetizer
- Time: About 45 minutes, not including making the Tofu Chicharrones or other tofu
- Gluten Free

....

Cool, crunchy cabbage slaw piled atop creamy warm yuca is a vegan riff on the Nicaraguan dish called *vigaron*, which serves as both a comfort and a fast food in its native land. Although the original version features pork, vegans get their choice of warmed Tofu Chicharrones, cooked chickpeas or fava beans, or even any baked tofu (Latin Baked Tofu is a standout here).

A salad that's a meal unto itself during winter months, when a leafy salad won't cut it, or in the summer, as an exceptional hearty entrée salad. In cool weather, replace underwhelming "winter" tomatoes with chunks of steamed winter squash.

Tip: Look for convenient bags of peeled, sliced frozen yuca in the freezer section of groceries that stock Latin American stuff.

Make-ahead Tip: Make Tofu Chicharrones and cook the yuca and fava beans (if using) up to three days in advance. Heat the tofu in a microwave or pan-fry again to reheat. Boil the cooked yuca for 5 to 7 minutes, until the center is hot, or steam in a microwave to reheat.

Dressing

    3 cloves garlic, minced or pressed
    1¼ teaspoons kosher or other coarse salt
    1 teaspoon dried oregano
    ½ teaspoon dried thyme
    ½ teaspoon ground sweet paprika
    3 tablespoons light olive or grapeseed oil
    ¼ cup freshly squeezed lime juice

Yuca and Salad

    1½ pounds yuca root
    1 small red onion, sliced into very thin rounds (⅛ inch)
    4 cups finely shredded green or red cabbage, or a combination of both
    4 tomatoes, seeded and diced
    1 cup shredded carrot
    ¼ cup finely chopped fresh cilantro
    1 recipe Tofu Chicharrones (page 101) or Latin Baked Tofu (page 103) sliced into thin strips, or 2 cups cooked chickpeas or fava beans, rinsed and drained
    Freshly ground black pepper

1. Trim ends of the yuca and use a sharp Y-shaped vegetable peeler to remove the waxed outside skin. With a heavy sharp chef's knife, split the root into two or three equal pieces horizontally, then cut each piece in half lengthwise. You should have four to six large, semicircular chunks of yuca. Slice each chunk into two or three more pieces.

2. Place in a large stockpot and pour in enough cold water to cover the yuca by at least 3 inches. Bring to a boil over high heat, partially cover the pot, and cook for 25 to 30 minutes, or until the yuca is very tender. Fully cooked yuca is ready when its white flesh has a semitranslucent appearance on the edges and it also flakes easily when pierced with a fork. Drain and let cool enough to handle. Separate the yuca into long pieces no thicker than 2 inches, but preferably a little less. Sometimes cooked yuca may have a thick rubbery skin on the outside edges of the root; this peels off easily, so remove and discard. Return the yuca to the pot and cover to keep warm.

3. While the yuca is boiling, prepare the dressing. In a large bowl, use a fork to mix together the garlic, salt, oregano, thyme, and paprika to form a paste. Whisk in the oil and lime juice, then set aside half of the dressing in a cup or small bowl. Combine the onion, cabbage, tomato, carrot, and cilantro, with the rest of the dressing in large bowl and toss to cover everything with dressing. If including legumes, also add these to the salad and toss with the other ingredients. Let the salad marinate for at least 20 minutes or up to 2 hours at room temperature.

4. When ready to serve, divide the warm yuca wedges among serving plates. Sprinkle each mound of yuca with Tofu Chicharrones or Latin Baked Tofu. Drizzle the reserved dressing on top of the yuca and tofu. Top each mound with an equal portion of salad. Sprinkle each with freshly ground black pepper and serve immediately.

SALVADORIAN MARINATED SLAW (CURDITO)

- **Makes 5 to 6 cups of slaw, depending on how long it's marinated**
- **Time: About 45 minutes**
- **Gluten Free, Soy Free**

Marinated cabbage slaws are found in many forms all over Central and South America. *Curdito* is my favorite, served with Salvadorian *pupusas* (page 162) and with any meal that could use a side of something tart, crunchy, and refreshing. It's also cheap, tasty, and easy to keep a little in the fridge for whenever the mood strikes. I make this in the morning when I know that I'll want *pupusas* for dinner, so that I'll have *curdito* ready when I get home!

Pressing the slaw is the traditional way to rapidly tenderize cabbage and is much simpler than other methods that require blanching the cabbage first. The longer this marinates, the less bulky the slaw becomes, so if you're serving it to lots of slaw lovers, consider making extra. An hour is the minimum marinating time, but if you're in dire need of *curtido*, you can squeeze the bagged slaw occasionally while chilling, to be ready in 30 minutes.

Tip: Buy a preshredded bag of cabbage and this slaw practically makes itself! Green is the most common cabbage color but tossing in a little red shredded cabbage creates a confetti-like effect.

> 1 to 1 1/2 pounds green or red cabbage, shredded very finely (8 to 10 cups of shredded cabbage)
> 1 to 2 pickled or raw jalapeños, seeded and finely chopped
> 1 large carrot, shredded
> 1/4 cup finely chopped fresh cilantro or parsley, or a combination of both
> 1 tablespoon coarse salt
> 2 teaspoons dried oregano
> 1/4 cup white vinegar, or more to taste

1. If you're shredding the cabbage—and lots of it—yourself, the best possible tool to use is a mandoline grater (a good-quality one works best and will keep those fingers safe!). Second best is a large food processor fitted with the shredding blade, but it's entirely possible to also thinly slice cabbage with a sharp heavy chef's knife and a cutting board. Slice the cabbage in half, remove and discard the core, slice the cabbage into chunks that can fit on your mandoline or into your food processor, and shred it all up. If you have any remaining odd-shaped pieces, chop them into fine shreds with a knife.

2. Combine the shredded cabbage and remaining ingredients in a large bowl and toss well to coat everything with the salt and vinegar. Stuff the *curdito* into a very large resealable plastic bag, at least 1 gallon or more. Press out all of the air and tightly seal the bag. From here you can either seal it into another bag, place on a shelf in the fridge, and place a heavy object on top, or place the bag in a large bowl, place a few heavy cans or a big bag of rice on top of the slaw, and transfer to the refrigerator. Chill for at least 1 hour or overnight; the longer the cabbage chills, the more tender and juicy it will become. To serve, lift up a handful of slaw and gently shake off any excess juices.

PERUVIAN RED CHILE–CORN SALAD WITH LIMAS AND CHERRY TOMATOES

- Serves 4 as a side or starter
- Time: About 30 minutes
- Soy Free

Not traditionally Peruvian, this salad makes good use of all the Latin American favorites:

corn, tomatoes, and lima beans, plus a gentle spicy kick from *ají panca* paste. Serve on a bed of baby spinach or arugula for worthy potluck fare or weeknight dinner. Canned or dried limas are often called "butter beans"—don't fear this un-vegan-sounding name; they are creamy and substantial. Look for canned organic limas, as they often have much less salt and taste sweeter and cleaner than nonorganic brands.

Tip: *Ají panca* is a chile popular in Peru and Bolivia. Like *ají amarillo*, it's often used in paste form. *Ají panca* has a brick red color with a mild heat level and complex notes of wood, smoke, and blackberries. See Ingredients for substitution suggestions.

> **2 cups fresh or frozen corn kernels, preferably white corn**
> **1 1/2 cups cooked white lima beans; if using canned, drain and rinse well**
> **1/2 pound cherry tomatoes, sliced in half**
> **1 small red onion, diced finely**
> **3 tablespoons finely chopped fresh cilantro**
> **3 tablespoons lime juice**
> **2 tablespoons *ají panca* paste**
> **2 tablespoons good-quality olive oil**
> **1/2 teaspoon agave syrup**
> **1 teaspoon dried oregano**
> **1/2 teaspoon salt, or more to taste**
> **Freshly cracked pepper**

1. In a 2-quart saucepan, bring 4 cups of water to a rolling boil. Stir in the corn kernels and cook for 2 to 3 minutes, or until the corn is cooked just enough so that it's no longer starchy but still crunchy. Drain the corn in a colander set over the sink and rinse with cold water to stop the cooking process. Shake the corn to rid it of excess water or let drain for 10 minutes. You may also cook the corn in a microwave by steaming with 3 tablespoons of water in a covered glass container. Drain and rinse the corn as directed. Place the corn in a large mixing bowl and add the rinsed lima beans. Add the cherry tomatoes to the corn and limas, and stir in the onion and cilantro.

2. In a large mixing cup, whisk together the lime juice, *ají panca* paste, olive oil, agave syrup, dried oregano, and salt until well mixed. Pour over the vegetable mixture, top with a few twists of fresh pepper, and use a large wooden spoon or rubber spatula to stir the vegetables until thoroughly coated with dressing. Cover and chill the salad for 20 minutes so that the flavors can blend.

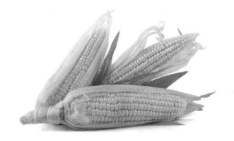

QUINOA SALAD WITH SPINACH, OLIVES, AND ROASTED PEANUTS

....

- Serves 4 as a side or starter
- Time: 45 minutes
- Soy Free

....

This nutritious salad is loaded with Latin America's greatest hits—corn, tomatoes, peanuts—and of course South American native supergrain, quinoa. Savor immediately to enjoy the amazing combination of the warm quinoa and cool vegetables. For an extra-awesome salad, substitute candied chile peanuts (see page 73) for the plain roasted peanuts.

1 cup uncooked quinoa, rinsed in a
    fine-mesh strainer
2 cups water
2 tablespoons lime juice
2 tablespoons good-quality olive oil
1 tablespoon red wine vinegar
1/2 teaspoon dried oregano
1 tablespoon *ají amarillo* or *ají panca* paste
3/4 teaspoon salt
1 red onion, finely chopped

1 bunch spinach (about 1/2 pound), well
    washed and sliced into thin ribbons
1 cup corn kernels, lightly blanched or
    roasted (see page 64)
1 large tomato, seeded and diced
2/3 cup kalamata olives, pitted and
    chopped
2/3 cup roasted unsalted peanuts,
    chopped

1. In a large pan over medium heat, warm the rinsed quinoa until dry and lightly toasted and fragrant, about 6 minutes, stirring constantly. Add the water, bring to a boil, and lower the heat to a simmer. Cover and cook for 20 minutes, or until all the water is absorbed and the quinoa grains are tender, plump, and translucent. Remove from the heat, fluff with a fork, and let cool, uncovered, for 20 minutes.

2. Meanwhile, in a mixing bowl, combine the lime juice, olive oil, wine vinegar, oregano, *ají* paste, salt, and onion. Let the onion marinate for the entire time the quinoa is cooking and cooling in the dressing so that it softens and becomes milder. When the quinoa has cooled, add the spinach, corn, tomato, olives, and peanuts. Serve immediately.

5

BEANS AND RICE,
LOS DOS AMIGOS

This chapter is dedicated to my lifelong best buddies, beans and rice. Try your hand at a few of the following recipes and you may find yourself inviting this dynamic duo over for dinner again and again.

The combination of beans and rice symbolizes what Latino *comida* is all about: a fusion of the Old World (rice) and the New (the common bean: black, pinto, and so on). Romantic imagery aside, the best thing is that a rice-and-beans meal always satisfies. The combination makes a nourishing complete protein, and you feel like you really ate *something*.

If you normally shy away from recipes that require a few steps, keep in mind that a batch of beans (and a double recipe of rice) will keep you set with brown bag lunches for at least three days. As a general rule, beans taste better the next day and will also considerably thicken as they cool. Make beans on a lazy Sunday night (simmering away on the back burner while eating faster fare such as tacos) and look forward to flavor-loaded beans for Monday dinner and delicious, almost-thick-as-refried beans by Wednesday. Just goes to show that beans are never boring!

BASIC BEANS FROM SCRATCH

- **Makes 5 to 6 cups of cooked beans with 2 to 3 cups of bean broth**
- **Time: 2 to 2½ hours, not including soaking**
- **Gluten Free, Soy Free**

This is a basic guide to cooking beans from scratch—if you've never tried it before, or had problems in the past, making a successful pot of beans from a bag of dried ones will change your life. Maybe not in the "I won the lottery" kind of way, although incredible flavor, perfect texture, easy-to-make, and insanely cheap are a winning combination.

Home-cooked beans made right just taste so much better than canned. In Latin cooking, the liquid that beans are prepared in—bean broth, if you will—is a flavorful ingredient in many dishes. In contrast, the cooking liquid that comes with canned beans tends to be insipid and too salty (which is why recipes using canned beans require them to be well rinsed and drained first). Make beans from scratch and you'll never have this problem; home-cooked bean liquid is silky, delicate tasting, and only as salty as you want it to be. Check out the Pantry section (page 13) for an overview of some popular Latin dried beans to look for.

1 pound dried beans, such as black beans, pintos, limas, garbanzos, white, Roman beans, bola roja, red, and so on

1 to 2 bay leaves

1/2 to 3/4 teaspoon salt

1 (3-inch) strip kombu (Japanese kelp), or 2 teaspoons dried epazote (optional)

1. The first step always with dried beans is to sort them to remove any stones, debris, or broken or off-looking beans. Spread the beans on a tabletop and pick out any random particle that doesn't belong there. I find it easiest as I go through the bean inspection process to sit at the table with a large bowl on my lap and sweep any proper-looking bean off the table and into the bowl.

2. Cover the beans with at least 6 inches of cold water and let sit on the kitchen counter for 8 hours or overnight. It can be helpful to start soaking the beans before you leave for work in the morning, then when you return in the early evening, the beans will be ready to cook.

3. Drain the soaking liquid from the beans, rinse the beans, and place in a large, heavy soup pot with a lid. Add about 5 cups of water or enough to cover the beans by about 4 inches. Stir in the salt and add the bay leaves and kombu or epazote, if using. Cover the pot and bring to a boil over high heat. Sometimes the beans will produce foam as they boil; if so, skim and discard the foam. Lower the heat to low, cover the pot, and simmer the beans for 2 to 2 1/2 hours. If the liquid level gets very low while the beans cook, stir in a cup of water or so at a time until done. Don't completely drown the beans in water, either (unless you are intentionally making a very brothy soup).

4. Perfectly cooked beans should be very soft with a tender interior and a soft exterior, and will mash easily when pressed with your tongue onto the roof of your mouth. Beans should never be very grainy or crunchy (they'll be hard to digest; see more next page). If your beans have that texture, keep cooking them until they are actually tender. If they still refuse to get tender, it could be that your beans are very old. Dried beans a year or more older can take a very long time to cook (or possibly never get tender).

5. To store cooked beans: Let them cool completely before pouring the beans with their liquid into containers. Cover tightly and store in the refrigerator for up to about 1¹/2 weeks. You can also freeze beans; I recommend separating them into smaller portions (even small resealable plastic bags) for easy thawing. Thaw beans in the refrigerator overnight, or, if using in soup, add small portions directly to the broth.

BEAN-COOKING TIPS

Let the beans properly soak for 8 hours instead of using any "quick soak" method. And always drain the soaking liquid from the beans and cook them in fresh water; the soaking liquid can contain the complex sugars that our belly has a tough time digesting (tough digesting now equals gassy times later!).

To avoid hard and grainy beans, never cook raw beans with an acidic food such as tomatoes, vinegar, peppers, *sofrito*, beer, wine, or citrus juices. It's okay to add these ingredients only after the raw beans are cooked and completely tender.

It's a myth that cooking beans with salt will make them tough. Cooking them with a little salt enhances the flavor and may even help tenderize the beans just a little faster.

For hard-core vegan bean cooking, try adding a 3-inch strip of dried kombu seaweed to the beans while they're simmering.

Kombu is said to help keep bean gasses in their place and hopefully out of your tummy. Or try adding a big pinch of dried epazote to beans while they're cooking; epazote is the Mexican answer to bean-gas control.

An easy home-cooked bean recipe is Onion-Flavored Beans: Ever have those very simple beans in Latin restaurants that don't have a chunk of vegetable in sight but are still sweet and flavorful? Try this technique for vegetable-free but tasty beans. Pour about 3 cups of beans into a large, deep skillet. Add 4 cups of liquid: either bean-cooking liquid, water, or a combination of

Canned Beans

Home-cooked beans are best but canned beans also work in most of these recipes. It's hard to deny the convenience of canned cooked beans, especially if you need only a handful for a salad or stuffed into *pupusas*. I try to switch calling for home-cooked dried and canned in these recipes, but really, you can always substitute canned for dried and vice versa.

As a general rule: Three 15-ounce cans of beans equal 1 pound (16 ounces) of uncooked dried beans. Of course, this can vary according to the size of the bean and variety; generally speaking, if I'm using smallish beans and it's a big soup, I may increase to four cans of beans, but if I'm making refried beans for a dinner for two, I might start with just half a pound of dried pintos. Experiment and listen to what your beany sense tells you.

the two. Peel a large yellow onion and slice in half, then place both halves, cut side down, into the beans. Bring the beans to a boil over high heat, lower the heat to low, and simmer uncovered, stirring occasionally, for 30 to 40 minutes, until the bean liquid has thickened to your desired consistency. Remove the onion and season the beans with salt and ground pepper to taste. You can discard the onion but some cooks consider the tender, juicy onion a delicacy . . . you might decide to slice it and serve on top of the beans!

HOME-STYLE REFRIED BEANS

- Makes about 4 cups
- Time: About 35 minutes, not including the precooking time needed if making from dried beans
- Gluten Free, Soy Free

In any *lucha libre* battle, Home-style Refried Beans will always drop-kick the canned stuff and win the championship belt of Best Refried Beans Ever. Homemade refried beans made with your favorite beans—pintos, black, or pink—are hall of fame–level comfort food. And they're relatively fast, leaving you with enough time to make some rice, heat some tortillas, and toss together a simple salad. Refried beans are simple to reheat, so make a double or triple batch for easy weeknight meals. Of course refried beans make an excellent à la carte dish paired with casseroles (any enchilada, for instance) or as a filling or topping for tacos or *sopes*.

2 tablespoons corn, peanut, or
  olive oil
3 cloves garlic, minced
1 small yellow onion (about 1/4 pound),
  diced small
1 to 2 jalapeño or serrano chiles, seeded
  and minced
1 teaspoon ground cumin
1/2 teaspoon dried oregano
1/2 teaspoon ground chile powder,
  such as ancho or a blend
2 (15-ounce) cans pinto or black or pink
  beans, drained and rinsed, or 31/2 to
  4 cups of cooked beans
1 bay leaf
2 cups water
Salt and fresh pepper

1. In a large, heavy cast-iron skillet, combine the oil and garlic and cook over medium heat. Allow the garlic to sizzle for 30 seconds, then add the onion and jalapeño. Using a wooden spoon to stir occasionally, fry until the onion turns translucent, about 10 minutes. Sprinkle in the cumin, oregano, and chile powder, and fry for another 30 seconds.

2. Stir in the beans, bay leaf, and water, and increase heat to medium-high. Bring the mixture to a boil, then lower the heat to medium again and allow to simmer for 20 minutes, or

until more than half the liquid has been absorbed but about an inch of liquid remains.

3. Remove the bay leaf and discard. Use a potato masher to mash the beans smooth, then stir to form a thick, moist paste, anywhere from 5 to 8 minutes. If refried beans appear to dry out, add a little water a few tablespoons at a time, until your desired consistency is reached. Serve immediately.

Make-ahead Tip: Make refried beans on the weekend and they'll keep tightly covered in the fridge for up a week. To reheat on the stovetop, place in a saucepan and add 2 to 3 tablespoons of water. Stir over low heat until hot and creamy. Reheat in a microwave the same way, adding a little less water and stirring occasionally until hot.

RED BEANS WITH DOMINICAN-STYLE SAZÓN

- Serves 6 to 8
- Time: About 2 hours precooking the dried beans, then 35 to 45 minutes cooking the dish
- Gluten Free, Soy Free

These red beans have a lively tropical flavor, thanks to a Dominican-style *sofrito* known as *sazón*, typically made with tons of finely chopped fresh sweet peppers, herbs, and vegetables. A little bit of fresh orange juice provides a sweet tangy twist, but leave it out if you prefer less fruity beans. If you can find them, use Dominican red beans, which look like a dark red, rippled version of pinto, or use Roman, cargamanto, or in a pinch red kidney beans.

Make-ahead Tip: You can freeze the freshly pureed *sazón* in a large resealable plastic bag for weeks prior to making these beans. To use, add frozen chunks of *sazón* to heated oil and proceed as directed.

Red Beans
  1 pound dried red beans, such as
     Dominican red, Roman, or kidney
  1 bay leaf
  3/4 teaspoon salt
  4 1/2 cups cold water

Sazón
  1/2 large green bell pepper, seeded
  1/2 large red bell pepper, seeded
  1 Cubanelle or yellow bell pepper,
     seeded
  1 small yellow or white onion
  6 cloves garlic
  1 cup fresh cilantro leaves, lightly packed
  1 stalk celery
  1/2 cup flat-leaf (Italian) parsley leaves,
     lightly packed, thick stems removed
  2 tablespoons white or red wine
     vinegar
  1 teaspoon dried oregano
  1/2 teaspoon ground cumin

1/2 teaspoon ground coriander

1 tablespoon hot sauce, or to taste

3 tablespoons olive oil

3/4 cup water

1/4 cup orange juice (optional, replace with water if desired)

Freshly ground pepper and salt

1. Prepare the basic beans first. Sort the red beans for any stones, broken beans, or random particles. Place the beans in a large glass or plastic bowl; add enough cold, fresh water to cover by at least 2 inches and let soak for 8 hours or overnight. Drain and rinse the beans of the soaking liquid. Place the beans and the 4 1/2 cups of fresh water, bay leaf, and salt in a large, heavy pot and bring to a rolling boil over high heat. Lower the heat to a simmer, skim off any foam, and partially cover the pot. Cook the beans for 1 1/2 to 2 hours, until tender, very soft, and easy to mash. Remove and discard the bay leaf.

2. While the beans are cooking, prepare the *sazón*. Chop the peppers, onions, garlic, cilantro, celery, and parsley into pieces small enough to lightly pack into your food processor bowl. Pulse until very fine, along with the vinegar, oregano, cumin, coriander, and hot sauce, doing so in two or more batches if it all doesn't fit at once.

3. Heat the olive oil in a large skillet over medium heat. Add the *sazón* and fry for 12 to 14 minutes, stirring constantly, until the color darkens and the mixture reduces by about a third. When the beans are tender, stir in the fried *sazón* (scraping in all of the juices), water, orange juice, freshly ground pepper, and salt.

4. Bring the beans to a boil again, lower the heat to a simmer, and partially cover. Cook for 30 to 35 minutes, stirring occasionally, until your desired consistency is reached. Add up to 1/2 cup of water to the beans if they appear too dry during the cooking, or continue to cook them for saucier, less soupy beans.

5. Serve hot with any flavored or plain white rice. Like many a bean dish, this tastes better the next day and reheats well in the microwave as well as on the stovetop.

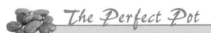 *The Perfect Pot*

To ensure that your beans are as gorgeous tasting as they look, consider the material and sturdiness of the pot you're using. Cast iron is fantastic for grilling and frying, but don't use it to cook beans if you'll be adding acidic ingredients (tomatoes, vinegar, citrus juices, beer) later, as they'll react with the uncoated iron to create undesirable off-flavors or color. Instead, use a stainless-steel pot for best results. To ensure even cooking, look for a pot with a thick, solid bottom. Avoid nonstick; it's not necessary as the beans contain so much water.

VENEZUELAN-STYLE BLACK BEANS (CARAOTAS)

....

- Serves 6 alongside rice and other sides
- Time: About 2 hours precooking the dried beans, then 35 to 45 minutes cooking the dish
- Gluten Free, Soy free

....

These are the beans I grew up with, a reminder of home with every bite. Black beans reign supreme in Venezuelan cuisine and are eaten any time of day with every kind of meal. Venezuelan food is mild, avoiding chiles and heavy spices in favor of the food's natural flavor. *Caraotas* are just that: black beans stewed with a touch of seasonings (*aleiños* in Venezuela) including onion and sometimes cumin, tomato, or a touch of natural brown sugar *papelón* (see *panela*, page 214).

Tip: Refry leftover *caraotas* to make them thick enough to be spread inside hot arepas or stuffed into empanadas.

    1 pound dried black beans
    5 cups cold water
    1/2 teaspoon salt
    1 bay leaf
    1 cup Basic Onion-Pepper Sofrito
        (page 32)
    1 large tomato, seeded and finely
        chopped, or 1/2 cup crushed
        canned tomatoes

1/2 teaspoon ground cumin
2 tablespoons *papelón*, grated
    and firmly packed, or dark brown sugar
Salt and ground pepper

1. Sort the black beans for any stones, broken beans, or random particles. Place the beans in a large glass or plastic bowl, add enough cold, fresh water to cover by at least 2 inches; and let soak for 8 hours or overnight.

2. Drain and rinse the beans of the soaking liquid. Place the beans, 5 cups of fresh cold water, salt, and the bay leaf in a large, heavy pot and bring to a rolling boil over high heat. Lower the heat to a simmer, partially cover the pot, and cook for 13/4 to 2 hours, until the beans are tender, very soft, and easy to mash on the tongue. Remove and discard the bay leaf.

3. Stir in the *sofrito*, tomato, cumin, *papelón*, and a little salt. Bring the beans to a boil again, lower the heat to medium, and cook, stirring occasionally, for 45 minutes to an hour, until your desired consistency is reached. Add 1/2 cup of water to the beans if they appear too dry. Season with pepper and more salt, if desired.

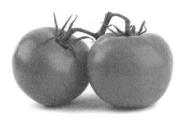

COLOMBIAN-STYLE RED BEANS

- Serves 4 to 6
- Time: About 35 to 45 minutes cooking the dish, not including the 2-hour precooking time if using dried beans
- Soy Free, Gluten Free

Beans in Colombian fare are kept simple but occasionally feature the addition of diced plantain. Green plantains are traditional but I like slightly ripe (but still firm) ones for a sweeter tropical flavor. Colombian bola roja beans—round red beans with a rich, sweet, nutty flavor—are ideal in this dish. Another bean to try is the Colombian favorite, cargamanto, also known as Roman beans. More brown than red, cargamantos look a little like pinto beans, and have a sweeter, earthier taste. Red kidney beans are tasty prepared this way, too.

Serve these beans with any rice, fried sweet plantains (sliced lengthwise down the center for two long pieces that will "frame" your dinner plate), a small arepa, a side of Tofu Chicharrones (page 101), and a crunchy cabbage-tomato salad for a meatless version of the Colombian national dish, Bandeja Paisa.

2 tablespoons olive oil
1/2 cup Basic Onion-Pepper Sofrito
   (page 32)

1 green or ripe but still firm plantain
1 small carrot, peeled and shredded
   (optional)
1 teaspoon ground cumin
1 1/2 teaspoons ground paprika
1 teaspoon dried oregano
4 cups cooked red beans,
   red kidney beans, or Colombian
   bola roja or cargamanto beans, or
   2 (15-ounce) cans red beans, drained
   and rinsed
2 1/2 cups vegetable broth or water
Salt and freshly ground pepper

1. In a large heavy pot, combine the olive oil and *sofrito* over medium-high heat. Fry for 2 minutes, then stir in the chopped plantain, shredded carrot if using, ground cumin, paprika, and oregano. Stir and continue to fry for another 5 minutes, until the plantain starts to turn yellow. Stir in the beans and vegetable broth. Bring the mixture to a boil, then lower the heat to medium-low and simmer for 35 to 40 minutes, stirring occasionally. Much of the liquid will have evaporated but the beans should be saucy. If not, continue to cook for another 10 minutes, until the desired consistency is reached. Remove from the heat and season with salt and freshly ground pepper. Allow the beans to cool for 15 minutes before serving, for best flavor and consistency.

DRUNKEN BEANS WITH SEITAN CHORIZO

....

- Serves 6 alongside rice and/or tortillas
- Time: About 2 hours precooking the dried beans and 45 minutes cooking the dish

....

These boozy beans are the *mas macho* of recipes but are perfect for the beer-loving lady (or guy) in your life. The ever-popular pinto bean gets a slow simmer in beer, a dash of tequila, roasted chiles, and seitan chorizo for a bold Tex-Mex-inspired pot o' beans that is best served with a side of Homemade Soft Corn Tortillas (page 165) for mopping up all those tasty juices. Or lighten things up with a simple green cabbage salad (page 71), if you like. If you think I'm going to tell you these beans taste even better the next day, then you just read my mind, or it could be the beer talking!

Tip: I like to keep these beans saucy rather than soupy. If the beans are looking too liquidy (more than 2 inches of liquid covering), remove a few cups of liquid from the pot before adding the beer.

1 pound dried pinto beans
4 1/2 cups cold water
A big pinch of dried epazote
1 teaspoon salt
3 tablespoons peanut oil
1 large yellow onion, peeled and diced
2 serranos or other hot chiles, roasted, seeded, and chopped

3 links Chorizo Seitan Sausages (page 36), diced finely
1 1/2 teaspoons dried Mexican oregano
2 teaspoons ground chile powder (a blend or a single chile)
1 teaspoon ground cumin
1 cup fresh or canned diced tomatoes
1 (12-ounce) bottle of Mexican beer, preferably lager-style
1 tablespoon tequila

Garnish

1 cup finely diced onion
3 tablespoons finely chopped cilantro
2 tablespoons lime juice
2 pickled jalapeños, chopped finely

1. Sort the pintos for any stones, broken beans, or random particles. Place the beans in a large glass or plastic bowl; add enough cold, fresh water to cover by at least 2 inches; and let soak for 8 hours or overnight.

2. Drain and rinse the beans of the soaking liquid. Place the beans, the 4 1/2 cups of fresh water, and the epazote in a large, heavy pot and bring to a rolling boil over high heat. Lower the heat to a simmer, partially cover the pot, and cook for 1 3/4 to 2 hours, until the beans are tender, very soft, and easy to mash on the tongue. Drain off about 2 cups of bean-cooking water and set aside.

3. About an hour into cooking the beans, heat the peanut oil in a cast-iron skillet over medium heat. Add the onion and serranos and fry for 5 minutes, until the onion is soft and translucent. Stir in the seitan chorizo and fry for 8 minutes, stirring frequently. Add the oregano, chile powder, cumin, and tomatoes, and fry for 6 to 8 minutes, until very soft. Set aside until the beans are completely soft, then stir the fried vegetables and chorizo into the beans, making sure to scrape in as much of the pan juices as possible. Stir in the beer; you should have enough liquid to cover the beans by about 2 inches; add more bean-cooking liquid as necessary. Simmer the beans over medium-low heat for 45 minutes, until thickened. Turn off heat, stir in the tequila, and let the beans cool for 15 minutes prior to serving.

4. To serve: Combine the diced onion, cilantro, lime juice, and jalapeño. Spoon the beans onto a serving plate and sprinkle with the onion garnish. Serve immediately with hot corn tortillas or any rice and a simple green cabbage salad. (If serving beans later, hold off on making the garnish until ready to serve.)

COSTA RICAN REFRIED RICE AND BEANS (GALLO PINTO)

....

- Serves 4 generously, or 6 as a side
- Time: Less than 30 minutes, not including precooking the rice and beans

....

The perfect combination of beans and rice has a different name and personality in most every Latin American country. Costa Rica and Nicaraguan *gallo pinto*—literally "painted rooster"—is a remarkably satiating mix of precooked rice and beans "refried" with extra vegetables, herbs, and spices. I could eat *gallo pinto* for breakfast, lunch, or dinner with avocado, cabbage salad, sweet fried plantains, or just a dash of hot sauce.

Home-cooked black beans or small red beans (look for Central American red beans) are the first choice for *gallo pinto*, because the cooking liquid gives the refried rice and beans the proper color, flavor, and consistency. This is a meal where the bean-cooking liquid is important to the final dish; if you must use canned beans, use a combination of organic brands with little or no added salt and plus a good-quality vegetable broth.

Tip: In Costa Rica, *gallo pinto* is often made with a healthy dollop of the regional favorite condiment, Salsa Lizano—a sweet, tangy sauce with plenty of cumin and tropical fruit. As of this writing, Salsa Lizano is vegan. If you don't have a Central American community nearby, it can be hard to find, so this recipe uses Worcestershire sauce and additional cumin to mimic the flavor. If you score a bottle of real Salsa Lizano, use it to replace the Worcestershire sauce (or add more to taste) and consider cutting the ground cumin in half.

3 tablespoons olive or other vegetable oil
3 cloves garlic, minced

1/4 pound (one small) onion, diced finely

1 small red or green hot chile, seeded and minced (optional)

1 red bell pepper, seeded and diced finely

2 cups cold cooked long-grain white or brown rice

1 teaspoon ground cumin

2 cups cooked black, red, or pink beans

1/2 cup bean-cooking liquid or vegetable broth, plus a little extra if necessary

1 tablespoon vegetarian Worcestershire sauce

1/2 teaspoon liquid smoke

1/2 teaspoon salt

1/2 teaspoon freshly ground pepper

1/2 cup finely chopped fresh cilantro

Hot sauce, for serving

1. In a large, deep cast-iron skillet, heat the olive oil and garlic over medium heat. When the garlic starts to sizzle, add the onion, chile (if using), and bell pepper, and fry for 6 to 8 minutes, or until the onion is soft and translucent. Stir in the rice and fry for 10 minutes, stirring frequently. Then stir in the cumin, beans, bean-cooking liquid, Worcestershire sauce, liquid smoke, salt, and ground pepper. Use a metal spatula to stir frequently, and occasionally mash some of the beans into the rice. Cook until most of the liquid is absorbed but the mixture is still moist, 10 to 15 minutes. If the mixture looks too dry, drizzle in 1 to 2 tablespoons of additional liquid until your desired consistency is reached.

2. Stir in the cilantro and remove from the heat. Serve mounded on a serving dish, or pack it lightly into a measuring cup or large ramekin and it turn upside down onto a serving dish for a cute timbale-style presentation. Serve with hot sauce, as desired.

Wake Up with the Painted Rooster

A simplified version of *gallo pinto* is a favorite protein- and fiber-packed breakfast of mine. It can be made in less than 20 minutes, if you have the two main ingredients prepared and ready to go in the fridge. Make it with brown rice and you probably won't be hungry until well into lunchtime!

Prepare a batch of Basic Beans from Scratch (page 81)—use black or your favorite red bean—and enough rice to make at least 4 cups. Keep the rice and the beans in two separate containers in the fridge until ready to use. Lightly oil a well-seasoned cast-iron pan and add a heaping 1/2 cup each of the rice and drained beans for each serving. Follow the basic procedure on page 90 for making *gallo pinto*, first frying together the beans and rice until hot and slightly browned and then pouring in 1/4 to 1/3 cup of bean-cooking liquid and several dashes of either vegetarian Worcestershire sauce or Salsa Lizano and your favorite hot sauce to taste. Cook until the liquid has evaporated and the mixture is sizzling. Serve with more hot sauce and sliced tomatoes, avocado, or diced tropical fruit.

CLASSIC STOVETOP LONG-GRAIN WHITE OR BROWN RICE

- Serves 4 as a side, about 3/4 cup per serving
- Time: Less than 30 minutes

Latin American cooking requires learning to make good long-grain rice. Long-grain white rice is standard, but brown rice is an increasingly popular alternative, so included here are suggestions for using brown rice plain or in recipes.

White Rice

    1 cup uncooked long-grain white rice
    1 1/2 cups water (but check the package directions for the suggested amount)
    1 tablespoon olive oil or nonhydrogenated vegan margarine
    1/2 teaspoon salt

Brown Rice

    1 cup uncooked long-grain brown rice
    2 cups water
    1 tablespoon olive oil or nonhydrogenated vegan margarine
    1/2 teaspoon salt

1. Rinse whichever rice you are using in a fine-mesh strainer. In a large, heavy-bottomed pot with a tight-fitting lid, combine the rice, water, oil, and salt. Cover and bring to a boil over high heat, stir the rice *only* once, and lower the heat to low. Cover the pot and cook for 20 to 25 minutes for white rice, or 40 to 45 minutes for brown rice, until all the water has been absorbed. Properly cooked rice is tender and slightly chewy with no crunchy cores.

2. Remove from the heat and let sit with the cover on for 5 minutes. Remove the lid, fluff the rice with a fork, and serve immediately.

A Few Important Things to Keep in Mind When Making Stovetop Rice

- The kind of pot you use can make or break your rice. Look for a medium-size, thick-walled, heavy-bottomed pot with a tight-fitting, heavy lid, as this will ensure proper steaming of the rice. And old-fashioned way to get a tight seal around the edge of your pot is to line the edges with foil, but if you invest in a quality pot this isn't really necessary.
- Never stir rice while it's cooking (only risotto gets to break this rule)! Just keep that lid on and check only after the minimum suggested cooking time. Latin-style rice should be firm and fluffy. Stirring rice while it's cooking can result in broken grains and make your rice mushy or sticky. Just stir once before simmering and fluff rice with a fork after the grains are done cooking.

- Not all brands of white rice are the same when it comes to how much liquid is needed during cooking. Read the directions on the package for the recommended water amounts and cooking times, and make adjustments accordingly with the liquid amounts and cooking times for these recipes. Long-grain brown rice is more predictable, with a fairly consistent 1-part-rice to 2-parts-water ratio.
- Using a gas range? Look for inexpensive metal heat diffusers that can be placed under pots to ensure more even cooking.

Easy Variations

Use your favorite vegetable broth instead of water. Omit the salt if your broth already contains salt.

Toss in 1 to 2 finely minced garlic cloves, along with the water or broth.

Sprinkle hot cooked rice with a few twists of freshly ground black pepper or lemon or lime juice.

Just before fluffing hot rice, sprinkle with finely chopped fresh cilantro, parsley, green onions, or chives, then use a fork to fluff the fresh herbs into rice.

Garnish hot rice with toasted pumpkin seeds (pepitas; see page 138 for how to toast) or pine nuts.

CILANTRO-LIME RICE

- Serves 4 as a side, about 3/4 cup per serving
- Time: Less than 30 minutes

A light and lovely rice to serve when just plain old rice isn't enough. Lime and fresh herbs make it a perfect complement to heavier stews and fried foods, and it's easy

About That Brown Rice

I love brown rice and eat it all the time, but Latin food sometimes makes me crave white rice. Call it a yearning for kid comforts, but there's *no problema* with the occasional indulgence . . . if you're eating your beans and veggies every day, you're still getting boatloads of fiber. That being said, many veggie cooks out there will want to use brown rice in these recipes.

When converting any white rice recipe to brown, follow these double rules: Double the total amount of liquid *and* double the cooking time. So if you're using 1 cup of brown rice, expect to use 2 cups of liquid and cook for *at least* 40 minutes (instead of 20), possibly more.

to put together, too, when three different things are cooking on the stovetop.

Tip: This rice works well with rice cookers. Simple toss everything except the last two ingredients into your cooker and follow the manufacturer's directions for white rice. Mix in the cilantro and green onion when done and leave it on the warm setting until ready to serve.

    1 cup uncooked long-grain white rice
    1 1/2 cups vegetable broth or water
    1 tablespoon olive oil
    2 tablespoons lime juice
    2 teaspoons grated lime zest
    1/2 teaspoon salt (only if you're using
        water)
    Freshly cracked pepper
    1/4 cup chopped cilantro, lightly packed
    1 green onion, green part only, sliced
        very thinly

1. In a heavy pot, combine the rice, vegetable stock, olive oil, lime juice and zest, salt (if using), and pepper to taste. Bring the mixture to a boil, lower the heat to a simmer, and cover the pot. Cook for 20 minutes, until the liquid is absorbed and the rice grains are tender.

2. Remove from the heat and sprinkle the rice with the cilantro and green onion. Fluff the rice, working in the chopped herbs. Serve immediately.

YELLOW RICE WITH GARLIC

- Serves 4 as a side, about 3/4 cup per serving
- Time: Less than 30 minutes

There's something about yellow rice that says, "Hey, Latino food alert!" It's a classic that goes perfectly with any bean or veggie or soy foods and seitan. Yellow rice has roots deep in Spanish rice flavored with saffron, which is influenced in turn by Arabic cuisine. Although the European Spanish version of yellow rice is typically colored with saffron, Latin American yellow rice's color usually comes from the uniquely New World achiote seed, making it a truly Creole creation.

Single-use packets of dry adobo seasonings are commonly used for coloring rice, but I prefer old-fashioned annatto (achiote) for the job. This way, you skip the artificial colors and MSG that practically all of those seasoning packets contain. Once you get in the habit of using annatto, it's a mystery why artificial color is even an option. Annatto provides a glorious yellow-orange hue, naturally and very cost effectively, too.

    2 tablespoons Annatto-Infused Oil
        (page 31)
    5 cloves garlic, chopped finely
    1 cup uncooked long-grain
        white rice

1 2/3 cups vegetable broth

Salt and freshly ground pepper

1/4 cup finely chopped fresh cilantro

1. In a large, heavy pot with a lid, combine the annatto oil and garlic over medium heat. Cook until the garlic is sizzling and fragrant, about 30 seconds. Stir in the rice and coat all of the grains with the oil. Pour in the vegetable broth, salt, and pepper and stir. Increase the heat and bring to a rolling boil, then lower the heat to medium-low. Cover and cook for 20 to 25 minutes, until the liquid is absorbed and the rice grains are tender.

2. Remove from the heat, fluff the rice with a fork, and serve garnished with the cilantro.

ARROZ CON COCO (SAVORY COCONUT RICE)

....

● **Serves 4 as a side, about 3/4 cup per serving**

● **Time: Less than 30 minutes**

....

Arroz con coco—rice with coconut milk—is a buttery and flavorful rice loved in many parts of Latin America. Sometimes it's cooked with raisins, but for those who may wonder why must everything have a dried grape in it, you can leave it out. A generous sprinkling of toasted coconut should win over any coconut fan in your life.

1 cup uncooked long-grain white rice

1 cup regular or lite coconut milk

2/3 cup water

1 tablespoon sugar

1/2 teaspoon salt

1/2 cup raisins or finely chopped fresh pineapple or mango (optional)

1. In a heavy pot, combine the rice, coconut milk, water, sugar, salt, and ground white pepper. If using raisins, add as well. Bring the mixture to a boil, lower the heat to a simmer, and cover the pot. Cook for 20 to 25 minutes, until the liquid is absorbed and the rice grains are tender.

2. When rice is done cooking, remove it from the heat and let sit with its cover on for 5 minutes. Remove the lid and fluff the rice with a fork. Add the chopped fruit, if using, fluff once more, and sprinkle the rice with the toasted coconut. Serve immediately.

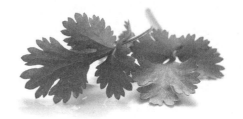

SAVORY ORANGE RICE, BRAZILIAN STYLE

....

- Serves 4 as a side, about 3/4 cup per serving
- Time: Less than 30 minutes

....

A fruity riff on the Brazilian classic way of preparing rice; white rice is gently toasted with onions and garlic prior to adding the liquid, which here includes orange juice. I like to serve with Feijoada (page 147) (you may want to double this recipe if you're serving an entire recipe of Feijoada for a big feast). Its delicate orange flavor goes go well with most any tropical Latin meal, but the variation for traditional Brazilian white rice that omits the orange is ideal for serving with anything.

2 tablespoons peanut or other light vegetable oil

1 small yellow onion, minced

2 cloves garlic, minced

1 cup uncooked long-grain white rice

1¼ cups very hot water or hot vegetable broth

1/3 cup freshly squeezed orange juice

Grated zest of 1 orange

1/2 teaspoon salt, or to taste

1 tablespoon minced fresh parsley or cilantro, for garnish

1. Heat the oil in a heavy-bottomed 2-quart pot over medium heat. Add the garlic and fry for 30 seconds, stirring, then add the onion. Cook until the onion is soft and translucent, 6 to 8 minutes. Add the rice and fry, stirring occasionally, until the rice turns a light tan color and some individual grains are golden brown, 4 to 5 minutes. Add the water, orange juice and zest, and salt, and stir.

2. Increase the heat and bring to a boil, stir once more, and lower the heat to a low simmer. Cover tightly and cook for 20 minutes, or until the rice is tender and all the liquid has been absorbed.

3. Remove from the heat, fluff the rice with a fork, sprinkle with the parsley or cilantro, and serve hot.

Variation

Brazilian-style White Rice: Replace the orange juice with more hot water or vegetable broth and omit the grated orange rind. Cook as directed.

6

VEGAN ASADO: TOFU, TEMPEH, AND SEITAN

Asado simply means "grilled" in Spanish but can loosely refer to any kind of grilled or roasted meat, depending on where you are in Latin America. Going against good grammar (and meaty traditions), it also refers to this collection of recipes featuring the beloved vegetarian trio of tofu, tempeh, and seitan. By now nearly all Americans (both North and South) have at least heard of tofu; it's the soft white bean curd that absorbs flavor readily and delivers high-quality protein. The other two—tempeh and seitan—have yet to acquire tofu's fame (or infamy?) but take readily to Latin-style preparation to expand the vegan scope of hearty protein foods.

Seitan is my favorite of the three for vegan Latin cooking: easy to make at home, looks great grilled or shredded, and makes convincing "meaty" dishes. It blends harmoniously with tomatoes, chiles, vinegars, and citrus juices and is perfect alongside standard fare such as beans, potatoes, or

plantains. I reserve tofu for the delicate seasoning used for seafood or roast pork, or for frying with plenty of oil (such as Tofu Chicharrones, page 101). Tempeh has a distinctive taste and texture that stands out (unlike blending in like tofu) and is great on the grill (for a true *asado*!).

The recipes in this chapter are designed to be paired with beans, a grain, and perhaps a vegetable for a fully rounded meal, so if you feel you want more than two slices of baked tofu (when serving multiple guests), go ahead and double or triple these recipes.

TOFU

Oh tofu, what to do with you? It's not a traditional part of the Latin American diet, but a vegan cookbook without tofu is like a tamale without a husk wrapper. Yet consider how Latin food is, in a way, "fusion" food—it's only a matter of time until tofu and other soy foods would find a place next to rice, beans, and plantains. It's all in how you prepare it: baking tofu smothered in herbs, roasting, or frying is a flattering fit for this humble and healthy protein source.

Putting on the (Tofu) Pressure

Pressing fresh firm (or extra firm) tofu prior to marinating makes tofu firmer, chewier, and less watery (better for soaking up marinades). You'll need an extra half hour to get best results (I skip this when in a rush) but the benefits are taste-worthy. Try it and see! To press tofu: Layer the tofu slices between paper towels and place on top of a folded kitchen towel. Place a dinner plate on top of the tofu, top with a heavy book or a few heavy cans, and press for at least 30 minutes. The towels will absorb the tofu's excess moisture.

CHIMICHURRI BAKED TOFU

....
- Serves 4, two slices each of tofu
- Time: About 55 minutes
- Gluten Free
....

This easy baked tofu is smothered in wonderful *chimichurri* sauce to form a dense, herby crust. The longer it bakes, the more the oven works at making the tofu dense and chewy. Use the downtime to make sides such as rice or potatoes and a big salad full of juicy tomatoes, shredded romaine,

and hearts of palm served with Cilantro-Citrus Vinaigrette (page 69).

Tip: For firmer baked tofu, try pressing it prior to adding the *chimichurri*. (See the tofu-pressing tip to the left.)

> 1 pound extra-firm tofu
> 2 tablespoons olive oil
> 1 tablespoon soy sauce
> Chimichurri Sauce with Smoked Paprika
>   (page 42)

1. Preheat the oven to 400ºF. Slice the tofu into eight 1/2-inch-thick slices and dab the slices dry with a paper towel or clean kitchen towel. In a shallow glass 9 by 12-inch baking dish, combine the olive oil and soy sauce. Lay a tofu slice in the baking dish, pressing it into the sauce mixture. Flip and press again to coat with the mixture. Repeat with the remaining slices and bake for 30 minutes, flipping once, until the slices are beginning to brown on the edges. Remove from the oven but don't turn the oven off.

2. With a rubber spatula or large spoon, spread about a third of the *chimichurri* sauce evenly and completely over the tops of the tofu. Flip the slices and spread another third or slightly more on top of the tofu. If desired, use a fork to poke holes through the tofu, pressing a little bit of the sauce into the center of the pieces. Bake for another 25 minutes, until the tofu is firm and the edges are golden brown. Bake longer if an even chewier texture is desired. Serve the tofu hot with remaining *chimichurri* sauce.

TOFU CHICHARRONES

- Makes about 2 cups
- Time: About 45 minutes, including pressing the tofu but not the overnight freezing/thawing
- Gluten Free

Chewy, smoky pan-fried tofu is a vegan stunt double for *chicharrones*, traditional deep-fried pork belly. Sprinkle it into Latin Caribbean dishes such as Mofongo (page 120) or into beans or knead into arepa dough for a special treat. You're not going to fool any die-hard original *chicharron* fans, but it has plenty of chewy, smoky, greasy character going for it.

Tip: This recipe requires an overnight freezing of the tofu, so plan at least 24 hours before you can have tofu *chicharrones*. Try speeding up the tofu thawing by placing the entire package in a large bowl of hot water.

1 pound firm Chinese-style tofu

Marinade
   3 tablespoons soy sauce
   1 tablespoon liquid smoke
   1 clove garlic, minced
   1 tablespoon red wine vinegar
   2 teaspoons agave syrup
   Peanut or other high-smoking-point vegetable oil, for frying
   Kosher salt

1. Freeze the entire unopened tofu package overnight until frozen solid; this will help the tofu form a special chewy texture that is exceptional when it comes to absorbing marinades. Remove from the freezer and place in a bowl of warm water, or leave in the fridge overnight to thaw. When completely thawed, remove the tofu from the package, drain, and slice into 1/4-inch-thick slices. Now, press the tofu: Layer the tofu slices between paper towels and place on top of a folded kitchen towel. Place a dinner plate on top of the tofu, top with a heavy book or a few heavy cans, and allow the tofu to press for at least 30 minutes. The tofu will flatten and most of its excess moisture will be removed.

2. Make the marinade: In a large plastic container with a lid, mix together the soy sauce, liquid smoke, crushed garlic, vinegar, and agave syrup. Remove the tofu from the pressing setup, tear into 1/4-inch or smaller bits (have fun and make the shapes a little uneven), and add to marinade. Tightly cover the container and shake vigorously to coat the tofu in the marinade, then set aside for 15 minutes. Shake the container occasionally to coat each piece with the marinade.

3. In heavy cast-iron pot, heat about 1/2 inch of peanut oil over medium heat. The oil is ready when a small piece of tofu sizzles instantly and browns within 30 seconds. Carefully lower a generous 1/2 cup of marinated tofu bits at a time into the hot oil. Use a slotted metal spatula to turn the tofu pieces to brown every side evenly, and occasionally press the frying tofu with the spatula. Remove the tofu when deep golden brown and crisped on the edges, 8 to 10 minutes. Ladle it onto a plate lined with paper towels or crumpled brown paper, to drain, and sprinkle with a little salt, if desired. Repeat with the remaining tofu. Let cool to room temperature before storing, chilled, in a tightly covered container.

ZESTY ORANGE MOJO BAKED TOFU

- Serves 3 to 4
- Time: About 55 minutes

This easy baked tofu in a perfectly tangy citrus marinade is inspired by the famous *mojo* sauces of Cuba. A long roasting gives this tofu a chewy outside with a creamy interior, for a very hearty yet light protein side. This loves to be served with Yuca with Cuban Garlic-Lime-Mojo Sauce (page 127).

1 pound extra-firm tofu
2 tablespoons olive oil
1 tablespoon soy sauce

Mojo Marinade
1/2 cup freshly squeezed orange juice
2 tablespoons lime juice
1 tablespoon olive oil
Grated zest of 1 orange
4 cloves garlic, chopped
1 teaspoon dried oregano
1/2 teaspoon ground cumin
1 teaspoon salt, or to taste
Freshly ground black pepper

1. Slice the tofu into eight 1/2-inch-thick slices and dab the slices dry with a paper towel or clean kitchen towel. Press the tofu as directed in the tip box (page 100) if desired. Preheat the oven to 400ºF. In a shallow glass 9 by 12-inch baking dish, combine the olive oil and soy sauce. Lay a tofu slice in the baking dish, pressing it into the sauce mixture. Flip and press again to coat with the mixture. Bake for 20 minutes; remove from the oven but don't turn the oven off. The tofu will be bubbling and juicy.

2. Combine all the marinade ingredients in a small bowl and stir well.

3. Flip each piece of tofu and pour the marinade over tofu; the marinade will nearly cover the top of the tofu. Bake for another 30 minutes until the tofu is firm and any remaining marinade has thickened up a little bit. Bake longer if an even chewier texture is desired. Serve the tofu hot and topped with any remaining marinade juices from the baking pan.

LATIN BAKED TOFU

- **Serves 4, two slices each of tofu**

A tangy red marinade soaks into baked tofu, for a versatile chewy protein for any Latin cuisine you're dishing up tonight. Use it to fill tacos (page 176) or arepas (page 177), sliced onto yuca-cabbage salad (page 78), or served with rice, beans, and of course fried plantains. For best results, press the tofu prior to marinating (see page 100).

1 pound extra-firm tofu
2 tablespoons olive oil
1 tablespoon soy sauce

Red Marinade
1/2 cup white wine, beer, or
   vegetable broth
2 tablespoons red wine vinegar
2 tablespoons olive or peanut oil
2 tablespoons tomato paste
1 tablespoon soy sauce
4 cloves garlic, grated
1 teaspoon ground cumin
1 teaspoon dried oregano

1. Slice the tofu into eight 1/2-inch-thick slices and dab the slices dry with a paper towel or clean kitchen towel. Press the tofu as directed in tip box (page 100) if desired. Preheat the oven to 400°F. In a shallow glass 9 by 12-inch baking dish, combine the olive oil and soy sauce. Lay each tofu slice in the baking dish, pressing it into the sauce mixture. Flip and press again to coat with the mixture. Bake for 20 minutes; remove from the oven but don't turn the oven off. Tofu will be bubbling and juicy.

2. Combine all the marinade ingredients in a small bowl and stir well.

3. Flip each piece of tofu and pour the marinade over the tofu; the marinade will nearly cover the top of the tofu. Bake for another 30 minutes, until the tofu is firm and any remaining marinade has thickened up a little bit. Bake longer if an even chewier texture is desired. Serve the tofu hot, topped with any remaining marinade juices from the baking pan.

Variations
Baked Tofu with Salsa de Maní: Bake the tofu as directed and prepare Peanut Sauce (page 41) while the tofu is baking. During the last 10 minutes of baking, top the tofu with half of the peanut sauce. Serve the tofu with the remaining peanut sauce.

Tofu in Sofrito: Bake the tofu as directed. During the last 20 minutes of baking spoon 1 cup of Basic Onion-Pepper Sofrito (page 32) over the tofu. Flip after 10 minutes and proceed as directed.

SEITÁN

Love how just an accent translates a word into another language? Seitan can be worked in just about every savory recipe in this book, but the following recipes especially highlight the chewy meaty satisfaction that seitan delivers.

MOJO OVEN-ROASTED SEITAN

- Serves 4, about 1 cup of sliced seitan per serving
- Time: Less than 20 minutes, not including making Steamed White Seitan

I developed this sizzling seitan for the fabulous Cubano Vegano Sandwich (page 66) but it's a worthy accompaniment to any fully dressed Latin platter, particularly ones with a Cuban or Caribbean flavor. The marinade is a classic tangy citrus *mojo*. Thin strips of seitan are then dressed in it and roasted just long enough to become tender, moist, and juicy. Double the recipe and you'll have enough to serve four tonight with an entrée platter and tomorrow in sandwiches.

1/2 recipe (2 loaves) Steamed White Seitan (page 35)

Marinade
1/2 cup freshly squeezed orange juice
3 tablespoons lime juice
3 cloves garlic, grated
3 tablespoons olive oil
1 teaspoon dried oregano
1/4 teaspoon ground cumin
1/4 teaspoon salt

1. Thinly slice the seitan into strips 1/4 inch thick or even thinner. Preheat the oven to 375ºF. In a glass 7 by 11-inch pan, whisk together all of the ingredients except for the seitan. Add the seitan strips and toss to coat thoroughly with the marinade. Roast for 14 to 16 minutes, flipping the seitan occasionally with tongs, until sizzling and most of the marinade has been absorbed. Don't overbake; the seitan should look juicy. Remove from the oven and serve immediately, or if using in sandwiches, briefly chop into thin strips and let cool enough to handle.

PERUVIAN SEITAN AND POTATO SKEWERS (SEITAN ANTICUCHOS)

- Serves 2 to 3 generously as a main dish, or 4 as an appetizer
- Time: About 45 minutes, including assembling the kebabs

Seitan kebabs go Peruvian in this meatless adaptation of the popular street food *anticuchos*, hearty grilled fare that was all the rage with the ancient Inca and remains that way today. The popular Peruvian *ají panca* gives this kebab's marinade its brick red color and woodsy, fruity flavor. It's a luscious dish to throw at sworn meat 'n' potato devotees that can hold its own on the grill.

Traditionally, these skewers are simply served with boiled potatoes. Here, pre-cooked potatoes get an additional flavor rush by brushing with extra marinade and grilling with the seitan. Tiny new potatoes work best for skewering, but chunks of cooked but firm waxy potato work. Keep the veggies to a minimum with these kebabs; if you must, add only a piece of onion and/or a slice of bell pepper.

Tip: No skewers? This recipe works also grilled "free form" in a cast-iron grill pan. Also, put those skewers on the grill pan for indoor grilling thrills.

½ recipe (two loaves) Steamed Red
    Seitan (page 34), or ¾ pound seitan

Marinade

5 cloves garlic

3 tablespoons *ají panca* paste, or
    3 teaspoons mild ground red chile
    powder, such as ancho

¼ cup red wine vinegar

3 tablespoons peanut oil or vegetable oil

1 tablespoon agave syrup or brown sugar

1 teaspoon ground cumin

1 teaspoon dried oregano

½ teaspoon smoked paprika

½ teaspoon salt

¼ teaspoon finely ground black pepper,
    or to taste

Skewers

1 pound waxy potatoes, preferably very
    small new potatoes (about the size of a
    Bing cherry or smaller)

1 bell pepper, red or green, seeded and
    sliced into 1-inch pieces (optional)

1 large yellow onion, sliced into 1-inch
    pieces (optional)

12 to 14 bamboo or metal skewers (if using
    bamboo, presoak skewers according to
    the package directions.)

1. Slice the seitan into bite-size cubes, about ½ inch across, and place in a large mixing bowl. If using onion or pepper slices, add along with the seitan. In another mixing bowl, use a Microplane grater to grate the garlic into the bowl. Add the *ají panca* paste, red wine vinegar, peanut oil, agave syrup, cumin, oregano, paprika, salt, and pepper and stir until smooth with a whisk or fork. Pour the mixture over the seitan cubes and veggies (if using) and toss to coat completely with marinade.

2. While the seitan is marinating, cook the potatoes. Thoroughly clean the potatoes first, leaving the skins on. If you're using potatoes other than small new ones, cut them into bite-size chunks; leave small new potatoes whole. Place in a large, heavy pot and add enough cold water to cover the potatoes. Bring to a

rolling boil over high heat, then lower the heat to a simmer and cook the potatoes until they are tender but still hold their shape, 12 to 14 minutes. Drain and spread the potatoes on a dish to cool enough to handle.

3. When the potatoes have finished cooling, preheat your grill according to the manufacturer's directions. Since these are quick-cooking ingredients, you want your grill to have an evenly hot, not blazing, heat that can crisp the outside of these skewers without overdrying the seitan. If you're using a grill pan, you'll probably need 6 to 8 minutes to get your grill ready to go over medium-high heat. Make sure to oil your grill well, as seitan and veggies (and even the marinade) don't contain loads of fat to keep things from sticking. I like to use those new high-smoking-point cooking sprays (including ones designed for grilling) just for this.

4. Prepare your *anticucho* by alternating pieces of marinated seitan with onions, peppers, and an occasional potato piece on the skewers. Brush with additional marinade, taking care to especially coat the potatoes. Place the kebabs on the preheated grill. Don't crowd the pan; leave enough room so the edges of the ingredients can cook evenly. Occasionally brush the cooking kebabs with leftover marinade. Cook on each side for 3 to 4 minutes, until the seitan and vegetables are browned on the edges and look juicy. If the ingredients stick to the grill, spray more oil onto the grilling surface. Take care not to overcook the skewers. Remove from the heat and serve immediately with a cold beer, any potato dish, and So Good, So Green Sauce, if desired.

Variation

Try substituting malt vinegar in place of red wine vinegar, for a slightly sharper marinade.

LATIN SHREDDED SEITAN

- **Serves 4 as part of an entrée with rice, beans, *tostones*, and so on; stuffed into arepas, serves up to 6**
- **Time: About 30 minutes, not including making Steamed Red Seitan**

North Americans like their ground beef; for most Latin American countries, seasoned and shredded beef is required. Seitan is what we use here in Veganzuela and therefore we'll have shredded *seitán, por favor.* Seitan doesn't exactly shred, so a little chopping is necessary to get a similar consistency. Don't worry about precision when slicing; you'll want a random look to those seitan "shreds." Just aim to get the thinnest slivers you can manage.

This shredded seitan recipe works in any cuisine. The variations that follow reflect the seasoning popular in some regional cuisines, to mix or match with Latin starches and sides.

½ recipe (two loaves) Steamed Red
  Seitan (page 34)
3 tablespoons olive or peanut oil
1 clove garlic, chopped
1 small yellow onion (about ¼ pound),
  chopped finely
½ red bell pepper, seeded, sliced in half,
  then sliced into very thin strips
½ teaspoon ground cumin
½ cup white or red cooking wine or
  vegetable broth
2 juicy tomatoes, seeded and chopped
  finely, or ½ cup crushed tomatoes
Salt and freshly ground pepper

1. With a sharp, heavy chef's knife, slice each portion of seitan into the thinnest medallions you can. Then stack two medallions together and quickly (but carefully) chop the seitan into very thin, irregularly shaped slivers. Repeat with the remaining seitan. You should have slivers of seitan that are at most ⅛ inch thick, but that can be the length of the original medallion or shorter.

2. In a large, heavy skillet, combine the olive oil and garlic and cook over medium heat until the garlic starts to sizzle, about 30 seconds. Add the onion and bell pepper, stirring occasionally and cooking until the onion is soft and translucent, 6 to 8 minutes. Stir in the cumin, cook for 1 minute, then pour in the wine and tomato; stir. Add the seitan, stir to coat with the sauce, and simmer for another 12 to 14 minutes. The seitan should look juicy; if it starts to

look dry, add a little more wine or even more tomato. Season with salt and pepper and serve immediately.

Variations

Give your shredded seitan some regional flavor by adding the following along with the seitan:

Cuban "Ropa Vieja" Style: Replace the red bell pepper with a green bell pepper, and along with the onion, add 1 teaspoon of dried oregano. Along with the seitan, add a bay leaf and an additional ½ cup of crushed tomatoes. Simmer until most of the liquid has been absorbed but the seitan is still a little bit saucy. Remove and discard the bay leaf when ready to serve.

Venezuelan "Mechada" Style: Add 2 tablespoons vegan Worcestershire sauce along with the seitan. Cook a little longer so that the seitan has a moist but not overly saucy consistency. You may want to use less salt in the final seasoning, so taste before you shake!

Mexican Chile-Braised Seitan: Split, seed, and toast 1 to 2 dried ancho or guajillo chiles, grind in a spice grinder, and add along with the tomatoes and wine. If you like, try substituting a light-colored Mexican beer for the wine. Serve garnished with a little chopped fresh cilantro.

Chipotle Adobo Seitan: Blend in a few chipotles in adobo sauce, plus a few tablespoons of their sauce, along with the tomato sauce.

Puerto Rican "Picadillo" Style: Though *picadillo* often features ground meat, slivered seitan works better here. Replace the red bell pepper with a green bell pepper. Use crushed tomatoes and increase to 1¼ cups; along with that, add ¼ cup of chopped green olives (stuffed with pimiento, if you like), ¼ cup of capers, 1 teaspoon of dried oregano, and 1 bay leaf. *Picadillo* should have a saucy consistency. Remove and discard the bay leaf when ready to serve, and season with 1 teaspoon of wine vinegar.

SEITAN SALTADO (PERUVIAN SEITAN AND POTATO STIR-FRY)

- Serves 4 with a side of rice, or 2 to 3 big servings as a main course
- Time: 45 minutes

Maybe one of the most un-Latin-seeming dishes is Peruvian *lomo saltado.* Influenced by the cuisine of Peru's Japanese and Chinese immigrants, *lomo saltado* is a Latin American stir-fry with slices of meat (seitan, in our case) and veggies seasoned with tangy soy-based sauce, along with tomatoes, *ají amarillo,* and french fries. Did she just say french fries?

That's right, *lomo saltado*'s contribution to the world of faster food is a stir-fry enriched with everyone's favorite potato-based edible, for a satisfying un-meat 'n' potatoes meal. Serve with plain steamed long-grain rice or a simple tomato cabbage salad, if one carb at a time is more your style.

Tip: *Lomo saltado* is a great way to use up leftover veggies. Just don't overdo it; add a few sliced mushrooms or slivers of red bell pepper. Seitan and potatoes should dominate with vegetables in a supporting role.

Tip: Frozen premade french fries or even leftover takeout fries are an excellent shortcut for this dish. Prepare the frozen fries as directed on the package, or give the leftover restaurant fries a brief reheating by baking them at 400°F for 8 to 10 minutes, or until hot and a little crisp on the edges. I like to toss individual portions of stir-fry and french fries just before serving, to help keep the potatoes crisp.

Baked Fries
    2 pounds russet or other high-starch
        potatoes, scrubbed clean, peeled
        (or leave unpeeled for a rustic look)
    2 tablespoons peanut or olive oil

Stir-fry
    ½ recipe (two loaves) Steamed Red or
        White Seitan (page 34 and 35), or slightly
        less than 2 pounds purchased seitan

4 tablespoons soy sauce

3 tablespoons red wine vinegar

3 cloves garlic, minced

1/2 teaspoon ground cumin

A generous pinch of dried oregano

1/2 pound yellow onions

1 to 2 tablespoons *ají amarillo* paste, or
    1 to 2 fresh or frozen amarillo or
    hot red chiles

3 tablespoons red cooking wine or
    vegetable broth

3 large, firm plum tomatoes

4 tablespoons peanut oil

Freshly ground pepper

Steamed long-grain white or brown rice,
    about 1 cup per serving (optional)

2 tablespoons finely chopped cilantro

1. Make the baked potato fries first. Preheat the oven to 400ºF. Slice the potatoes into french fry sticks about 1/2 inch thick, pour the 2 tablespoons of oil onto a large, rimmed baking sheet, add the sliced potatoes, and toss thoroughly with the oil. Don't crowd the pan; use two pans if the fries are overlapping. Bake the fries for 20 to 24 minutes, flipping once halfway through the baking, until the potatoes are golden and the edges are crisp and browned. Sprinkle with a little salt, if desired. Turn off the oven, open the oven door just a little, and leave the baking sheet in the oven to keep the fries warm.

2. Prepare the seitan and prepare the stir-fry ingredients: Slice the seitan into 1/4 by

1-inch strips. In a large bowl, combine the soy sauce and the red wine vinegar, garlic, cumin, and oregano. Add the seitan strips and use tongs to toss and coat the seitan completely with the marinade. While the seitan is marinating, peel the onion, slice it in half, then slice it into thin strips. If using fresh *ají amarillo* or other chiles, remove the seeds and mince. Slice the plum tomatoes in half, remove the seeds, and slice into thin strips. Measure the cooking wine and have it handy in a small cup.

3. In a 12-inch nonstick skillet (or wok, if you have one), heat 2 tablespoons of the peanut oil over medium-high heat. Add half of the seitan strips and fry on each side for about 2 minutes. The seitan should be browned on the edges but still juicy. Transfer the seitan from the pan to a dish and repeat with the remaining seitan. Add the remaining 2 tablespoons of oil to the pan and add the onions. Stirring, fry the onions for 3 to 4 minutes, until they begin to soften and turn golden on the edges. If using minced chiles, stir into the onions and fry for 1 minute. If using *ají amarillo* paste, whisk into wine.

4. Pour the wine over the onion mixture and stir to deglaze the pan (dissolving any browned bits from the bottom of the pan). Scrape in any remaining seitan marinade. Using tongs, stir in the tomato strips to coat them in the bubbling wine mixture. Sprinkle within remaining tablespoon of soy sauce and season with plenty of freshly ground pepper. Add the seitan strips and continue using tongs to coat them with the

sauce, then turn off heat. Have ready serving dishes and mound a serving of rice into the dishes, if using.

5. To put everything together: place a serving of baked french fries in a large mixing bowl (maybe even the one you used to marinate the seitan with . . . it's okay because it's vegan!). Use tongs to add a portion of stir-fried seitan and vegetables on top of fries and drizzle a little bit of the pan juices over the whole thing. Toss the fries with the stir-fry, taking care to coat the potatoes with the seitan juices. Slide onto a serving dish, sprinkle with some chopped cilantro, and serve immediately.

TEMPEH

Tempeh is perhaps the most misunderstood of the vegan protein power trio. It should be prepared a little differently from both tofu and seitan, for maximum enjoyment. Unlike tofu, tempeh possesses an attitude of its own, with a light yeasty-mushroom flavor and a firm, sliceable texture. Tempeh may be an acquired taste but it's an institution in the American vegan diet. The following recipes are simple ways that make the most of tempeh's charms and are quickly put together for any weeknight meal.

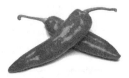

TEMPEH ASADO

- Serves 2 to 3 as a main course, or 4 served with lots of sides or in a taco
- Time: Less than 30 minutes

Mexican-inspired flavors plus grilling turns tempeh into a fast and tasty protein to stack alongside rice, beans, and salad for an easy weeknight meal. Grill or pan-fry tempeh for equally yummy results. It's a quick filling for tacos topped with any salsa, shredded cabbage, and a dollop of Cashew Crema (page 51).

Tip: Steaming tempeh in a microwave is fast and less messy. Place the sliced tempeh in a glass microwave-safe bowl with a lid and add ½ cup of water. Toss the tempeh to moisten with the water. Cover and microwave on high for 5 to 6 minutes, or until the tempeh is has softened and has absorbed some of the liquid. Drain the excess water. Your tempeh is now ready to marinate!

1 (8-ounce) cake tempeh

Marinade
⅓ cup light-colored Mexican beer or vegetable broth
3 tablespoons freshly squeezed lime juice
1 tablespoon soy sauce
2 tablespoons peanut oil
2 cloves garlic, crushed or finely grated
½ rounded teaspoon ground cumin

½ teaspoon dried Mexican oregano, crumbled by rubbing between your palms (releases flavor and eliminates any coarse leaves)

1. Slice the entire tempeh cake in half lengthwise, then slice it into thirds. From here, you can either slice each third on a diagonal to form triangles (good if serving as an entrée) or leave as rectangles for use in sandwiches or tacos. Steam the tempeh in either a steamer basket, a covered saucepan with 1 cup of water over high heat, or a microwave as directed above. Be sure to drain it of any excess water before adding to marinade.

2. In a square pan or glass baking dish, whisk all of the marinade ingredients together. Add the tempeh and flip each piece over a few times to help it absorb the marinade. Let sit for 10 minutes at room temperature. While this is going on, you can heat a cast-iron grill pan over medium high heat. If pan-frying the tempeh, generously oil the pan with peanut oil or high-smoking-point canola oil. Using metal tongs, place the pieces of tempeh onto your grill or pan, taking care not to crowd the pan. Brush with some of the extra marinade. Grill on each side for 3 to 4 minutes, flip and keep brushing with marinade, using up the rest of the marinade on the tempeh as it cooks. Tempeh should not cook for more than 6 to 7 minutes total, or it may become too dry.

3. Serve the hot tempeh immediately. To serve in tacos, cut the tempeh into squares as directed above, grill, and coarsely chop the hot tempeh into bite-size bits. Serve in soft corn tortillas with sliced radishes, chopped cabbage, salsa, and a sprinkle of lime juice.

Variation

Ancho Chile–Tempeh Asado: Whisk into the marinade 1 tablespoon of ground ancho chile powder. Or try a blend of several of your favorite chile powders.

Tempeh Asado with Oaxacan-style Mole: Serve grilled hot tempeh with a generous side of warm Chocolate-Chile Mole Sauce (page 51), along with your favorite grain or Calabacitas (page 122).

YELLOW CHILE GRILLED TEMPEH (WITH AJÍ AMARILLO)

....

- **Serves 2 to 4**
- **Time: Less than 30 minutes**

....

Ají amarillo gives tempeh a rich golden color and a fruity, sweet heat. Serve with any Peruvian-style feast or good old beans and rice.

1 (8-ounce) cake tempeh

Marinade
½ cup vegetable broth
2 cloves garlic, grated or crushed

1 heaping tablespoon *ají amarillo* paste
1 teaspoon dried oregano
1/2 teaspoon ground cumin
2 tablespoons olive oil
1 tablespoon lime juice
1 teaspoon soy sauce
1/4 teaspoon salt

1. Slice the entire tempeh cake in half lengthwise, then slice it into thirds. From here, you can either slice each third on a diagonal to form triangles (good if serving as an entrée) or leave as rectangles for use in sandwiches or tacos. Steam the tempeh in either a steamer basket, a covered saucepan with 1 cup of water, or a microwave as directed above. Be sure to drain of any excess water before adding to marinade.

2. In a square pan or glass baking dish, whisk all the marinade ingredients together. Add the tempeh and flip each piece over a few times to help it absorb the marinade. Let sit for 10 minutes at room temperature. While this is going on, you can heat a cast-iron grill pan over medium-high heat. If pan-frying the tempeh, generously oil the pan with peanut or high-smoking-point canola oil.

3. Using metal tongs, place the pieces of tempeh on your grill or pan, taking care not to crowd the pan. Brush with some of the extra marinade. Grill on each side for 3 to 4 minutes, flip and keep brushing with the marinade, using up the rest of the marinade on the tempeh as it cooks. The tempeh should not cook for more than 6 to 7 minutes total, or it may become too dry. Serve the hot tempeh immediately.

PAN-FRIED TEMPEH WITH SOFRITO

- Serves 2 to 4
- Time: Less than 30 minutes, not including making Basic Onion-Pepper Sofrito

This toothsome tempeh benefits from an initial generously done pan-fry, then a second "smothering" in *sofrito* for a saucy Latin flavor. A solid accompaniment to Rice with Pigeon Peas (page 140) or Yuca with Cuban Garlic-Lime-Mojo Sauce (page 127).

1 (8-ounce) cake of tempeh
2 tablespoons soy sauce
Vegetable oil, for pan-frying
1/2 cup Basic Onion-Pepper Sofrito (page 32)
2 plum tomatoes, seeded and minced
1 tablespoon red wine vinegar
1 tablespoon finely chopped fresh cilantro
1 teaspoon ground cumin
1/2 cup white wine, vegetable broth, or beer
Olive oil, for pan-frying

1. Slice the entire tempeh cake in half lengthwise, then slice it into thirds. Steam the tempeh in either a steamer basket, a covered saucepan with 1 cup of water, or a microwave

as directed above. Be sure to drain of any excess water before adding to marinade. Place in a square pan or glass baking dish and sprinkle both sides of the tempeh with the soy sauce.

2. Generously oil a cast-iron pan with olive oil and heat over medium heat. Add half of the tempeh and pan-fry for 8 to 10 minutes, flipping frequently until golden. Slide the tempeh onto a plate. Fry the remaining tempeh, adding more oil as necessary, and remove from the pan. Add the *sofrito*, tomatoes, wine vinegar, cilantro, and cumin and fry until the tomatoes are soft, 6 to 8 minutes. Add the tempeh and fry for 5 minutes, stirring occasionally. Pour the wine over the tempeh and fry for another 5 minutes, until most of the liquid is absorbed but the tempeh is still saucy. Serve immediately.

7

COMPLETE YOUR PLATE: VEGETABLES, PLANTAINS, AND GRAINS

*L*atin cuisine is all about vegetables . . . but maybe in slightly different way than what you may be used to. Latin home cooking typically puts those vegetables into *things* rather than serves them on the side. Expect your veggies to be simmering in a hearty soup or stew, tucked into an entrée, or tossed in a fresh salad. But that doesn't mean vegetable sides don't exist; they are essential to any well-dressed *plato tipico*. Starchy sides such as potatoes, yuca (also known as cassava or manioc), and plantains (big cousin to bananas) are fried, boiled, roasted, or sauced for a unique experience every time.

There are so many flavors you probably already associate with Latin food: aromatic cilantro; the savory-to-sweet range of plantains; starchy, nutty yuca. (If these names mean nothing to you, flip your way immediately to the Pantry section, pages 7–22, before you start wondering what the heck

I'm asking you to write down on your next shopping list!) A trip to the Latin market can reveal these veggies and many more for use in the following recipes. And not every traditional Latin vegetable may be unfamiliar . . . the humble South American native the potato is an everyday veggie, no matter which America you live in.

FRIED SWEET PLANTAINS

- ● **Makes 1 serving per plantain**
- ● **Time: 20 minutes or less**
- ● **Gluten Free, Soy Free**

Sweet plantains, lightly caramelized, fried golden-brown on the outside and meltingly tender on the inside. Got your attention, no? Fried sweet plantains, known as *plátanos maduros* or sometimes just *maduros*, are a classic side to any Latin dinner plate. Along with the beans, rice, main protein, and veggies, the fried *plátano maduro* makes up what's often nicknamed a *bandera* ("flag") in many regions, maybe because the whole ensemble resembles the stripes of a particularly tasty flag. One large plantain makes one side or appetizer portion per person.

Ripe plantains (1 plantain per serving)
Vegetable oil for frying, such as canola
   or a blend
Lime juice or salt (optional)

1. When those plantains are ready and ripe, generously pour enough oil into a cast-iron or large nonstick skillet to cover the bottom by 1/4 inch and preheat over medium-high heat. The idea is to pan-fry—not deep-fry—the plantains. On a cutting board, slice both ends off a plantain and use a sharp paring knife to slice a shallow cut—just deep enough to slice through the skin only—from one end of the plantain to the other. Use your thumbs to peel off the skin, working your nail under the peel. This should be considerably easier than removing the skin from a green plantain. If the plantain is insanely ripe it may be very mushy, but that's okay; just gently remove the peel and place the flesh on the cutting board.

2. There are many options for slicing up a *plátano maduro* for frying; try a few to see which suits your entrée or meal best.

- Slice diagonally on a 45-degree angle into 1- to 1 1/2-inch-thick slices for easy-to-fry *plátanos*.
- Or, slice the entire plantain horizontally into two long pieces for a long, plantain shape that looks great along the edges of dinner plates.

How to Ripen a Plantain

The most important part of this recipe is to first make sure your plantains are really ripe. Many Latin markets sell both green (unripe) and yellow-black (ripe) plantains; occasionally ripe ones are priced slightly higher. Although these "ripe" plantains may have yellow peels, sometimes they are not quite ready for properly made *maduros*. A really fry-worthy ripe plantain should have a primarily black peel and feel soft when gently pressed. It should still look fairly plump and not withered.

If your plantain seems too firm, let it sit for one to three more days to get really ripe. The ripening trick of putting it in a paper bag (fold the top) can be helpful for speeding up the process. I often buy a bunch of plantains both green and "ripe" to have them ready for different stages of frying when needed. The great thing about plantains is that even if you forget about them for a week (or two), chances are they haven't gone rotten . . . they've only gotten better! That blackened fruit at the bottom of your fruit bowl has potential!

- Or, slice in half, then slice each *plátano* again in half, horizontally.

3. Any way you cut it, slide the slices into the hot oil and fry for 10 to 14 minutes, flipping a few times, until the *maduros* are golden-brown and caramelized. Do not overcrowd the pan. If you like, gently press down on the plantains when they're very soft from cooking, to help them spread slightly and encourage further browning. Add a little more oil to your pan if *maduros* start to stick or don't seem to be caramelizing enough.

4. To serve: slide the hot plantains directly onto a serving plate and sprinkle with a little lime juice or nothing at all. Draining fried sweet plantains is optional; I like them best when they're just a little greasy, but you can always gently blot them with a paper towel, if desired.

SWEET AND NUTTY ROASTED STUFFED PLANTAINS

- Serves 4
- Time: About 45 minutes
- Gluten Free, Soy Free

Slow roasting is another way to savor sweet ripe plantains and with little oil or effort. A typically Latin method for enhancing roasted ripe plantains is to stuff them with grated *panela* (unrefined brown sugar) and fresh white cheese and bake until everything

is melted and caramelized. Here, I've stuffed them with a blend of finely ground walnuts, brown sugar, lime juice, and a touch of cayenne for a nutty, sweet, salty wonder. A little white vegan cheese on top elevates these to perfection. One stuffed baked plantain makes a luscious and filling side dish or an exotic weekend breakfast treat.

4 soft ripe plantains

Filling
1/2 cup walnuts
3 tablespoons brown sugar or freshly grated *panela* (see page 214)
1 1/4 teaspoons salt
1/4 teaspoon ground cayenne, or to taste
3 tablespoons lime juice
Shredded mozzarella or Monterey Jack vegan cheese, preferably one that melts (optional)

As with the Fried Sweet Plantains (page 115), your plantains must be really ripe—with almost an entirely black peel—for them to roast properly. See page 116 for how to ripen them.

1. Preheat the oven to 375ºF. Lightly oil a glass 7 by 11-inch baking pan and tear off a length of foil that can tightly cover the top of the pan. On a cutting board, slice both ends off a plantain and use a sharp paring knife to slice a shallow cut—just deep enough to slice through the skin only—from one end of the plantain to the other. Use your thumbs to peel off the skin, working your nail under the peel. Cut a slit down the center of each plantain, taking care not to slice entirely through.

2. Lightly spray or rub the outsides of the plantains with vegetable oil, place in the pan slit side up, tightly cover the top with foil, and bake for 30 minutes. Remove from the oven and take off the foil.

3. While the plantains are roasting, pulse the walnuts, brown sugar, salt, and cayenne together in a food processor into fine crumbs. Divide the mixture equally and stuff it down the center of the roasted plantains. Sprinkle the lime juice on top of the filling and, if using vegan cheese, place a thin layer on top of the filling. Leaving the pan uncovered, bake it for 10 to 12 minutes, until the topping is browned. If desired, broil (on a low setting, if possible) for an additional 3 to 5 minutes, to further brown the top and help melt the vegan cheese if using, watching carefully so it doesn't burn.

Just Roasted Plantains

Roasting ripe plantains is a great way to enjoy them without a drop of oil. Simply follow directions for roasting in Sweet and Nutty Roasted Stuffed Plantains (page 117). Optionally, you can slice down the middle, fill with vegan cheese or a sprinkle of lime juice, and bake as directed. If desired, try broiling the fully cooked plantains for 4 to 6 minute to brown lightly, being careful not to overcook.

4. Serve immediately with an additional sprinkle of lime juice.

CRISPY FRIED GREEN PLANTAINS (TOSTONES)

- **1 serving per fried plantain**
- **Time: Less than 30 minutes, not including the optional soaking**
- **Gluten Free, Soy Free**

Crunchy slabs of fried green plantains pull together most any Latin meal. They also make addictive snacking or appetizers served lightly salted or with a garlicky *mojo* (page 128), Spicy Salsa Golf (page 53), veggie ceviche (pages 59–61), or even dipped in Chocolate-Chile Mole Sauce (page 51). Fried plantains have different names (*tostones, patacones, tajadas, mariquitas*) and shapes depending on the country—this version is for the wildly popular (in New York City at least) *tostones* style, a twice-fried green slice that's smushed down just prior to a second frying to create a thinner and extra-crunchy treat. *Tostones* are a huge feature of Latin Caribbean cuisine and can even be found floating in soups or transformed further into Mofongo (page 120).

Tip: For best results, use very green and firm plantains. If they have softened, then leave them alone for a few more days and make Fried Sweet Plantains (page 115).

How to Crush a Tostone

There are many methods for crushing *tostones* for their second frying. The idea is to use a heavy, flat object to evenly apply enough pressure to the cooked plantain to flatten it, but not so much that it falls apart. Start with one end of the cooled fried plantain, slice it, then gently but firmly press enough to flatten it to about 1/2 inch thick without breaking it. Soup cans, large coffee cans, tortilla presses, even a rolling pin can work. There's a special Latin kitchen tool called a *tostonera* that is designed just for this and does the job perfectly. They range from supercheap unfinished wood (very flimsy) to excellent-quality bamboo or plastic (pricey); but if you love *tostones*, you'll love using a *tostonera* just as much (see Kitchen Tools, page 26).

Vegetable oil, such as peanut or high-heat canola blend, for deep-frying
1 very green and firm plantain per serving
Salt

1. Pour at least 2 inches of oil into a large, heavy pot (a cast-iron Dutch oven is ideal) and preheat over medium-high heat. Cover a large plate with paper towels or crumpled brown paper, for draining the hot *tostones*. The oil is hot enough when a very small piece of raw plantain placed in the hot oil immediately starts to bubble and fry rapidly and quickly; the idea is to use very hot (but never smoking) oil so that the *tostones* cook evenly without soaking up too much grease.

2. Use plantains that are deep green, very firm, and with no yellow spots. On a cutting board, use a sharp paring knife to slice both ends off a plantain and slice a shallow cut—just through the skin only—from one end of the plantain to the other. If the skin seems particularly hard, run another cut opposite the first. Use your thumbs or the edge of a butter knife to pry off the skin, working your fingers or the dull blade under the peel. Green plantain skins can be a little stubborn at times; if any tiny bits of peel remain, remove them.

3. Diagonally slice the plantain into 11/2-inch-thick pieces. The greater the angle you slice, the longer and the bigger your final *tostones* will be. Slide into the hot oil and fry for 4 to 5 minutes, flipping once. Remove from the oil and place on the paper-lined plate to drain for about 2 minutes. I usually fry one plantain at a time this way, putting in new slices while the formerly frying ones rest.

4. When the fried slices are just cool enough to handle (after 2 to 3 minutes), gently but firmly flatten them so that they are about 3/8 inch thick. See tip box above for suggested methods and tools. Use metal tongs to return the flattened plantains to the frying oil. Fry for another 3 to 4 minutes, turning once, until golden and crisp along the edges. Return to the paper to drain, sprinkle the hot *tostones* with salt, and serve immediately.

Variation

Even Crispier Tostones: After slicing the raw plantains, place them in a large bowl, cover with warm water, and stir in a little bit of salt. Soak the plantains for 15 minutes to half an hour. When ready to fry, remove from the water, blot the plantains thoroughly with a clean kitchen towel or paper towel (don't skip this or the *tostones* could splatter when fried), and fry as directed. If desired, after it's been flattened, you may also dip the plantain briefly in the salted water and blot, for an even crispier finish. The oil may splatter, so be sure to step back when dropping plantains into the hot oil.

MOFONGO

- **Makes about 2 cups, 1/2 cup serving each**
- **Time: Less than 15 minutes, not including preparing the *tostones***
- **Gluten Free, Soy Free (if tofu omitted)**

Mofongo, via Puerto Rico (with variations in the Dominican Republic and Cuba), makes something already delicious—fried green plantains—even better. *Mofongo* is a tasty stuffinglike mash of crushed *tostones* seasoned with plenty of garlic, moistened with a little broth and superfried tofu for a blast of smoky flavor. For best results, use firm green plantains or ones just starting to turn yellow. *Mofongo* is also a useful way to use up crumbly *tostones* that may have fallen apart after the second frying step.

Mofongo for presentation is usually pressed into appealing shapes with either a bowl or a cup. Surround your unmolded *mofongo* with a small pool of warm vegetable broth just before serving, for additional juiciness.

Tip: I like to use a pastry cutter (the thing with several thin curved blades encasing a handle grip) or a mezzaluna (curved chopping blade) for "mashing" up *tostones* for mofongo. The thin blades slice into the fried plantains quickly and the grip provides plenty of control.

Make-ahead Tip: Prepare the *tostones* up to two days in advance. Chop right before frying.

4 large green plantains, prepared as tostones (page 118)
1 tablespoon olive oil
3 cloves garlic, minced
1 recipe Tofu Chicharrones (page 101) (optional but very good)
1/2 teaspoon liquid smoke
1/2 cup warm vegetable broth, or more
Salt and freshly ground pepper

1. Prepare plantains as if making *tostones* (page 118), frying, pressing, and frying again. Chop the warm *tostones* into fine, stuffing-like bits with a mezzaluna, pastry cutter, or a heavy, sharp knife.

2. In a large nonstick skillet, heat the olive oil and minced garlic over medium heat until the garlic is sizzling and fragrant, about 30 seconds. Stir in the Tofu Chicharrones and fry for 1 minute, if using. Stir in the mashed *tostones* and liquid smoke, then pour in 1/2 cup vegetable broth and simmer for 1 minute to deglaze the bottom of the skillet for 3 to 4 minutes, then turn off the heat. Mofongo should resemble a moist stuffing; if too dry, dribble in warm vegetable broth, a tablespoon at a time, until desired consistency is reached. Season with salt and pepper.

3. To serve: pack 1/2 to 1 cup of *mofongo* in a measuring cup, ramekin, or small bowl, top with the serving plate, and flip. Remove the object you just used as a mold. There you have it, a shapely serving of *mofongo*. Or if you don't like flipping plates, just serve in a free-form pile, like stuffing. Drizzle a little extra warmed vegetable broth onto each serving if more moistness is desired, and serve the hot *mofongo* immediately.

BRAISED BRAZILIAN SHREDDED KALE

- Serves 4 as a side
- Time: 30 minutes
- Gluten Free, Soy Free

Kale is a popular leafy green veggie in South America, and in Brazil it's often served as a side (with *feijoada*) or in soups. Brazilian kale is typically sliced very finely so that it's enjoyed as a mound of juicy skinny shreds (rather than ribbons or leaves). Liquid smoke replicates the bacon or ham that is sometimes paired with kale—you can leave it out, but you'll miss out on something delicious!

Tip: Use kale with large, flat leaves (such as Lacinato, also called "dinosaur" kale) for easy preparation. If all you have is ruffled kale, no problem, just gather a bunch of leaves, firmly press them down into the cutting board, and try to keep everything in a neat bunch as you chop away. Collard greens can be substituted for kale, also.

1 pound kale, well washed, tough thick
    stems removed, leaves kept intact
2 tablespoons peanut or unprocessed
    coconut oil
4 cloves garlic, finely minced
1 small yellow onion, sliced in half and
    diced finely
1/4 cup water or vegetable broth
1/2 teaspoon liquid smoke (optional)
1/2 teaspoon salt, or to taste

1. Stack several leaves of kale on a cutting board. Tightly roll up the leaves to form a tube, then use a sharp, heavy knife to slice the kale tube into very thin shreds (1/8 inch or thinner). Place the shredded kale in a large bowl and set aside.

2. Combine the oil and garlic in a large nonstick skillet over medium heat, stirring until the garlic is sizzling and fragrant, about 30 seconds. Add the onion and cook until soft and translucent, 6 to 8 minutes. Add a big handful of kale and stir with tongs (silicone tipped is best for use with nonstick cookware), until the shreds wilt enough to create room in the pan. Continue to add the kale, a handful at a time, until all of the kale is finally incorporated, about 10 minutes or so. Continue to cook the kale until it has wilted a little more and released some juices, about 5 minutes. Sprinkle the water and liquid smoke over the kale, cover the pan and steam the kale for 4 to 6 minutes, or until the kale is tender and juicy. Season with salt and serve hot as a mound on serving plates.

CALABACITAS (MIXED SQUASH SAUTÉ)

....
- Serves 4 as a side, 2 as an entrée
- Time: About 45 minutes
- Gluten Free, Soy Free
....

A lighter take on the traditional Mexican preparation of squash made better with a dual-season dose of zucchini and pumpkin. Use butternut or calabaza pumpkin for your winter squash and add the best-quality summer squash you can find; pick small young squash for the most flavor and most tender texture. *Calabacitas* makes a whole meal, served with any salsa and some Homemade Soft Corn Tortillas (page 165) or Whole Wheat Flour Tortillas with Chia (page 166).

Tip: Have too much summer corn to deal with? Toss it into this juicy sauté!

1 pound summer squash: zucchini, yellow squash, pattypan, and so on, ends trimmed, cut into 1/2-inch slices
1 teaspoon salt, or to taste
1 small onion, sliced into thin slivers
2 cloves garlic, minced
1 tablespoon olive or peanut oil
1 pound calabaza pumpkin, butternut squash, or any sweet winter squash, peeled, seeded, and cut into 1/2-inch cubes
1 teaspoon dried oregano
1/4 teaspoon ground cumin
1 tablespoon lime juice
2 plum tomatoes, seeded and diced into 1/2-inch pieces
1 cup fresh corn kernels (optional)
Freshly ground black pepper

1. Place the summer squash in a bowl, sprinkle with 1/2 teaspoon of the salt, and let sit for 15 minutes. The squash will release excess water; when ready to use, rinse and drain well. While the squash is draining, sauté the onion and garlic with the peanut oil in a large, deep nonstick skillet over medium heat until the onion is soft and translucent, 6 to 8 minutes. Add the calabaza pumpkin and 1/4 cup of water. Cover and steam for 10 to 12 minutes, until the

pumpkin is easily pierced with a fork. Remove the lid and add the drained summer squash, oregano, cumin, lime juice, tomatoes, corn (if using), and the remaining 1/2 teaspoon of salt. Cook and stir occasionally until the summer squash reaches your desired tenderness, 8 to 10 minutes. Season with freshly ground black pepper and serve.

Variation

Add 1 to 2 stemmed and finely chopped fresh green or red chiles to the frying garlic. Remove seeds if you want less heat, or keep them for more fire!

SWISS CHARD WITH RAISINS AND CAPERS

- Serves 4 as a side
- Time: Less than 20 minutes
- Gluten Free, Soy Free

Tender Swiss chard pairs beautifully with the classic Spanish combination of sweet raisins and salty capers. This is an easy side that's good with just about anything, especially rice or quinoa, for absorbing the chard's savory juices. Red chard looks particularly pretty but green, yellow, or rainbow chard is fresh and summery.

1 large bunch chard (over 1/2 pound or a little more)

2 tablespoons olive oil
2 cloves garlic
2 tablespoons capers
1/4 cup dark raisins
2 tablespoons cooking wine, vegetable broth, or water
Salt and pepper

1. Wash the chard, then trim away the dried-out–looking parts of the ends of the stems. Remove and dice the stems into 1/2-inch chunks. Roll up a few leaves and slice into 1/2-inch ribbons. Keep the stems and leaves separate for now.

2. Over medium heat in a large, heavy skillet, heat together the olive oil and garlic until sizzling. Stir in the capers and fry for about 30 seconds, then stir in the raisins and chard stems. Stirring occasionally, cook for 4 to 6 minutes, or until the chard stems start to become tender but are still firm. Toss in the chard leaves, stirring to coat with the oil, and cook until the leaves start to wilt, about 1 1/2 minutes. Stir in the cooking wine to deglaze the pan and then remove from the heat.

3. Season the chard with salt and pepper and serve immediately, making sure to ladle some of the chardy juices onto the serving plates.

Variation

Use spinach instead of chard, or a mixture of both!

PAN-GRILLED VEGETABLES IN CHILE-LIME BEER

- Serves 4 as a side
- Time: 20 minutes or less
- Soy Free

Vegetables and beer were meant to be good friends. A quick dip in a simple Mexican-style beer marinade adds flavor and depth to such tender crunchy vegetables as summer squash, asparagus, or even okra for grilling in a cast-iron skillet or grill pan. Just a little beer goes a long way in flavoring these vegetables, so there's no need to raid the keg for this delicious and easy summer vegetable side.

2/3 cup Mexican beer
2 tablespoons lime juice
1/2 teaspoon salt
1 clove garlic, crushed or grated on a
    Microplane grater
1/2 teaspoon ground chile powder
1 teaspoon olive oil
2 pounds summer squash (such as
    zucchini, yellow squash, pattypan),
    asparagus, or whole okra pods
Additional vegetable oil, for grilling

1. Preheat a cast-iron skillet or grilling pan over medium heat. In a shallow bowl, whisk together the beer, lime juice, salt, garlic, chili powder, and olive oil. If using squash, slice it into long, 1/4-inch-thick strips. Asparagus only needs to be trimmed. If okra pods are very large, slice in half lengthwise; leave small pods whole.

2. Place the vegetables in the beer marinade and marinate for 5 minutes, stirring frequently. Lightly oil the preheated pan and add one-third of the vegetables. Don't crowd the pan; leave enough room that vegetables can be easily flipped. Drizzle the vegetables with 1 to 2 tablespoons of marinade and grill for 4 to 8 minutes, flipping occasionally, until they are browned and tender. If necessary, add a little more oil to keep the vegetables from sticking. Remove from the pan, add a little more oil, and repeat with the remaining vegetables.

3. Serve hot or at room temperature.

Variations

Properly trimmed nopales paddles that have had their spines removed (see Noteworthy Nopales) love this marinade. Either slice into 1/2-inch-wide strips or slice each paddle into "fingers" but leave the strips attached at the base of the paddle. Marinate the nopales and drizzle or brush frequently with beer marinade as they cook on the grill or skillet.

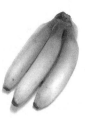

Noteworthy Nopales

Nopales are the thick fleshy paddles from a cactuslike plant enjoyed in Mexico and Central America, grilled or pickled for eating in tacos, tortas, and most every food in between. Although they're covered with long thorns and tiny transparent spines and look like a cartoon cactus, properly peeled and prepared nopales "paddles" are delicious. They have a fresh, grassy, asparagus-like crunch with a bit of the slipperiness of okra.

I love nopales but I really don't like removing the spines. At all. I go as far as to recommend that unless you find handling spines somehow relaxing (maybe you wrestle porcupines or juggle sea urchins on the weekends?), it may be in your best interest to either enjoy them pickled or seek out prepeeled, spine- and thorn-free paddles at your local Mexican produce vendor.

PERUVIAN POTATOES WITH SPICY "CHEEZY" SAUCE

- Makes a little over 2 cups of sauce to serve with 4 to 6 servings of potatoes
- Time: Less than 20 minutes, not including cooking the potatoes

Peruvians enjoy yellow cheese sauce just as North Americans do, but it's spicy and usually served on boiled or fried potatoes or yuca. Known as *salsa a la Huancaína*, named for the Huancayo region of Peru, it's spiked with their beloved yellow chile (*ají amarillo*) that gives it a spicy, slightly sweet punch and deep yellow color. This dairy-free *Huancaína* gets its "cheeziness" from nutritional yeast (page 11)—a hardworking vegan multitasker if there ever was one—and nothing else will do. *Salsa a la Huancaína* is eaten hot over cooked veggies, or try it at room temperature served as a dip.

Tip: Use purple potatoes for an exciting contrast of yellow sauce and inky purple-blue potatoes peeking though.

1½ cups mild vegetable broth

3 tablespoons garbanzo flour

2 tablespoons *ají amarillo* paste

4 teaspoons peanut or vegetable oil

1 clove garlic, chopped

1 small yellow onion, chopped finely

½ teaspoon salt, or to taste

⅔ cup nutritional yeast flakes

¾ cup heavy cream substitute or rich nondairy milk

2 tablespoons lemon juice

¼ cup plain cracker crumbs (such as water crackers or saltines)

2 pounds red, purple, or yellow waxy potatoes or yuca, boiled and kept warm

10 pitted black kalamata olives, for garnish

1. In a large liquid measuring cup or mixing bowl, whisk together the vegetable broth and garbanzo flour until blended, then stir in the *ají*

amarillo paste and set aside. In a large saucepan, heat the peanut oil and garlic over medium heat until the garlic starts to sizzle, about 30 seconds. Stir in the onion and fry until soft, about 4 minutes. Whisk the vegetable broth mixture one more time, then pour it into the saucepan. Continue to whisk the mixture over medium heat for 4 to 6 minutes, or until the garbanzo flour cooks and thickens the mixture. Stir in the salt, nutritional yeast flakes, heavy cream substitute, lemon juice, and cracker crumbs. Simmer the mixture for another 2 to 3 minutes to completely soften the cracker crumbs.

2. Remove from the heat and pulse with an immersion blender to create a smooth texture. The sauce should be creamy and have the consistency of very thick gravy. Taste and adjust for salt and add a little more lemon juice, if desired.

3. Serve immediately, spooned on top of hot cooked potatoes or yuca. Traditionally, *salsa a la Huancaína* is draped on food so that it forms a concealing blanket of sauce, but I prefer to drizzle it or serve it on the side for dipping. The sauce will continue to thicken as it cools; thin with more vegetable broth or nondairy milk, as needed, to your desired consistency. Garnish each serving with a few black olives.

Variation

Salsa a la Huancaína Verde: Sometimes Huancaína sauce is blended with the unique Peruvian herb *huacatay,* "black mint," for a green, herb–flecked sauce. Black mint has a flavor strongly reminiscent of tarragon, with hints of mint, cilantro, and oregano. Peruvian markets may stock black mint either in jars as a puree or whole leaves packed frozen; add 1 to 2 tablespoons of puree or 2 to 3 tablespoons of chopped frozen leaves to the sauce just before blending.

To make a fresh herb substitute for fresh black mint, add to the *Huancaína* sauce just before blending: 2 tablespoons finely chopped fresh tarragon, 1 tablespoon each chopped fresh mint and chopped fresh cilantro, and a pinch of dried oregano.

CRUNCHY FRIED YUCA (YUCA FRITA)

- **Serves 4 as a side or appetizer**
- **Time: About 45 minutes**

Flaky, crunchy on the outside, and creamy inside, fried yuca is delicious comfort food at its calorie-laden best. Once you're hooked, this may have you seriously reconsidering french fries. Enjoy as a decadent side or appetizer served piping hot with a sprinkle of good salt and a twist of lime.

Make-ahead Tip: Yuca must be fully cooked by boiling before frying. Boil the yuca, break into pieces, and store in a tightly covered container in the fridge for up to three days until ready to fry.

2 pounds yuca (one really big fat yuca
　　root about 9 inches long by 3 to
　　4 inches wide)
Peanut, canola, or corn oil, for deep-frying
Salt
Lime wedges

1. Trim the ends of the yuca and use a Y-shaped vegetable peeler to remove the waxy skin. With a heavy, sharp chef's knife, split the root horizontally into two or three equal pieces, then cut each piece in half lengthwise. You should have 4 to 6 large, semi-circular chunks of yuca. Slice each chunk into two or three more pieces. Place in a large stockpot and pour in enough cold water to cover the yuca by at least 3 inches.

2. Bring to a boil over high heat, partially cover the pot, and cook for 25 to 30 minutes, or until the yuca is very tender. Fully cooked yuca is ready when its white flesh has a semi-translucent appearance on the edges and it also flakes easily when pierced with a fork. Drain and set aside to cool.

3. Pour the frying oil into a large, heavy pot (cast iron is best) and preheat over medium-high heat. Make sure that there are at least 2 inches of oil in the pan. Cover a large plate with paper towels or crumpled brown paper, for draining the hot fried yuca. The oil is hot enough when a very small piece of yuca placed in the hot oil immediately starts to bubble rapidly and fry quickly; the idea is to use very hot (but never smoking) oil so that the yuca pieces cook evenly without soaking up too much grease.

4. When cool enough to handle, separate the yuca into long pieces no thicker than 2 inches but preferably a little less. Sometimes cooked yuca may have a thick, rubbery skin on the outside edges of the root; this peels off easily, so remove and discard it. Place a few chunks in the oil at a time, taking care not to crowd the pan. Fry for 8 to 10 minutes, turning each piece occasionally with metal tongs or a slotted spoon. The yuca is ready when it's firm and crisp looking with slight golden bits on the edges. Remove from the oil, very carefully shake off any excess, and place on the paper-lined plate to drain. Transfer to a serving plate and sprinkle with salt.

5. Serve with lime wedges and eat while hot.

YUCA WITH CUBAN GARLIC-LIME-MOJO SAUCE

- **Serves 4 as a side or more as an appetizer**
- **Time: About 45 minutes**

This laid-back Cuban method of preparing yuca is sure to bring requests for more. Tangy garlicky seasoned olive oil sauce makes simple boiled yuca irresistible. Serve as an appetizer on a big platter or arrange individual servings as a side with any Caribbean or tropical entrée.

2 pounds yuca, fresh or frozen chunks

Tangy Mojo Sauce
  1/2 **cup olive oil**
  6 to 8 cloves garlic, minced finely
  **1 small yellow onion, cut in half and
    sliced thinly**
  1 teaspoon salt
  1/2 **teaspoon ground cumin**
  1/4 **cup freshly squeezed lime juice**
  Freshly ground black pepper

1. Trim the ends of the yuca and use a Y-shaped vegetable peeler to remove the waxy skin. With a heavy, sharp chef's knife, split the root horizontally into two or three equal pieces, then cut each piece in half lengthwise. You should have four to six large, semicircular chunks of yuca. Slice each chunk into two or three more pieces. Place in a large stockpot and pour in enough cold water to cover the yuca by at least 3 inches.

2. Bring to a boil over high heat, partially cover the pot, and cook for 25 to 30 minutes, or until the yuca is very tender. Fully cooked yuca is ready when its white flesh has a semi-translucent appearance on the edges and it also flakes easily when pierced with a fork.

3. Prepare the *mojo* sauce: In a large saucepan, combine the olive oil, garlic, and onion and bring to a gentle simmer over medium heat, then lower the heat to low. Simmer for 12 to 14 minutes, or until the garlic and onion are very

soft and just starting to turn golden. Remove from the heat and stir in the salt and ground cumin . . . resist the urge to drink the luscious-smelling cumin-garlicky oil right away and set it aside for 2 minutes to cool slightly. Gently stir in the lime juice and a few twists of freshly ground pepper.

4. To serve: Drain the hot yuca from the pot. Sometimes cooked yuca may have a thick, rubbery skin on the outside edges of the root; this peels off easily, so remove and discard it. Arrange the yuca in a mound on a serving platter, drizzle with the sauce, and pile the onions on top of the yuca. Serve immediately.

Variation

Mojo Sauce with Tostones: Prepare the *mojo* sauce (without the yuca), let cool slightly, and with an immersion blender puree enough to finely chop the onions, for a delicious garlicky dip for tostones.

AMARANTH POLENTA WITH ROASTED CHILES

- **Serves 4, generous 1-cup servings**
- **Time: Less than 30 minutes**

This hearty polenta is a perfect storm of ancient amaranth (a nutritious Central American native grain), corn, and roasted green chiles and offers a greater nutritional boost and pleasantly crunchy texture over standard polenta. Serve it hot, or chill it, slice, and lightly pan fry for a savory, alternative breakfast.

1 Anaheim or poblano chile
1 to 2 hot green chiles, such as serrano or jalapeño
2 tablespoons olive oil
2 cloves garlic, minced or grated
1 green onion, chopped finely
1/2 cup uncooked amaranth grain
4 cups water or vegetable broth
3/4 teaspoon salt (use just a pinch if using vegetable stock)
2/3 cup polenta-style cornmeal
1 tablespoon fresh lime juice

1. Roast all the whole, unsliced chiles on a gas stove until well charred. Place the chiles in a bowl, cover the bowl with plastic wrap or a plate, and set aside for 5 minutes or longer. Remove the green chiles' skin. Remove the seeds from the Anaheim or poblano; you can leave the seeds in the green chiles if you're craving a spicy polenta. Finely chop the chiles and set aside.

2. In a large, heavy saucepan, heat the olive oil over medium heat. Stir in the garlic and green onion and fry until the green onion is softened, about 2 minutes. Stir in amaranth and fry for 1 minute, stirring to coat with the oil. Pour in the water, stir, and add the salt. Increase the heat to bring the mixture to a boil

and then lower the heat to low. Partially cover and cook for 10 to 12 minutes, until the amaranth grains are tender and look transparent (and resemble miniature cooked quinoa grains).

3. Increase the heat and bring the liquid to a gentle boil, then pour in a little bit of the cornmeal at a time while stirring constantly with a wire whisk to eliminate any lumps. A few minutes into stirring the polenta, you'll want to switch to using a wooden spoon to stir, as the mixture will continue to thicken. Stir in the chopped chiles and continue to stir the polenta for 12 to 14 minutes, or until your desired thickened, creamy consistency is reached.

4. When ready to serve, stir in the lime juice and scoop onto serving plates.

5. To prepare polenta for frying: Pour the hot polenta into a small glass or metal loaf pan rinsed first with cold water. Spread the top of polenta as evenly as possible and chill overnight or until very firm. Slice into 1-inch-thick pieces and gently place in a preheated, well-oiled cast-iron pan. Chilled amaranth polenta is softer than regular polenta, so use a wide spatula to gently flip; add a little more oil if it starts to stick. Fry until hot and serve immediately.

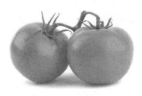

QUINOA–OYSTER MUSHROOM RISOTTO (QUINOTTO)

- Makes four 1-cup side servings, or serves 2 to 3 as a main course
- Time: About 45 minutes

Quinoa risottos are nothing new, but is a basic recipe that can be adapted for whatever mood you're in with any vegetables, herbs, and faux meats. *Quinotto*—as it's sometimes called in quinoa-lovin' countries such as Peru, Ecuador, and Bolivia—is less like rice risotto and instead an intensely flavorful change of pace from pilaf-style quinoa. It's a tasty introduction for people who may not be excited by plain-Jane boiled quinoa.

Tip: Look for flavorful, light-colored broths or a mushroom broth. I didn't include salt in this recipe as most veggie broths have plenty.

1/2 pound oyster or cremini mushrooms
3 tablespoons olive oil
2 cloves garlic, chopped finely
3 large shallots, chopped finely
1 cup dried quinoa, rinsed in a
   fine-mesh strainer
1/2 cup white wine
1/2 teaspoon dried thyme, crumbled
1/2 teaspoon dried oregano
1 tablespoon *ají amarillo* or *ají panca* paste (optional)
3 cups hot vegetable broth (use a lightly flavored stock or a "chicken"-flavored one, for best results)
1 tablespoon lime juice
Freshly ground black pepper to taste
Finely chopped fresh cilantro or
   flat-leaf (Italian) parsley

1. Lightly brush mushrooms with a clean dishcloth to remove any debris. Cut off and discard any tough stems, then slice into thin strips. In a large, heavy saucepan, heat 2 tablespoons of the olive oil over medium heat. Add the mushrooms and sauté for 4 to 5 minutes, or until golden. Remove the mushrooms; set aside a few strips of mushroom for garnishing later.

2. Add the remaining tablespoon of olive oil to the pan. Add the chopped garlic and shallots and fry, stirring occasionally, until golden and fragrant, about 5 minutes. Add the quinoa and fry, stirring occasionally, until it turns slightly golden, 2 to 3 minutes. Pour in the white wine and stir to deglaze the bottom of the pot and dissolve any browned bits. Stir in the dried thyme, oregano, and *ají* paste and simmer for 1 minute.

3. Pour in 1 cup of broth and continue to stir a little more frequently. After the liquid has been absorbed, pour in a little more broth. Continue like this, adding more broth after the

quinoa has absorbed most of the liquid, stirring, cooking for 30 to 35 minutes total. The *quinotto* is done when the quinoa grains are tender and plump and the mixture is very moist but all of the liquid has been absorbed. Remove the pan from the heat, cover, and let the *quinotto* sit for 10 minutes.

4. Remove the cover, add the lime juice, and season with ground pepper. Gently stir with a fork. Scoop onto individual serving plates, garnish with a few strips of sautéed mushroom, and sprinkle with cilantro or parsley.

●　●　●

8

ONE-POT STEWS, CASSEROLES, AND CAZUELAS

*T*here are so many Latin comfort foods—tamales, tortillas, yellow rice—who doesn't love all these things? But some of the most comforting are the hearty stews eaten all over Central and South America. These *cazuelas*—also a general name for the big pots they're cooked or served in—are indeed one-pot meals, brimming with vegetables, grains, and proteins. Eat a serving or two and you're set for the rest of the day or until the next *cazuela*, of course.

Casseroles are enjoyed in South America as casual family meals just as much as they are up north. I've included a few American-friendly concoctions crafted out of Latin ingredients, and my favorite recipe for vegan chiles rellenos. While not exactly a casserole, it's delicious and can feed an army of *relleno* fanatics.

• • •

POTATO-CHICKPEA ENCHILADAS WITH GREEN TOMATILLO SAUCE

- Serves 4 to 6
- Time: About 1 1/2 hours, not including making Tomatillo Sauce and Pine Nut Crema
- Gluten Free

I'll take an enchilada over a taco or burrito any day, but that's just me. Also it's my favorite way to get that recommended daily dose of chile sauce (there is an RDA for that, right?), and this enchilada is drenched in Tomatillo Sauce. The sublimely dairy-like Pine Nut Crema recalls classic *enchiladas suizas*, which spares the chicken in favor of creamy chickpeas. Enchiladas are ideal make-ahead meals and are superstars when it comes to being reheated. Cilantro-Lime Rice (page 95) and Mango-Jicama

Chopped Salad (page 77) are my favorite sides to serve here.

Make-ahead Tip: Enchiladas can be labor intensive but are easier if the components are prepared in advance. The Tomatillo Sauce, Pine Nut Crema, and potato filling can all be refrigerated in tightly sealed containers for up to a week. Try making them over the course of three weeknights, and by the midweek just open the fridge, bring out the components and a stack of corn tortillas, and have enchiladas in about 45 minutes. While they bake, it's easy to make a salad, rice, or even both.

1 recipe Green Tomatillo Sauce (page 40)
1 recipe Pine Nut Crema (page 45)

Filling
1 pound white or yellow-skinned waxy
potatoes
4 cloves garlic, minced
2 tablespoons peanut or olive oil
2 jalapeño or serrano chiles, roasted and
chopped finely
1/2 pound red onion, diced
2 teaspoons dried Mexican oregano
1 teaspoon ground cumin
A big pinch of dried epazote (optional)
1 cup vegetable broth, preferably
"chicken" flavored
2 cups cooked chickpeas, or 1 (15-ounce)
can, well rinsed, chopped coarsely
1/2 teaspoon salt, or more to taste
Freshly ground pepper

For Assembly
12 corn tortillas

1. Make the Green Tomatillo Sauce and the Pine Nut Crema first and have them handy. You can prepare them up to 2 days in advance before preparing the enchiladas.

2. Prepare the filling: Clean, peel (or don't, if you like the skin), and dice the potatoes into 1/4-inch cubes. Place in a large pot, add enough cold water to cover, and bring the water to a rolling boil over high heat. Cook the potatoes until a fork easily pierces a chunk, about 20 minutes. Drain and set aside. Preheat the oven to 375ºF. Lightly oil a casserole dish, about 12 by 8 by 2 inches or slightly larger. Have ready enough aluminum foil to cover the top of the casserole.

3. In a large skillet over medium heat, fry the chopped garlic in the peanut oil until the garlic starts to sizzle, about 30 seconds. Add the chiles, onion, oregano, cumin, and epazote and fry, stirring occasionally, for 5 minutes, or until the onion turns soft and translucent. Add the vegetable broth, cooked potatoes, chopped chickpeas, and salt. Cook the mixture, stirring occasionally, until most of the broth has reduced but the mixture is still moist. Mash the potatoes just enough to create a chunky texture; taste and add freshly ground pepper and additional salt as desired.

4. Create an enchilada assembly line: Have ready a pie plate filled with about 3/4 cup of

Green Tomatillo Sauce, the prepared casserole dish, a stack of corn tortillas, a lightly greased cast-iron pan set over medium heat, and the filling. Ladle a little bit of the sauce on the bottom of the casserole dish and spread it around. Take a corn tortilla, place it on the heated pan for 30 seconds, then flip it over and heat until the tortilla has become soft and pliable. Drop the softened tortilla into the pie plate filled with the sauce; allow it to get completely covered in sauce, flip it over, and coat the other side. Now place that saucy tortilla in the casserole dish. Spoon 3 to 4 tablespoons of the filling down the middle and roll the enchilada tightly. Continue with the rest of the tortillas, tightly packing the enchiladas next to one another in the casserole in a single layer only.

5. Pour about a cup of sauce over the enchiladas, spreading it evenly over the whole casserole. Don't worry about having extra sauce left over; you'll want to serve this with the enchiladas when they're done. When done assembling the enchiladas, spoon generous dollops of Pine Nut Crema on top of the casserole. It looks best if you don't try to spread it evenly; rather, leave some spots uncovered to let the Green Tomatillo Sauce show through. Cover tightly with the foil and bake for 25 minutes. Remove the foil and bake for another 15 to 20 minutes, until the edges of the tortillas are slightly browned. If you like, set the oven to broil on high for an additional 2 to 3 minutes, to further brown the Pine Nut Crema; watch carefully so it doesn't burn.

6. Let the enchiladas cool for 5 minutes before eating. Top individual servings with the remaining warmed Green Tortilla Sauce.

Variations

Finely chop one loaf of Steamed White Seitan (page 35) and add to the filling, along with the chickpeas.

Red Chile Enchiladas: Replace the Green Tomatillo Sauce with Red Chile Sauce, and the chickpeas with two loaves of Steamed Red Seitan (page 34), chopped finely. Proceed as directed.

The Whole Enchilada

Use this enchilada recipe as a template to make any kind of enchilada anytime out of most any kind of filling. Enchiladas fit the bill of great foods that transform leftovers into—I'm going to say it—*look forwards*. Chop up steamed bits of veggies, random beans, stray seitan, or lonely tofu, roll in tortillas, and smother with your favorite sauce . . . enchiladas are up to your most demanding leftover recycling needs and ready to do it up in style.

QUICK RED POSOLE WITH BEANS

- Serves 4, or 2 to 3 really hungry hombres
- Time: About 30 minutes
- Gluten Free, Soy Free

Posole is a Mexican long-simmered stew chock full of history, endless variations of ingredients, and the common thread of hominy. And sometimes you need hot posole stew and you need it . . . almost now! Posole loves to be topped with lots of saladlike ingredients—crunchy cabbage, radishes, avocado—that coolly contrast with the soothing, warm tomato stew below.

I'm a fan of canned hominy for fast and easy posole making. The canned stuff just requires a brief rinse to use, is cheap, and is ready for whenever you need this quick-cooking posole.

Tip: If you have a little more time, try roasting any dried red chile (or two or three) for really flavorful posole. Follow the chile-roasting directions used in the Red Chile Sauce (page 45).

2 tablespoons olive oil
1 large yellow onion, peeled and diced
4 cloves garlic, minced
1 large poblano chile or green Cubanelle pepper
1 teaspoon ground cumin
1½ teaspoons dried Mexican oregano
1 teaspoon red chile powder, such as ancho or guajillo
1 (24-ounce) can diced tomatoes with juice, or 2 pounds very juicy fresh plum tomatoes, seeded and chopped
1 (15-ounce) can pinto or black beans, drained and rinsed, or 2 cups cooked
1 (15-ounce) can white cooked hominy, drained and rinsed, or 2 cups cooked
1 cup Mexican light-colored beer or vegetable broth
¼ teaspoon salt, or to taste
1 tablespoon lime juice
Freshly ground pepper

Optional Garnishes

Large tortilla chips or fried tortilla strips
Chopped fresh cilantro
Thinly sliced white radishes
Chopped fresh tomato
Finely diced fresh onion
Finely shredded white cabbage or a crunchy lettuce such as romaine
Slices of ripe avocado
Lime wedge

1. In a large pot, combine the oil and garlic over medium heat. Cook until the garlic is fragrant, about 30 seconds, then add the onion and poblano chile. Stir and cook until the vegetables are softened and the onion is translucent, 8 to 10 minutes. Add the cumin, oregano, and chile powder and fry for another minute. Now add the diced tomatoes with juice, beans,

hominy, beer, and salt. If using fresh tomatoes, you may want to add more beer, water, or vegetable broth if the tomatoes alone don't provide enough liquid to create a stew. Stir, increase the heat, and bring the mixture to a gentle boil. Lower the heat to medium-low and simmer for 25 minutes, or until the vegetables are tender. Turn off the heat, stir in the lime juice, and season with freshly ground pepper. Let the posole sit for about 10 minutes prior to serving, to cool slightly and allow the flavors to meld.

2. Ladle into large individual serving bowls and either decorate with separate mounds of cilantro, lettuce, and so on or place each garnish in its own serving bowl and have guests pass the bowls around. Serve with hot corn tortillas.

GREEN POSOLE SEITAN STEW WITH CHARD AND WHITE BEANS

- Serves 4 to 6 generously
- Time: About 1½ hours
- Soy Free

Green posole is another variety of this popular Mexican stew, making use of tomatillos instead of tomatoes to create the broth base. Thing get even greener in this posole with the addition of chard (or spinach, if you prefer) and toasted ground green pumpkin seeds. I'm crazy for this combination of white beans, hominy, and Steamed White Seitan in this tangy tomatillo-based broth. Serve with hot, freshly made Homemade Soft Corn Tortillas (page 165)

This intense stew is one of my favorite recipes—some guests might be left guessing at exactly what they're dipping their tortillas into, but they'll all agree it's just *fabuloso*.

1 pound tomatillos, husks removed, washed
4 tablespoons peanut or other light vegetable oil
½ recipe (2 loaves) Steamed White Seitan (page 35), diced into ½-inch cubes
¼ cup shelled pumpkin seeds (pepitas)
2 cloves garlic, chopped
2 jalapeños, serranos, or other green chiles, washed, sliced in half, and seeded if a milder posole is desired
1 medium-size onion, chopped
½ cup fresh cilantro leaves, lightly packed
1½ teaspoons dried oregano or epazote
1 teaspoon ground cumin
2 cups vegetable broth
½ cup Mexican light-colored beer or vegetable broth
1 (15-ounce) can white beans (cannellini or navy, for example), drained and rinsed, or 2 cups cooked
1 (15-ounce) can white cooked hominy, drained and rinsed, or 2 cups cooked
½ pound Swiss chard, thick stems removed, sliced into thin ribbons
½ teaspoon salt, or more to taste

Optional Garnishes

Large tortilla chips or fried tortilla strips
Lime wedges
Thinly sliced white radishes
Slices of avocado
Large white corn tortilla chips

1. Fill a large pot with enough water to allow the tomatillos to float, cover with a lid, turn the heat to high, and bring the water to a rolling boil. Add the tomatillos, stir them occasionally, and cook for 10 minutes, or until the skins start to split and the tomatillos' bright green color begins to fade. Use a slotted spoon to transfer the cooked tomatillos to a bowl to cool for 20 minutes. The cooked tomatillos may collapse and release some juices while they cool.

2. In a large, heavy-bottomed soup pot, heat 2 tablespoons of the oil over medium heat and add the diced seitan. Sauté for 10 to 12 minutes, stirring occasionally, until the seitan is browned. Remove from the pot and set aside. In a cast-iron skillet over medium heat, toast the pumpkin seeds until lightly browned, 3 to 4 minutes, watching carefully so they don't burn. Pour the seeds into a food processor and pulse to finely grind, then set aside.

3. In a blender jar, pulse the cooled tomatillos with their juices, garlic, chiles, onion, cilantro, oregano, and cumin to form a thick sauce. In the large soup pot used to sauté the seitan, heat the remaining 2 tablespoons of oil over medium heat. Add the blended tomatillos and cook for

10 minutes, until the sauce turns darker (no longer bright green) and thickens slightly. Slowly stir in vegetable broth, beer, and ground pumpkin seeds and bring to a boil again, then lower the heat to a simmer. Add the sautéed seitan, beans, and hominy. Partially cover and simmer for 25 minutes.

4. Stir in the shredded chard, partially cover again, and simmer for another 10 to 12 minutes, or until the chard is completely wilted and tender. Add salt to taste.

5. When ready to serve, ladle into large, deep soup bowls and top with several white tortilla chips stuck into the stew, plus a small pile each of sliced radish and avocado and a slice of lime. Serve hot with a stack of hot corn tortillas.

Variation

Omit the seitan and instead soak 1 cup of chunk-style TVP in boiling water for 10 minutes, drain well, then add to the posole with the beans and hominy.

CREAMY POTATO PEANUT STEW (GUATITA)

- **Makes about 6 cups; serves 4 to 6**
- **Time: About 1½ hours**

This amazing peanut-laced concoction is a riff on *guatita*, a hearty (and usually very meaty) stew popular in Ecuador and Chile. Origins aside, cows everywhere would applaud if they could about your choice of using TVP, seitan, Soy Curls, or soy-free chickpeas in this meatless adaptation. For best results, choose thin-skinned red potatoes for a handsome stew.

Serve with the traditional condiment of Pickled Red Onions, white or brown rice, avocado, and *tostones* or keep it simple with a pile of steamed kale sprinkled with lime juice.

1½ pounds red- or yellow-skinned
    waxy potatoes
1 cup dried TVP chunks or Soy Curls
2 tablespoons peanut or olive oil
4 cloves garlic, peeled and minced
1 large (about ½ pound) onion, diced
1 red bell pepper, seeded and diced
¼ cup white wine or beer
2 teaspoons dried oregano
1½ teaspoons ground cumin
1 teaspoon ground paprika
1 teaspoon Annatto-Infused Oil (page 31)
2½ cups vegetable broth
½ cup creamy natural peanut butter
2/3 cup crushed tomatoes with juices,
    or 3 fresh plum tomatoes, seeded and
    chopped finely
½ cup unsweetened soy milk, almond milk,
    or other unsweetened nondairy milk
2 tablespoons lime juice
1 teaspoon salt, or to taste
Freshly ground pepper
½ cup finely chopped fresh cilantro

Optional Garnishes
  Pickled Red Onions (page 43)
  Slices of avocado and/or tomato
  Your favorite hot sauce (Ecuadorean
    sauces are a fine choice here)
  1 cup of hot steamed white or brown rice
    per serving
  Freshly steamed torn kale

1. Scrub the potatoes and remove any buds or eyes. Without peeling, slice the potatoes into ½-inch pieces and place in a bowl of cold water to prevent browning (drain the water just before using). Place the TVP in a small bowl and cover with boiling water. Soak for 5 minutes, then drain.

2. In a heavy-bottomed soup pot, heat the oil and garlic over medium heat. Fry until the garlic just starts to sizzle, about 30 seconds. Add the chopped onions and red pepper and fry until soft, at least 12 minutes. Deglaze the pan with wine and add the oregano, ground cumin, paprika, and annatto oil. Cook for 2 minutes, then add the drained potatoes, TVP, and vegetable broth. Increase the heat to medium-high and bring the mixture to a boil, then lower the heat to low, partially cover the pot, and simmer for 20 to 25 minutes, stirring occasionally, until the potatoes are tender.

3. Ladle about ½ cup of the hot broth into a small bowl. Add the peanut butter to the bowl and stir to emulsify the peanut butter to a creamy, smooth mixture, adding more broth if

necessary. Spoon this mixture back into the pot. Add the crushed tomatoes, nondairy milk, lime juice, and salt to the stew, and stir. Taste and adjust the flavor with more lime juice or salt, if necessary. Turn off the heat, season the *guatita* with freshly ground pepper, cover the pot, and allow the stew to sit for 15 minutes before serving.

4. To serve: Mound 1 cup of hot rice per person in a large, wide serving bowl, ladle the stew around the rice, and sprinkle with chopped cilantro. Serve with a generous side of Pickled Red Onions and generous shakes of your favorite hot sauce.

Variations

Replace the TVP with 2 to 3 cups any steamed seitan or purchased seitan, sliced into ½-inch cubes.

Replace the TVP with 3 or 4 cups of cooked chickpeas; use more for a heartier stew. If using canned chickpeas, rinse well and drain before using.

RICE WITH PIGEON PEAS (ARROZ CON GANDULES)

- Serves 6 generously
- Time: 45 to 55 minutes, not including making the *sofrito*
- Gluten Free, Soy Free

Puerto Rican rice and beans can be a meal unto itself. This recipe includes three variations to suit every demanding vegan palate: traditional white rice, brown rice for the healthy minded, or a "deluxe" *habichuelas* version loaded with pumpkin, capers, and more for a rich and festive dish. Serve Arroz con Gandules with hot sauce and a simple salad or steamed green veggie for a hearty meal. A side of hot, crisp *tostones* (page 118) makes this a proper Puerto Rican repast.

Look for pigeon peas (*gandules*) where Latin groceries are carried. I like frozen *gandules* the best for their excellent flavor and zero added salt; don't thaw them first, just add the frozen peas directly to the rice when directed. Canned *gandules* work, too; as with any canned bean, rinse first to remove the excess sodium. Or, if you really love *gandules*, experiment with cooking your own from scratch with dried beans (see page 83).

Tip: When preparing large amounts of complex rice dishes (ones that contain large amounts of moist ingredients), I prefer to bake the rice in the oven instead of on the stovetop. I highly recommend it if you're new to cooking rice. I also think baking rice works better than rice cookers for elaborate Latin-style rice. Baking the rice prevents accidental burning and encourages more even cooking. Especially if you are attempting the brown rice or *habichuelas* version, baking will prevent things from getting mushy and give you fluffy, perfect rice every time!

Note: If you're using precooked Basic Sofrito, you're halfway there already! If you don't want to be bothered, you can substitute 1 green bell pepper, 1 large yellow onion, 2 cloves of garlic, all chopped finely and sautéed in 3 tablespoons of olive oil until very soft, at least 20 minutes.

2 cups uncooked long-grain white rice
2 cups frozen *gandules* (pigeon peas), or 1 (15-ounce) can, drained and rinsed
2 bay leaves
3 cups boiling water or vegetable broth
1 cup Basic Onion-Pepper Sofrito (page 32), the tomato or cilantro variation
1 cup diced canned tomato, drained of juices, or 1/2 pound fresh tomato, diced
1 tablespoon tomato paste
2 tablespoons Annatto-Infused Oil (page 31)
2 teaspoons salt (omit if using salted vegetable broth)
1 1/2 teaspoons ground cumin
1 teaspoon dried oregano
1 teaspoon liquid smoke
1/2 teaspoon freshly ground pepper
1/2 cup finely chopped fresh cilantro

1. Preheat the oven to 350°F. Have ready a lasagne-type baking pan that measures about 14 by 17 inches by at least 4 inches deep. Pour the rice, *gandules*, and bay leaves into the pan. Pour the boiling water over the rice, then stir in the sofrito, tomato, tomato paste, oil, salt, cumin, oregano, liquid smoke, and freshly ground pepper. Stir well to combine all of the ingredients, then cover the pan with aluminum foil as follows: Tear off two or three sheets of foil, each longer than the pan by at least 4 inches. Overlap the sheets and tightly crimp the edges to secure a tight fit over the pan. Bake for 40 to 45 minutes, or until all of the liquid is absorbed by the rice.

2. Remove from the oven, let sit covered for 15 minutes, sprinkle with chopped cilantro, then fluff the rice with a fork to redistribute the peas and seasonings evenly. Remove the bay leaf. Serve with hot sauce, slices of avocado, and fried or baked plantains, if desired.

Variations
In place of white rice, use 2 cups of uncooked long-grain brown rice and increase the total amount of liquid to 4 cups of boiling water or broth. Increase the cooking time to 55 to 65 minutes.

Arroz con Gandules easily gets dressed up for parties, holidays or just big family dinners with a few tasty add-ins! Prepare as directed, up until you're ready to cover the pan with the foil. Before doing that, stir in the following:

1/3 cup capers, drained
1/2 cup sliced green olives or sliced green olives stuffed with pimientos, drained
1 (6-ounce) jar pimientos, drained and

diced (you may skip these if you're
using green olives stuffed with
pimientos)

1/2 pound calabaza pumpkin or winter
squash, seeded, peeled, and cut into
1-inch cubes

1/4 pound of commercially prepared
smoked tofu or vegan chorizo sausage,
1/2 recipe Latin Baked Tofu (page 103),
or one to two loaves of Steamed Red or
White Seitan, sliced into 1/2-inch cubes

1. Cover the pan tightly with foil and bake as directed. Fluff the rice to evenly distribute everything. Serve with *tostones* (page 118).

SPICY TORTILLA CASSEROLE WITH ROASTED POBLANOS

....

- Serves 6, or 4 to 5 generously
- Time: About 1 1/2 hours
- Gluten Free

....

This saucy, spicy casserole with an all-natural "cheezy" topping is like a deconstructed chiles rellenos meets lazy, no-roll enchiladas with a lasagne-vibe. Either way, it's a treat for a weeknight meal or a filling brunch. The poblanos and the serranos/jalapeños can build up the spice level substantially, so trust your gut (and tongue) as to how many chiles you want to add.

Slightly stale tortillas (store-bought or homemade) are ideal here as they hold their shape and texture better than fresh ones. This recipe is perfect after a weeklong bout of taco-making leaves you with plenty of extra tortillas to use up.

Make-ahead Tip: Roast the poblanos and boil the potatoes the day before. You can even make the Pine Nut Crema and tomato sauce up to 3 days in advance and store them tightly covered in the fridge. If you're making this for a brunch, it becomes a snap to assemble all of the precooked ingredients an hour before serving, making it easy enough for you to roll out of bed and look like a genius to your sleepy-eyed brunchers.

1 1/2 pounds white potatoes, peeled

1 pound poblano chiles
(about 4 large chiles)

1 small white onion, minced

1 (28-ounce) can diced tomatoes

2 to 3 serrano or jalapeño chiles,
stemmed, seeded (if less heat is
desired), and chopped

2 cloves garlic, chopped

1 teaspoon ground cumin

1 teaspoon dried Mexican oregano

1/2 teaspoon salt

2 tablespoons peanut oil

1 cup vegetable broth

1 pound corn tortillas, preferably a few
days old (14 to 16 tortillas)

1 recipe Pine Nut Crema (page 45)

2 tablespoons pumpkin seeds
(pepitas) or pine nuts

Chopped fresh cilantro and thinly sliced onions and lime wedges, for garnish

1. Roughly chop the potatoes, place them in a large saucepan, and fill with enough cold water to cover. Bring to a boil over high heat, partially cover, and cook for 14 to 16 minutes, or until tender. Drain and set aside. When the potatoes are cool enough to handle, press into large crumbles.

2. Meanwhile, over a gas burner, roast each whole, intact poblano chile. Use metal tongs to turn the chile several times over the flame until its skin is blackened, sizzling, and blistered, 3 to 5 minutes. Place the roasted chile into a tightly covered container or a sealed paper bag. Repeat with the remaining chiles. Alternatively, you can roast all the chiles on a rimmed baking sheet at 450°F for 15 to 20 minutes, or until their skin is blackened and the chiles have collapsed. Allow the chiles to cool enough to be handled. Gently remove their skin, split open, cut away the stem and seed base, and remove any excess seeds. Chop the chiles into 1/2-inch strips and set aside.

3. Make the tomato sauce: In a blender jar, pulse together the onion, diced tomatoes with their juice, chopped serrano chiles, garlic, cumin, oregano, and salt, to blend an almost smooth salsa (some fine chunks are okay). In a large saucepan, heat the oil over medium heat and carefully pour in the salsa. It may splatter a little but that's all right, just keep stirring. In-

crease the heat and bring the mixture to a boil, lower the heat, and simmer for 10 minutes. Stir in the vegetable broth and simmer for an additional 5 minutes. While the sauce is simmering, preheat the oven to 375°F and have ready a 13 by 9 by 2-inch pan and a sheet of foil large enough to tightly cover the pan.

4. Assemble the casserole: Pour 1/2 cup of the sauce into the bottom of the pan and tilt it to spread it around. Using tongs, dip a tortilla into the pot of sauce and place it on the bottom of the pan. Continue with five more tortillas, dipping them in the sauce and overlapping them, spreading their edges a little up the sides of the pan. Top with about half the crumbled potatoes and sliced poblanos, then ladle another 1/2 cup of sauce on top. Dip another tortilla in the sauce, layer it on top of potatoes, and continue as before with five more tortillas. Finally, sprinkle the remaining potatoes and poblano strips on top. Tear any remaining tortillas into thick strips, dip them into the sauce, and spread them on top of the casserole. Pour any remaining sauce evenly over the casserole and cover with the foil, crimping the edges tightly. Bake for 20 minutes. Remove from the oven and take off the foil. Increase the oven temperature to 400°F.

5. Spread dollops of the Pine Nut Crema over the top of the steaming hot casserole. You don't have to be even about it; a few bits of the casserole showing underneath are fine. Sprinkle the pumpkin seeds over the *crema*. Return

the pan to the oven and bake for 20 minutes, until the top of the *crema* is golden and the seeds are toasted. If desired, broil the casserole for 4 to 5 minutes to continue browning spots of the *crema*, but watch carefully as not to burn the seeds.

6. Serve the casserole hot, sprinkled with cilantro and onions. Pass around lime wedges for squeezing on top of each serving. This casserole heats up well the next day in the microwave.

CREAMY CORN-CRUSTED TEMPEH POT-PIE (PASTEL DE CHOCLO)

● Serves 4 to 6

Oye shepherd's pie fans! This twist on the Chilean comfort food *pastel de choclo* (literally, "corn pie") bears a striking similarity to your favorite deep-dish pie. The meatless *pastel* is a savory tempeh stew flecked with that superbly Spanish tag team of raisins and green olives, but the top "crust," a delicate corn pudding–style topping spiked with fresh basil, steals the show. *Pastel de choclo* is often made in deep individual serving bowls but works just as well in any large casserole dish, preferably glass or ceramic.

Tip: Use fresh corn from the cob (white corn, if possible) for making the topping, for best flavor and firmest texture. If that's not an option, use frozen corn. To get rid of frozen corn's excess water, thaw it in a colander over the sink to drain completely.

Filling
- 8 ounces tempeh, sliced into ½-inch cubes
- 2 tablespoons peanut oil or olive oil
- 2 medium-size yellow onions (½ pound), chopped finely
- 1 large carrot, diced
- 2 tablespoons white or red wine or vegetable broth
- 1 teaspoon ground cumin
- 1½ teaspoons dried oregano
- 1 teaspoon ground sweet paprika
- ½ pound potato or yuca, peeled, cooked, and diced into ¼-inch cubes
- 1 cup vegetable broth
- 2 tablespoons soy sauce
- ¼ cup dark raisins
- ½ cup sliced green olives
- Freshly ground pepper

Corn Topping
- 3½ cups fresh or frozen corn kernels (thawed and drained, if frozen)
- 3 tablespoons cornstarch
- ⅔ cup soy creamer or heavy cream substitute, or a combination of the two
- 1 clove garlic, chopped
- ½ teaspoon salt
- Freshly ground pepper

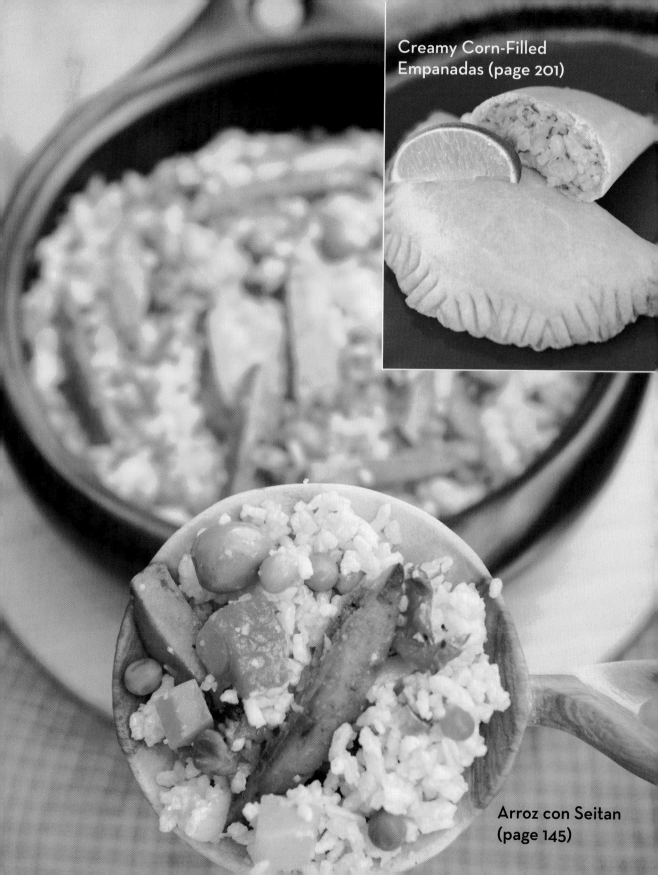

Creamy Corn-Filled
Empanadas (page 201)

Arroz con Seitan
(page 145)

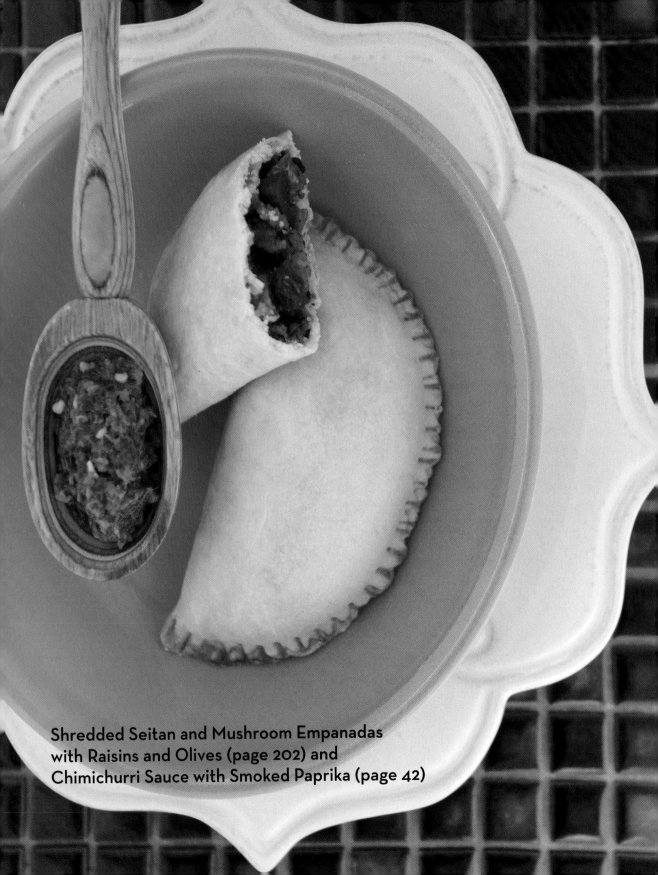

Shredded Seitan and Mushroom Empanadas
with Raisins and Olives (page 202) and
Chimichurri Sauce with Smoked Paprika (page 42)

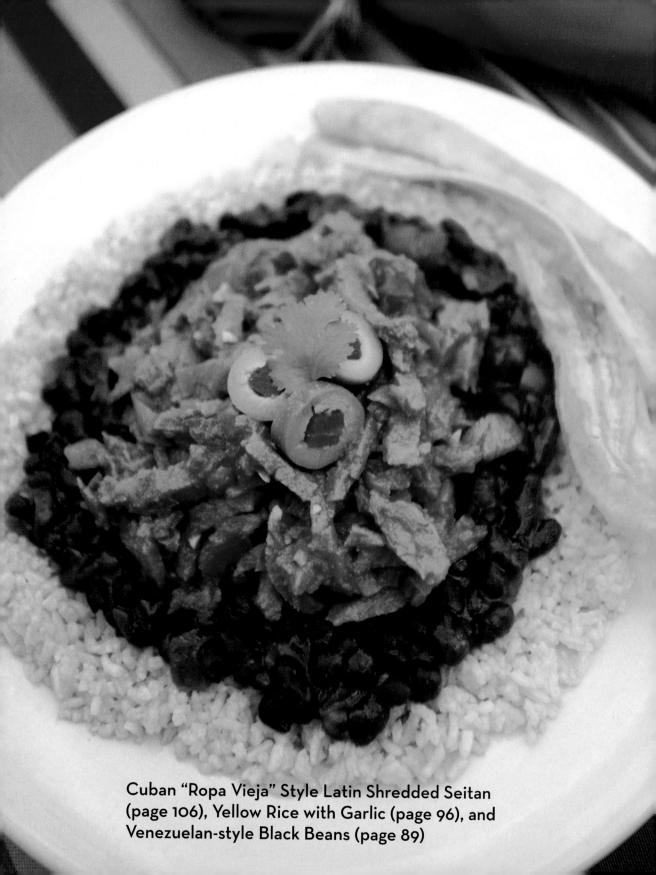

Cuban "Ropa Vieja" Style Latin Shredded Seitan
(page 106), Yellow Rice with Garlic (page 96), and
Venezuelan-style Black Beans (page 89)

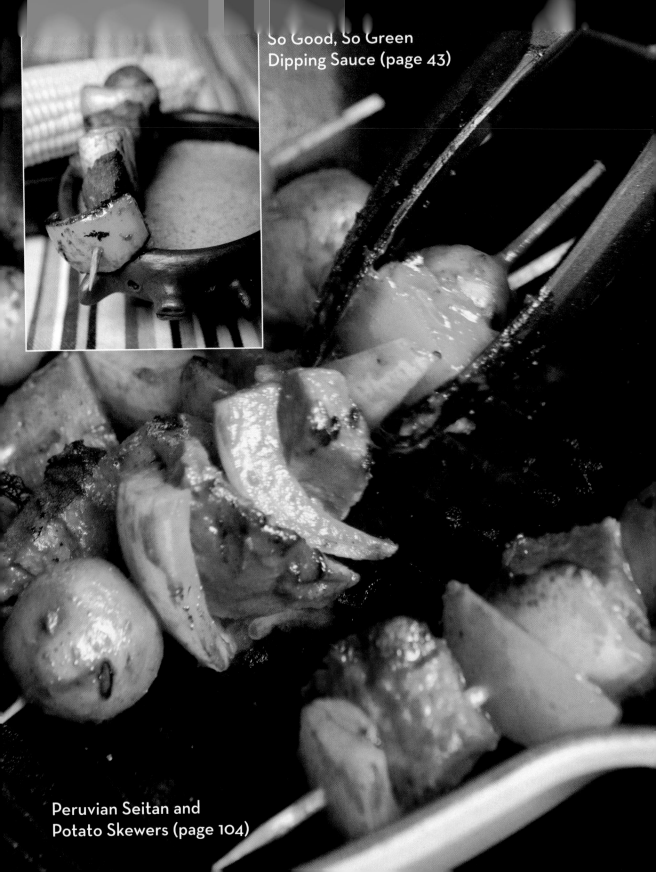

So Good, So Green
Dipping Sauce (page 43)

Peruvian Seitan and
Potato Skewers (page 104)

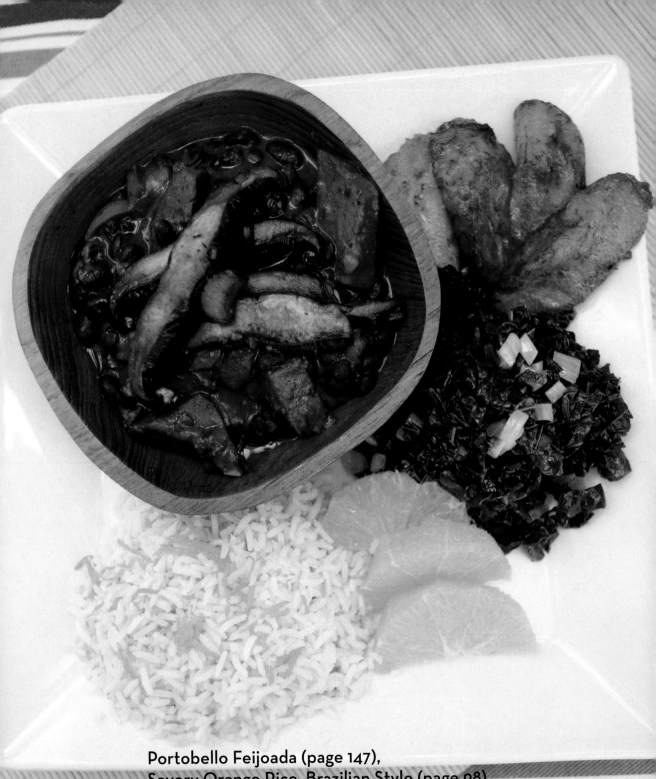

Portobello Feijoada (page 147),
Savory Orange Rice, Brazilian Style (page 98),
Braised Brazilian Shredded Kale (page 121), and
Fried Sweet Plantains (page 115)

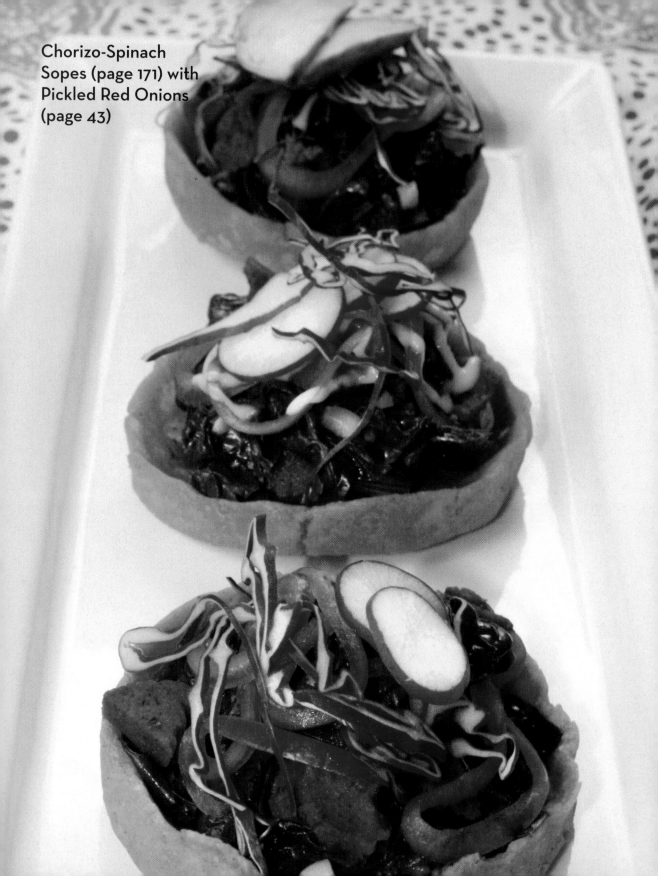

Chorizo-Spinach
Sopes (page 171) with
Pickled Red Onions
(page 43)

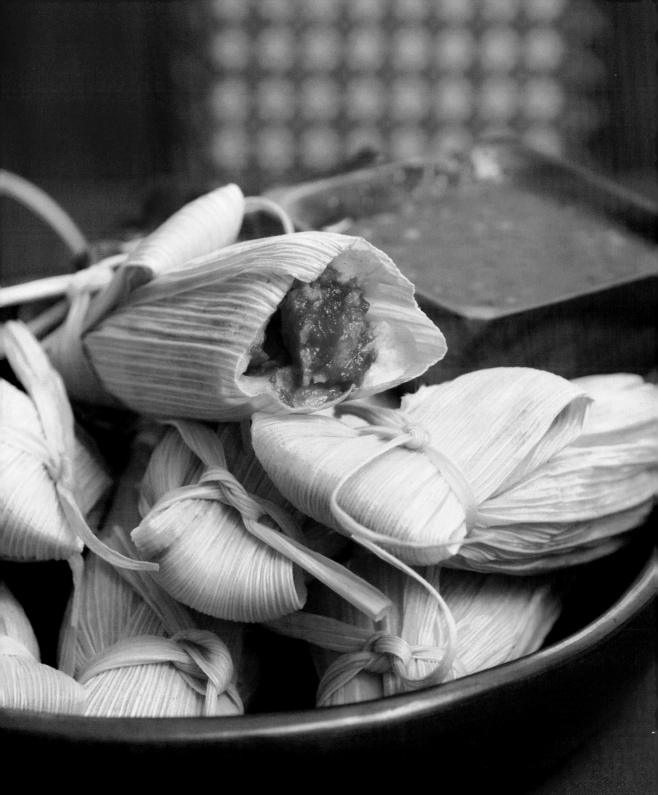

Red Chile–Seitan Tamales
(page 191)

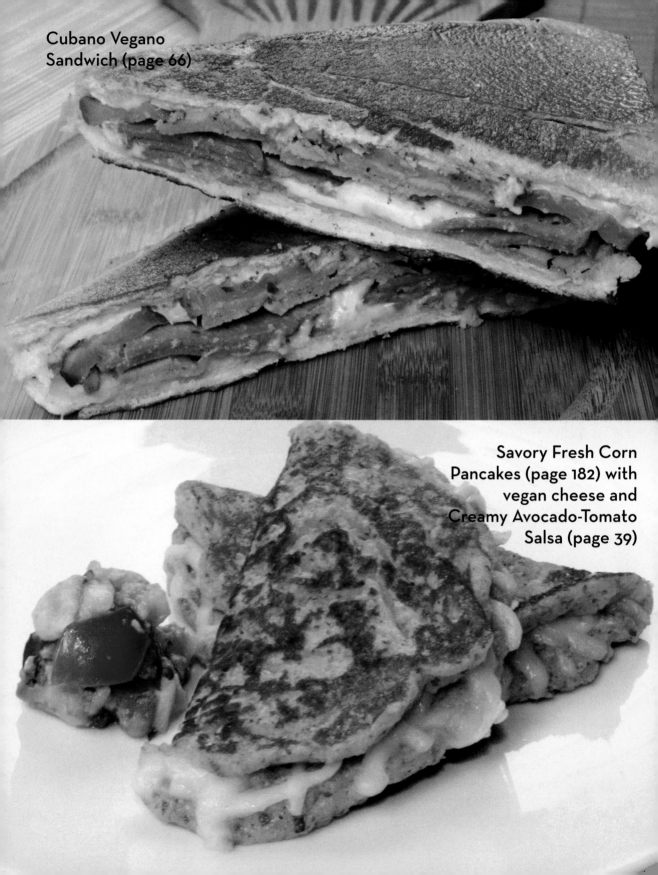

Cubano Vegano
Sandwich (page 66)

Savory Fresh Corn
Pancakes (page 182) with
vegan cheese and
Creamy Avocado-Tomato
Salsa (page 39)

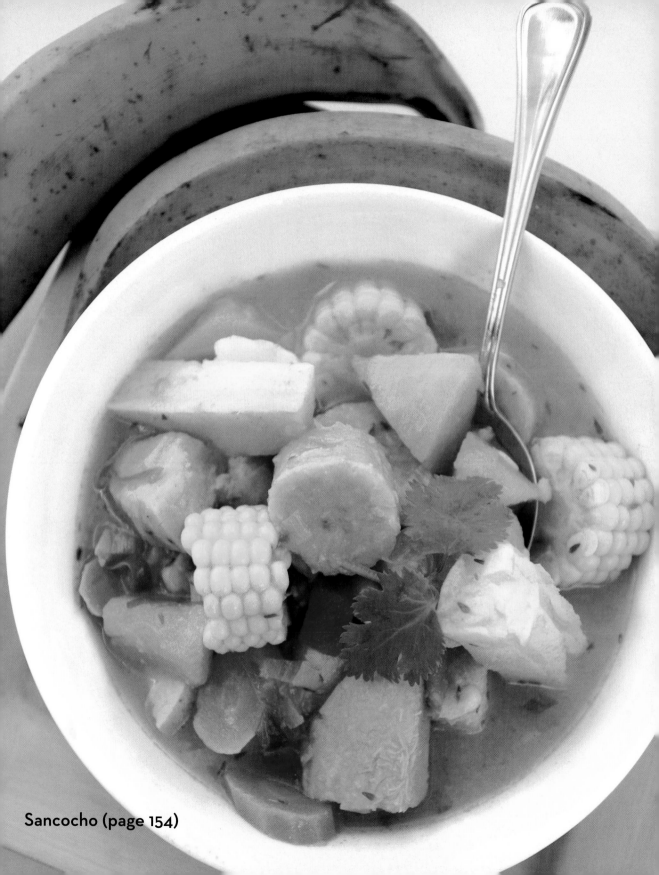

Sancocho (page 154)

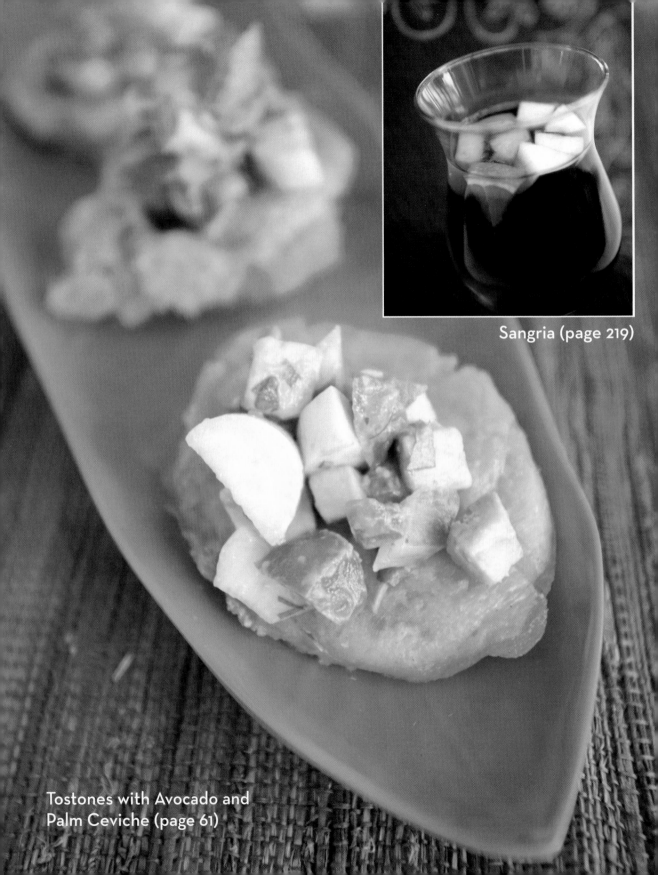

Sangria (page 219)

Tostones with Avocado and
Palm Ceviche (page 61)

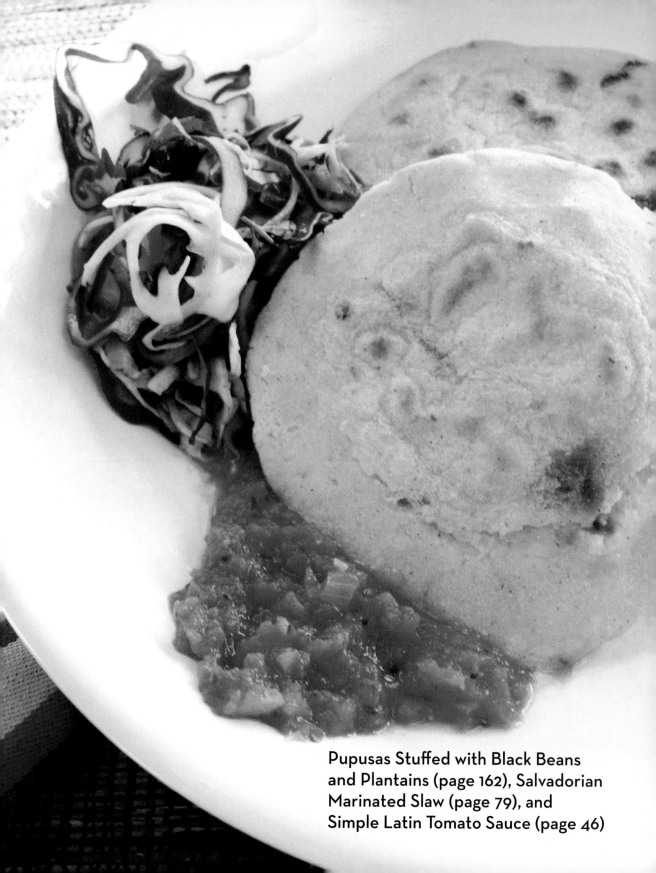

Pupusas Stuffed with Black Beans and Plantains (page 162), Salvadorian Marinated Slaw (page 79), and Simple Latin Tomato Sauce (page 46)

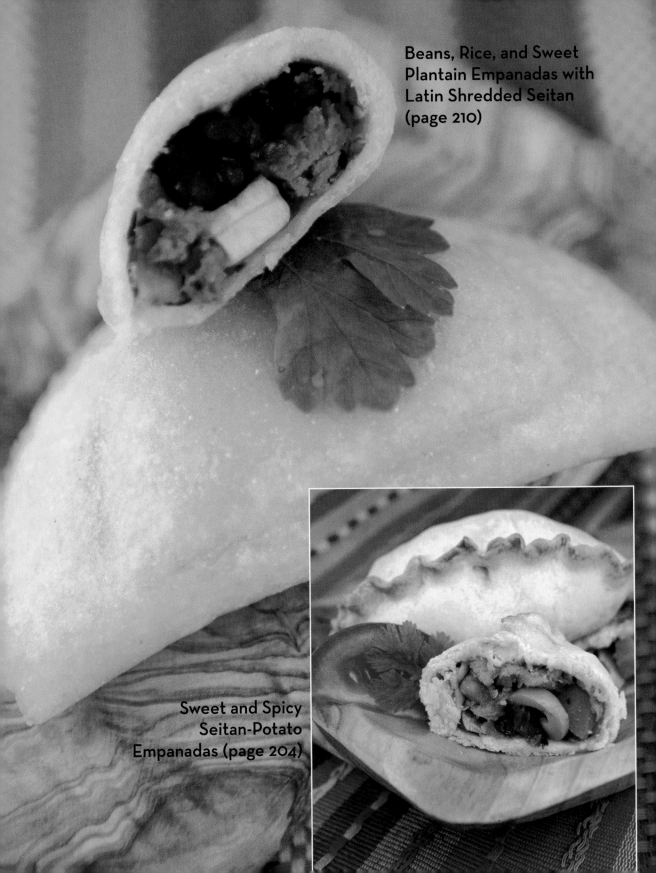

Beans, Rice, and Sweet Plantain Empanadas with Latin Shredded Seitan (page 210)

Sweet and Spicy Seitan-Potato Empanadas (page 204)

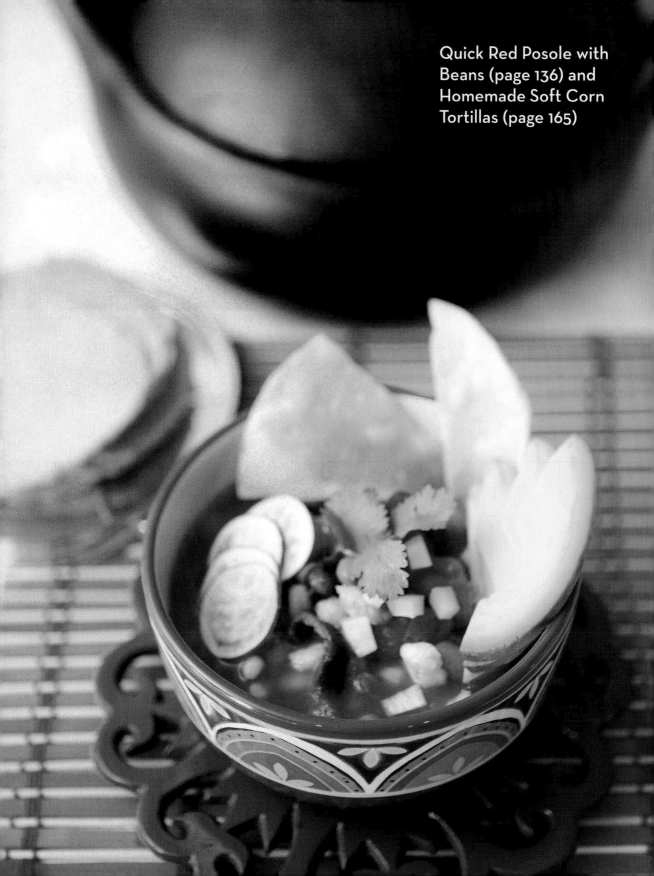

Quick Red Posole with Beans (page 136) and Homemade Soft Corn Tortillas (page 165)

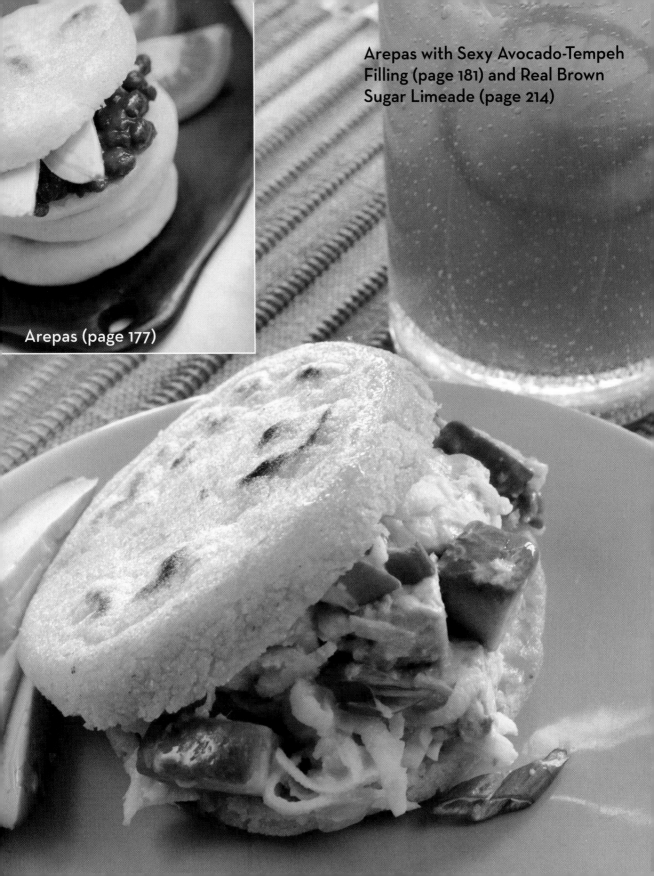

Arepas with Sexy Avocado-Tempeh Filling (page 181) and Real Brown Sugar Limeade (page 214)

Arepas (page 177)

Churros (page 223) and
Chocolate para Churros
(page 225)

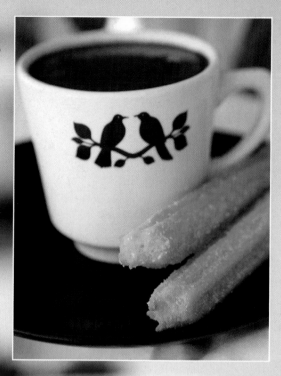

Coconut Tres Leches Cake
(page 230)

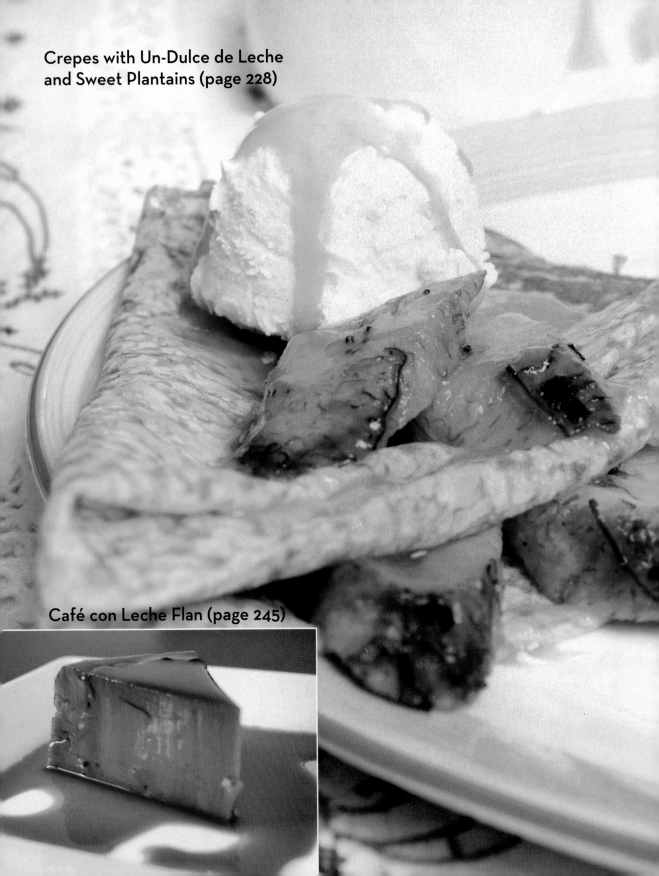

Crepes with Un-Dulce de Leche
and Sweet Plantains (page 228)

Café con Leche Flan (page 245)

3 tablespoons peanut oil

8 to 10 large fresh basil leaves, chopped finely

1 tablespoon sugar, or about 1 teaspoon of sugar per individual pie

1. Cook the tempeh for 10 minutes, either by steaming in a steamer basket or microwaving for 8 minutes in a covered glass bowl with 1 cup of water. Drain the cooked tempeh if necessary and crumble when cool enough to handle. Lightly oil a glass or ceramic 11 by 7-inch baking dish that measures at least 3 inches deep, or use four 2-cup ovenproof individual ceramic casserole dishes.

2. In a large skillet over medium heat, heat the oil, add the onions and carrot, and sauté for 10 to 12 minutes, or until the onions are very soft and translucent. Add the wine, stir, and bring to a simmer. Add the cumin, oregano, and paprika and stir. Add the crumbled tempeh, potato, vegetable broth, soy sauce, raisins, olives, and a few twists of freshly ground pepper. Simmer the mixture for 5 minutes, stirring occasionally. Taste and adjust the seasonings with more ground pepper as desired. Remove from the heat and ladle into the prepared casserole dish(es).

3. Preheat the oven to 400°F and make the corn topping. In a blender jar, pulse the corn kernels, cornstarch, soy creamer, garlic, salt, and pepper until thick and creamy. In a large saucepan, heat the oil over medium heat, then pour in the corn mixture, stirring occasionally with a silicone spatula or a wooden spoon, until the mixture thickens to the consistency of thick cooked oatmeal. Remove from the heat, stir in the basil, and spread evenly over the filling. Sprinkle the top of the pie(s) evenly with the sugar.

4. Place a baking sheet with a rim under the pie in case the filling bubbles over the edges of dish. Bake for 45 minutes, or until the corn topping is golden and the filling is bubbling. If desired, broil on high for an additional 3 to 4 minutes, to create dark brown spots on the corn topping, to give your *pastel de choclo* a much-desired, traditional well-browned look. Let the pie(s) cool for at least 15 minutes before serving; the filling and topping will be very hot!

Variation

For a soy-free variation, replace the tempeh with 4 cups of cooked chickpeas, chopped coarsely.

ARROZ CON SEITAN

Serves 4 to 6 generously
Time: About 1½ hours

A veggie tribute to the enduring Hispanic dish (*arroz con pollo*) that lets the chicken cross the road for yet another day. Steamed White Seitan (page 35) or purchased seitan is lightly browned and cradled in lively yellow rice pilaf. Beer adds depth and richness to this dish but it's not essential; veggie broth will do the job just as well. Serve with a green or cabbage salad.

Tip: If you think you can cheat and use Basic Onion-Pepper Sofrito (page 32) to start this recipe, then you are *correcto*! Substitute half of the Basic Onion-Pepper Sofrito recipe (about 1 cup) for the garlic, onion, and bell pepper.

Seitan

- 1/2 recipe (two loaves) Steamed White Seitan (page 35), or 12 ounces commercially prepared seitan, sliced into thick strips about 3 or 4 inches long
- 1 tablespoon lime juice
- 2 tablespoons olive oil
- Big pinch dried oregano

Sofrito and Arroz

- 2 tablespoons Annatto-Infused Oil (page 31)
- 1 tablespoon olive oil
- 5 large cloves garlic, minced
- 1/2 pound yellow onion, finely chopped
- 1/2 pound green bell pepper, seeded and finely chopped
- 2/3 cup plain tomato sauce
- 1 cup light-colored Mexican beer or vegetable broth
- 1 1/2 teaspoons dried oregano
- 1 teaspoon ground cumin
- 1 bay leaf
- 1/4 teaspoon salt, or more as desired
- 1 1/2 cups long-grain white rice
- 1 1/4 cups water or vegetable broth or a combination of the two
- 1 cup fresh or frozen small green peas (*petit pois*, small sweet peas are best)
- 1 carrot, peeled and diced small
- 1/2 cup sliced pimiento stuffed green olives
- 1/4 cup capers (optional)
- 1/4 cup finely chopped cilantro
- Freshly ground black pepper

1. Prepare the seared seitan: In a large bowl whisk together lime juice, olive oil, and dried oregano. Add the seitan strips, using tongs to toss and coat them with the marinade. Marinate for 10 minutes, tossing occasionally. Heat a cast-iron skillet or grill pan over medium-high heat and generously coat with cooking spray or brush with peanut oil. Add a layer of marinated seitan strips, taking care not to crowd the pan. Fry seitan on each side for 1 to 2 minutes, flipping once (metal tongs work nicely here). Seitan should be crisp and dark on the edges but still look juicy. Remove from pan and set aside.

2. While preparing the seitan, prepare the sofrito: In a large Dutch oven or enamel-glazed cast-iron pot with a tight-fitting lid, combine Annatto-Infused Oil, olive oil, and garlic over medium heat. Fry until the garlic is fragrant (about 30 seconds). Add the onion and bell pepper and fry uncovered, stirring occasion-

ally, until vegetables are very soft and juicy, about 12 to 14 minutes.

3. Stir in the tomato sauce, beer (or vegetable broth), dried oregano, cumin, and bay leaf and simmer for 4 minutes. Stir in the salt, rice, water or vegetable broth, peas, and carrots; cover the pot, and bring the mixture to a boil. Remove the lid, reduce the heat to a low simmer, and push seared seitan strips down into the rice mixture. Sprinkle sliced olives and capers, if using, over everything, cover the pot, and cook for 30 to 35 minutes or until rice is tender, fluffy, and all of the liquid is absorbed.

4. Remove from heat, keeping the pot covered, and set it aside for 10 minutes to cool slightly. Add chopped cilantro and gently fluff the rice. Sprinkle with freshly ground pepper and serve right away.

PORTOBELLO FEIJOADA (BRAZILIAN BLACK BEAN STEW WITH PORTOBELLO MUSHROOMS)

....

Serves 6 to 8 generously
Time: About 3 hours (not including soaking
   beans), mostly simmering on stove

....

Feijoada is a very rich black bean stew much beloved in Brazil. Typically this thick concoction is very meaty and is served with a lush spread of fried plantains, sliced fresh oranges, braised kale, *chicharron*, and rice. This veggie incarnation uses large chunks of TVP (Textured Vegetable Protein, but everyone calls it TVP), an old school vegetable protein that expertly soaks up the rich bean broth. Long strips of Portobello mushrooms add variety and are a succulent contrast to the chewy TVP.

A simple way to serve this feijoada is with a side of lightly chopped steamed kale, white rice, and slices of fresh orange. Better yet, serve with Savory Orange Rice, Brazilian Style (page 98). Feijoada tastes even better the day after it's made.

Tip: Substitute 2 cups of diced red or white seitan for the dry TVP chunks. Do not presoak; just add to the stew along with the mushrooms.

2 cups dried black beans, sorted
1 teaspoon salt
2 bay leaves
1 generous cup large chunk TVP
2 cups boiling water
1/4 cup olive oil
4 cloves garlic, peeled and chopped
1 pound yellow onions, finely diced
1/3 cup red wine, light-colored Mexican
   beer, or vegetable broth
1/2 pound Portobello mushrooms, stems
   removed, caps sliced into 1/2-inch strips
1 teaspoon liquid smoke
1 1/2 teaspoons cumin
1 teaspoon dried thyme

1/2 teaspoon crushed red pepper flakes (optional)
2 cups vegetable broth
Salt and freshly ground pepper

1. Place black beans in a large glass or plastic bowl. Cover with 4 inches of fresh cold water and soak for 8 hours or overnight until beans have doubled in size. Drain beans and briefly rinse. Place beans in a 4-quart soup pot and add 5 cups of cold water, salt, and bay leaves. Bring to a boil over high heat, reduce to simmer, and cook for 2 to 2 1/2 hours or until beans are tender. Remove bay leaves from beans and discard.

2. While the beans are cooking, prepare the TVP and the sofrito: In a glass or metal mixing bowl combine the TVP and boiling water. Let TVP soak for 15 minutes; as it absorbs the boiling water it will double in size. When the TVP is cool enough to touch, drain it, gently squeeze out the excess liquid, and set aside. Combine the olive oil and garlic in a heavy 4-quart stainless steel or enamel-glazed pot. Fry the garlic over medium heat until it starts to sizzle and becomes fragrant, about 30 seconds. Add the diced onion and fry, stirring occasionally until the onion is translucent and tender, about 6 to 8 minutes. Add the wine (or beer or broth) and bring the mixture to a simmer, stirring to deglaze the pot. Stir in the mushrooms; liquid smoke; ground cumin; dried thyme; red pepper flakes, if using; and drained TVP chunks, and simmer for 10 minutes.

3. From the pot of black beans, scoop out 2 cups of beans and bean broth. Puree the beans with an immersion blender or a blender jar and set aside. Add the remaining beans and the rest of the bean broth to the simmering stew. Stir in the vegetable broth, then the pureed beans. Partially cover and bring feijoada to a rapid simmer, stirring occasionally. Cook feijoada until it reaches a chunky consistency but still has plenty of thick sauce, about 30 to 40 minutes. Season with salt and lots of freshly ground black pepper as desired. Remove from heat and let feijoada sit for 15 minutes to cool slightly and for the flavors to develop.

4. Serve feijoada in large but shallow bowls. Place a cup of rice on one side of the bowl and ladle the stew around the rice. Add some chopped, steamed kale (or Braised Brazilian Shredded Kale, page 121) and garnish with a few orange slices. Warm Tofu Chicharrones (page 101) make a great addition here, too; sprinkle a few on the stew and serve.

9

SUPER FANTÁSTICO
LATIN SOUPS!

Soup is serious food all over Latin America, often eaten as a whole meal instead of just an appetizer or first course. That's why Latin soups are so incredibly badass to behold. Flavorful broth bathes bold chunks of corn on the cob, vegetables, or even plantains. Thick stews are lavishly garnished with sliced avocados, crisp raw vegetables, or nuts. These soups are designed with maximum satisfaction in mind.

Vegetables are not commonly served as side dishes in Latin cuisine, perhaps because veggies are preoccupied with spending quality time in so many wonderful soups and stews. You are likely to get almost all of the daily vegetables you need with an average (and big) bowl of Latin soup. Sturdy ingredients such as potatoes, beans, and quinoa play an enormous role in making soup that really does eat like a meal. Vegan versions of these soups are then a natural extension, so don't delay if you need some real food today!

CREAMY POTATO SOUP WITH AVOCADO (LOCRO)

- Serves 4 to 6
- Time: About 45 minutes
- Gluten Free

Soothing potato soups are welcome anywhere there is cool weather and this Andean delight will feel familiar to even those way up north. Golden-hued *locros* have roots that stretch back to the ancient Incas, so you know they've got to be good. Of course, dozens of regional variations exist. This animal-free recipe has a garnish of ripe avocado that provides the perfect complement to the silky soup. The heavy cream substitute or nondairy milk is entirely optional but adds a sublime finish.

Tip: If serving four people, prepare two avocados for topping; for three or fewer people, just one avocado.

4 cloves garlic, minced

2 tablespoons peanut oil

1 large (about 1 pound) sweet white onion,
diced

2 tablespoons Annatto-Infused Oil
(page 31)

3 tablespoons white cooking wine or
vegetable broth

1/2 teaspoon ground cumin

2 1/2 pounds waxy potatoes, peeled and
diced into 1/2-inch cubes

4 cups water or vegetable broth, or a
combination of both

1/3 cup unsweetened heavy cream
substitute or nondairy milk

Salt and pepper

Garnishes

1/2 cup finely chopped fresh cilantro

1/2 cup minced red onion

2 tablespoons lime juice

2 ripe avocados, peeled, pitted,
and diced

1. In a large heavy pot over medium heat, combine the garlic, peanut oil, onion, and Annatto-Infused Oil. Fry until the onion is soft and transparent, 8 to 10 minutes. Add the white wine and deglaze the bottom of the pot, then stir in the ground cumin, potatoes, and water. Increase the heat to high and bring to a boil, stir, then cover and lower the heat to low. Simmer until the potatoes are tender and easily mash when pressed with a wooden spoon, about 30 minutes, and turn off the heat.

2. Remove about 1 1/2 cups of soup and puree, then stir back into the rest of the soup (blend more for a creamier soup, but leave a little bit of soup unblended for some texture). Stir in the cream substitute and season with salt and pepper to taste. Ladle the hot soup into large serving bowls.

3. For the garnish, toss together the cilantro, red onion, and lime juice. Sprinkle on top of each serving of soup, then top with the diced avocado and serve immediately.

CUBAN BLACK BEAN SOUP

- Serves 6 or more
- Time: 2 1/2 to 3 hours, most of that being inactive while the soup simmers. Does not include bean overnight soak time.

This delicious, classic Cuban soup features antioxidant-loaded black beans. This soup is practically a meal—serve on a mound of hot white rice in the center each serving, for just that.

Most preparations of this soup are robust but not exactly spicy. Knowing that many folks crave the spice, I've included a Caribbean-style variation with habanero pepper, to suit anyone looking for flavorful additional heat.

Tip: Shortcut this recipe by substituting 1/2 recipe of Basic Onion-Pepper Sofrito for the onion and green pepper. Or use the Sofrito con Tomate variation. Heat the *sofrito* in the pot over medium heat, add the garlic and tomatoes, and proceed as directed. If the *sofrito* looks a little dry, add 1 extra tablespoon of olive oil.

1 pound dried black beans

6 cups cold water

1 teaspoon kosher salt or sea salt

2 bay leaves

2 tablespoons olive oil

6 cloves garlic, minced

1/2 pound white onion, chopped finely

1/2 pound green bell pepper, seeded and diced finely

1/2 pound ripe tomatoes, seeded and diced finely, or 1 cup diced canned tomatoes with juice

1/2 cup red wine or vegetable broth

1 1/2 teaspoons dried oregano

1 teaspoon ground cumin

1 teaspoon liquid smoke (optional but yummy)

2 tablespoons red wine vinegar or lime juice

Salt and freshly ground pepper

Garnishes

A generous dollop of Cashew Crema (page 51)

1 tablespoon finely minced sweet white onion

1 tablespoon finely minced cilantro

1 cup hot long-grain white rice per serving

1. Sort through the beans and remove any random particles or broken beans and place in a large bowl. Add cold, fresh water to cover by 4 inches and soak for 8 hours or overnight. After the beans have doubled in size, drain, rinse briefly, and place in a 3-quart soup pot. Add the 6 cups of fresh, cold water, bay leaves, and kosher salt. Partially cover and bring to a rolling boil over high heat. Skim off and discard any foam. Lower the heat to low, stir, and cover. Stirring occasionally, cook for 2 to 2 1/2 hours, or until the beans are very tender. A perfectly cooked bean should mash easily when pressed with your tongue toward the roof of your mouth. You should have about 5 cups of liquid when all is said and done, but feel free to add a little more water or even vegetable broth if necessary (or if you like a thinner soup).

2. While beans are cooking, prepare the *sofrito*. In a large skillet, combine the olive oil and garlic and bring to a sizzle over medium heat, cooking the garlic for 30 seconds. Add the chopped onion, green bell pepper, and tomato. Stirring frequently, cook until the mixture is very soft and liquid has mostly evaporated, about 15 minutes. Add the red wine vinegar, oregano, and cumin, and simmer for 1 minute, stirring constantly. Remove from the heat and set aside.

3. When the beans are completely tender, stir in the cooked *sofrito*, making sure to scrape every bit into the pot. Add the liquid smoke,

stir, and partially cover. Bring to a boil over medium heat, lower the heat to a simmer, and cook for 30 to 35 minutes, until the soup has slightly reduced, then remove the bay leaves and discard. If desired, ladle 2 cups of soup into a blender jar, puree until smooth, and stir back into the soup to create a thicker, smoother consistency. Likewise, you can use your immersion blender directly in the soup and puree as desired. Season the soup with more red wine vinegar if desired and salt and pepper to taste. To serve: Ladle the soup into individual bowls, swirl with a dollop of Cashew Crema, and sprinkle with minced onion and cilantro. Serve with the hot rice.

Variations

As with many Latin bean dishes, you can also reduce the total amount of liquid used, so it's less soupy and more suitable as an entrée. Skip pureeing the beans and keep cooking them until they've reached your desired consistency. Serve the beans alongside the hot rice. This soup will continue to thicken as it sits overnight and will also be more flavorful the next day.

Black Bean Soup Habanero: This is a typical technique of using habanero pepper in soup. You'll likely only need one pepper per soup; because habanero pepper can very in size, experiment with smaller peppers for less of a punch. Take a whole unsliced habanero pepper and gently poke a few tiny holes along its sides with the tip of a very sharp knife. The larger the holes, the hotter your soup will become, so poke lightly! Add the pepper to the soup after it's reached a boil (after the *sofrito* has been added), and simmer as directed. Remove the pepper prior to seasoning with the vinegar and salt and pepper. The longer you leave the pepper in, the hotter the soup will become. Discard the pepper when you're done.

HEARTY PUMPKIN AND CRANBERRY BEAN STEW (POROTOS GRANADOS)

- Serves 6 or more generously
- Time: 2½ to 3 hours, most of that being inactive while the soup simmers. Does not include bean overnight soak time.
- Gluten Free, Soy Free

An earthy Chilean soup that often is accidentally vegan! Smooth, chestnut-flavored cranberry beans (called *porotos* in Chile) make sweet soupy music simmered with pumpkin and corn. The result is a soup that maybe won't win beauty contests but it's another hardworking, belly-filling Latin soup that soothes whether eaten out of a thermos at your office desk or on an Andean mountainside. There seems to be some dispute as to whether tomatoes belong, but they're included here because tomatoes make everything better.

Tip: I use an old trick to help break down the beans faster. A tiny pinch of baking soda added to the cooking beans hastens the breakdown of the beans' cell walls, resulting in a softer, creamier texture that mimics long hours over the fire. My mom usually adds this to her beans but I do this only occasionally, as apparently baking soda may destroy some of the B vitamins present in the beans. If you're eating plenty of veggies and whole grains daily then you can flirt with the occasional baking soda bean.

1 pound dried cranberry beans,
    Roman beans, navy beans, or any small
    white bean
6 cups cold water, plus 2 cups water or
    vegetable broth
2 bay leaves
A pinch of baking soda (less than
    1/8 teaspoon)
2 tablespoons peanut, olive, or
    vegetable oil
1 large (1/2 pound) yellow onion,
    chopped finely
1 hot green chile, seeded and minced
    (optional)
3 teaspoons sweet ground paprika
2 teaspoons dried oregano
1 teaspoon ground cumin
1 teaspoon dried basil
3 plum tomatoes (about 1/2 pound),
    seeded and diced
1 pound calabaza pumpkin, peeled,
    seeded, and diced into 1/2-inch cubes

2 cups fresh or frozen corn kernels
    (thawed and drained, if frozen)
1 1/2 teaspoons salt, or to taste
1/4 cup fresh basil leaves, rinsed and
    lightly packed

1. Sort through the beans and remove any random particles or broken beans and place in a large bowl. Add cold, fresh water to cover by 4 inches and soak for 8 hours or overnight. Drain, rinse, and place in a 3-quart soup pot. Add the 6 cups of fresh, cold water, bay leaves, and the pinch of baking soda. Partially cover the pot and bring to a rolling boil over high heat. Skim and discard any foam. Reduce the heat to low, stir, and cover the pot. Stirring occasionally, cook for 1 1/2 to 2 hours, or until the beans are very tender. A perfectly cooked bean should mash easily when pressed with your tongue toward the roof of your mouth. You should have about 5 cups of liquid when all is said and done, but feel free to add a little more water or even vegetable broth if necessary (or if you like a thinner soup).

2. While the beans are cooking, in a nonstick large skillet, heat the oil over medium heat, add the minced onions and chile pepper, and stir. Cook for 10 minutes, or until the onions are soft and transparent. Sprinkle in the paprika, oregano, cumin, and dried basil, stir, cook for 30 seconds, and turn off heat. When beans are completely tender, add the onion mixture, making sure to scrape every bit into the pot. Then stir in the additional 2 cups of water, diced tomatoes, and diced pumpkin.

3. Puree the corn kernels to a chunky consistency with a blender or immersion blender and stir into the stew. Bring the stew to a boil again over high heat, stir, and lower heat to a low simmer. Cook for 30 to 40 minutes, until the pumpkin is very soft and easily mashes if pressed against the side of the pot with a wooden spoon. If desired, create a creamier consistency by mashing more beans and pumpkin this way, or scoop out a few cups of soup, puree until smooth, and stir into soup.

4. Allow the soup to cool for 15 minutes before ladling into individual serving bowls. To use fresh basil for garnish, layer a few leaves on top of one another, roll into a tight cylinder, and slice thinly to create thin shreds. Sprinkle a few on top of the soup or even stir directly into the soup. Like all bean soups, this soup becomes more thickened and flavorful the next day.

SANCOCHO (VEGETABLE, ROOTS, AND PLANTAIN SOUP)

- Serves at least 6
- Time: About 1 hour, most of that being inactive while the soup simmers

Sancocho is a big, comforting soup that features delectable chunks of vegetables, root vegetables, and yuca—long simmered until the broth is gently thickened and rendered sweet and mild. Whole pieces of corn on the cob make this soup visually interesting and fun to eat. A little hot white rice on the side is just the thing, if you're in need of something extra.

There's room for variation when using potatoes, green plantains, or other Latin root vegetables such as *ñame* (pronounced nyah-meh) or anything that falls under the huge category of "yam" (*yautia* in Spanish). In New York City, these tropical root vegetables can often be found in even the most humble supermarket for prices that rival that of potatoes, making it easy to experiment and try something new.

Tip: For a boost of protein, I like to toss in 1 to 2 cups of reconstituted TVP or sautéed seitan. Or frozen green fava beans (not traditional, but this large, meaty bean goes great with the hearty veggies) or even chickpeas.

2 tablespoons olive oil or peanut oil

2 tablespoons Annatto-Infused Oil (page 31)

1 hot chile or habanero pepper (optional)

1 large leek, well washed, trimmed, and
　sliced into thin rings

4 shallots, sliced into thin rings

1 large red onion, sliced in half and cut into
　1/4-inch semicircles

6 green onions, white part separated
　from green, both parts chopped into
　1/4-inch slices

2 teaspoons dried oregano

1 teaspoon ground cumin

1/2 pound yuca, peeled and sliced into
　1-inch rounds, then into quarters

1 large carrot, sliced into very thin rounds, about 1/8 inch

1 pound calabaza pumpkin, peeled, seeded, and cut into 1-inch cubes

1/2 pound tropical tuber, such as *ñame* or waxy or green plantains, peeled and sliced into 1/2-inch rounds

2 tomatoes, seeded and diced, or 1/2 cup crushed tomatoes

2 ears of corn on the cob, cut into 2-inch pieces (a total of 8 to 10 pieces)

6 cups well-seasoned vegetable broth or bouillon

6 sprigs fresh thyme

2 bay leaves

1 to 2 cups reconstituted TVP, sautéed seitan, or frozen fava beans, lima beans, or chickpeas (optional)

3 tablespoons lime juice

Salt and freshly ground pepper

1 cup coarsely chopped cilantro

1. In a large soup pot, heat the olive oil, Annatto-Infused Oil, chile pepper, leek, shallots, onions, and white part of the green onions over medium-high heat (set aside green parts for later). Stirring, cook until the onions and leek are tender, about 6 minutes. Add the oregano, cumin, carrots, yuca, pumpkin, tubers, tomatoes, corn, vegetable broth, thyme, and bay leaves. If using fava beans or TVP, add here as well. Cover and bring to a boil, then lower the heat and bring the soup to a simmer.

2. Cook for 35 to 40 minutes, stirring occasionally, until the root vegetables and pumpkin are very tender. Turn off the heat and season the soup with lime juice, salt, and pepper to taste. Stir in the cilantro and reserved green part of the green onions before serving. Include a chunk of corn cob in each bowl of soup; to eat it, just scoop it up with your spoon, grab, and eat!

SWEET POTATO–CHIPOTLE BISQUE

- Serves 4 to 5
- Time: About 45 minutes, most of that being inactive while the potatoes cook
- Gluten Free

Chipotles and sweet potatoes deserve to be one of those cutting-edge flavor combos in the future. You'll be able to say, "I was there," as you sip this sophisticated "Nuevo Latino"–style, creamy dairy-free bisque. For best color and flavor, use common orange-fleshed sweet potato. Serve with warm tortillas or your favorite American-style corn bread.

Tip: The heavy cream substitute can be your choice of unflavored soy creamer, nut-based nondairy cream (such as Mimic-Creme), coconut milk, or even just your favorite rich nondairy milk. Each one of these choices will yield a slightly different taste but delicious results.

2 tablespoons olive or peanut oil

3 cloves garlic, minced

1/2 pound yellow onion, diced

1/2 teaspoon ground cumin

1/2 teaspoon dried oregano or epazote, crumbled

4 cups water or vegetable broth, or a combination of both

1/2 pound white waxy potatoes, scrubbed, peeled, and diced into 1-inch chunks

1 1/2 pounds sweet potatoes, scrubbed, peeled, and diced into 1-inch chunks

1 or more canned chipotles in adobo, sliced open and seeded, plus 1 to 2 tablespoons of the sauce

1/4 cup heavy cream substitute

1 tablespoon lime juice

Salt and freshly ground pepper

1/2 cup finely chopped fresh cilantro

Cashew Crema, for garnish (page 51) (optional)

1. Combine the oil and garlic in a large soup pot over medium heat, stirring occasionally, until the garlic starts to sizzle, about 30 seconds. Add the onion and sauté until tender and translucent, about 8 minutes. Stir in the cumin and oregano. Pour in the water and add the chopped potatoes and sweet potatoes. Partially cover and bring to a rolling boil over high heat. Lower the heat to a simmer and cook for 25 to 30 minutes, or until both the white and sweet potatoes easily mash when pressed against the side of the pot with a wooden spoon. Remove from the heat.

2. With an immersion blender, carefully puree the soup until it is very smooth and silky. If you prefer to use a blender, make sure to let the soup cool slightly first. Add the chipotle and adobo sauce and puree until completely incorporated; if you're unsure about how much heat you prefer, start with just 1 chipotle and a drizzle of sauce. The soup should now have pretty little red flecks of chipotle. Return the soup to the pot, bring to a simmer over low heat, and stir in the cream substitute, lime juice, salt, and pepper. Taste and adjust with more lime juice, salt, and pepper if desired. Stir in the cilantro, garnish with a swirl of Cashew Crema, if desired, and serve hot.

QUINOA-CORN "CHOWDER" WITH LIMAS AND AJÍ

- Serves 6
- Time: About 1 hour, most of that being inactive while the soup simmers

Make this filling soup when summer sweet corn is at its peak and your thoughts drift to chowder. Quinoa is often used to boost nutrition and flavor in soups in South America, particularly in regions around Bolivia, Ecuador, and Peru.

Top with avocados and roasted peanuts and you'll have a full meal, so do it right and serve in large, deep bowls. Choose your *ají* for different results: amarillo makes a golden soup with moderate fruity heat; panca imparts mild yet smoky, berrylike flavors; rocoto paste will make this soup very hot, so go easy until desired fire is achieved.

2 tablespoons peanut, corn, or other vegetable oil

2 cloves garlic, minced

1 large yellow onion, diced

1/2 cup uncooked quinoa, rinsed and drained (red quinoa looks great here)

2 tablespoons *ají* paste, such as amarillo, panca, or rocoto

11/2 teaspoons dried oregano

11/2 teaspoons dried basil

1 teaspoon ground cumin

1/2 teaspoon ground sweet paprika

1/2 pound waxy red potatoes, cleaned and diced small

3 cups fresh or frozen corn kernels (thawed and drained, if frozen)

One (14-ounce) can white lima beans (also called butter beans), drained and rinsed, or 2 cups cooked beans

4 cups water or vegetable broth, or a combination of both

2 plum tomatoes, seeded and diced small

1/3 cup heavy cream substitute or unsweetened nondairy milk

1 tablespoon red wine vinegar

3/4 teaspoon salt, or to taste

Freshly ground pepper

Garnishes

1/2 cup finely chopped fresh cilantro or parsley, or shredded basil

Chopped ripe avocado

Roasted chopped peanuts

Diced red onion or green onion

1. In a large soup pot, combine the oil and minced garlic over medium heat. Cook the garlic until fragrant, about 30 seconds, add the onion, and fry until the onion is softened and translucent, 6 to 8 minutes. Add the quinoa and stir occasionally, toasting the quinoa for 3 to 4 minutes, or until just starting to turn golden. Add the *ají* paste, oregano, basil, cumin, and paprika and fry for 1 to 2 minutes, or until fragrant. Now stir in the potatoes, corn, limas, and water. Increase the heat and bring the mixture to a gentle boil. Lower the heat to medium-low, cover, and simmer, stirring occasionally, for 30 to 40 minutes, or until the potatoes are very tender and the quinoa is tender and translucent. Stir in the tomatoes, cream substitute, vinegar, and salt, partially cover, and simmer for another 10 minutes, stirring occasionally. This soup should be thick, but if it appears too thick, stir in 1/2 cup to a full cup of water or broth along with the cream substitute, until the desired consistency is reached. Remove from the heat and season with ground pepper to taste.

2. Cover the soup and let it rest for about 15 minutes prior to serving, to allow it to cool slightly and for the flavors to meld. Ladle into deep serving bowls and top with chopped cilantro, avocado, peanuts, and onions as desired. Like any hearty soup, this tastes even better the next day; just store in tightly covered containers (without the toppings) in the refrigerator.

TROPICAL PUMPKIN SOUP

- Serves 4
- Time: 45 minutes
- Soy Free (if a nonsoy cream substitute used)

North Americans have a love affair with pumpkin that's only expressed in the fall months, but in Latin American it's a year-long romance. Tropical pumpkins look and taste a little different than the pumpkin pie–type pumpkins. Calabaza pumpkin is a Latin variety commonly found in markets in the United States. It's a huge winter squash that's often sold precut into smaller chunks, making it convenient for making soup or adding fresh pumpkin into recipes at a whim.

The first time I had this soup at fourteen years old, I was mesmerized by how my aunt transformed *auyama* (Venezuelan pumpkin) into a creamy soup with just three ingredients: squash, potato, and stock. Since then I've added a few more ingredients with a Caribbean flair. Try it with coconut oil at least once; I guarantee you'll love it. Just about any orange-flesh winter squash can also be substituted for the calabaza, too.

2 tablespoons unrefined (virgin) coconut oil or vegetable oil
1 large leek, well washed, ends trimmed, and chopped
1/2 teaspoon ground cumin
2 tablespoons white cooking wine or water
4 cups vegetable broth
11/2 pounds calabaza pumpkin, peeled, seeded, and chopped into 1-inch pieces
1/2 pound waxy white potatoes, peeled and chopped coarsely
2 sprigs fresh thyme, or 1 teaspoon dried
1 tablespoon lime juice
1/3 cup heavy cream substitute or coconut milk (optional, for extra supercreamy soup)
Salt and pepper
2 tablespoons finely chopped fresh cilantro
1 tablespoon finely chopped fresh mint

1. In a large soup pot over medium-high heat, add coconut oil and leek and fry until the leek is soft, about 6 minutes, stirring occasionally. Add the cumin and wine and simmer for about a minute, stirring occasionally. Pour in the vegetable broth and add the pumpkin, potatoes, and thyme. Cover and bring the soup to a boil over medium heat, then lower the heat to low and simmer the soup for 20 to 25 minutes, or until the pumpkin and potatoes are very tender and mash easily with the back of a wooden spoon.

2. Remove the thyme sprigs, if using. Use an immersion blender to puree the soup to a silky-smooth consistency. If you want to use a blender, allow soup to cool for at least 15 minutes, puree, then return to the soup pot. Season the soup with lime juice, heavy cream substitute (if using),

salt, and pepper and over low heat warm the soup as desired. Ladle the soup into serving bowls, sprinkle each serving with chopped cilantro and chopped mint, and serve immediately.

Make-ahead Tip: Make the entire soup up to two days in advance, minus the cilantro-mint topping. Make that just before heating and serving the soup.

POTATO-KALE SOUP WITH SIZZLING CHORIZO

- Serves 6
- Time: About 45 minutes

Potatoes and hearty greens always go great together as in this Brazilian-inspired soup by way of Portugal (*caldo verde*). The contrast of red or yellow potato skins and brilliant greens makes this a handsome soup, too. Topped with sizzling hot sautéed Seitan Chorizo Sausages (page 36), it gets ridiculously good. Considering how hearty this soup tastes, it's also pretty healthy. Skip the modest drizzle of olive oil (or just use less) and fry the chunks of chorizo with some nonstick cooking spray, for a nearly fat-free but satisfying soup.

2 pounds red or yellow waxy potatoes
1 large yellow onion (about 1 pound), diced
6 cloves garlic, chopped coarsely
1 teaspoon dried thyme
1 teaspoon dried oregano
6 cups water or vegetable broth, or a combination of both
1/2 pound kale, thick stems removed, chopped into bite-size pieces
2 tablespoons olive oil
1 1/2 teaspoons salt, or to taste
Freshly ground pepper
White wine vinegar

Fried Chorizo Topping
3 tablespoons Annatto-Infused Oil (page 31)
3 links of Seitan Chorizo Sausages (page 36)

1. Clean and remove any eyes or skin discoloration from the potatoes, then chop into bite-size chunks. In a large soup pot, combine the potatoes, onions, garlic, thyme, oregano, and water. Cover the pot and bring to a boil over high heat, then lower the heat to low. Simmer for 25 to 30 minutes, until the potatoes are extremely tender and easy to mash when pressed with a spoon.

2. Turn off the heat and use a potato masher or a wooden spoon to break up and lightly mash the potato chunks; leave some chunks intact. Turn on the heat to medium again. Stir a handful of kale into the soup at a time, allowing it to wilt, until all of the kale has been incorporated into the soup. Stir and cook until the kale is tender but still bright green, about 5 minutes.

Add the olive oil and season with salt, pepper, and a few dashes of white wine vinegar to taste. Turn off the heat, cover, and let the soup sit for 15 minutes prior to serving, to allow the flavors to meld.

3. While the soup is resting, heat the Annatto-Infused Oil in a small skillet over medium heat. Slice the Seitan Chorizo links in half lengthwise, then chop each piece into bite-size pieces. Sauté the chorizo until hot and lightly browned, about 5 minutes. Ladle the soup into large soup bowls. Top each serving of soup with pieces of hot chorizo and a drizzle of a little bit of the annatto oil. Serve the soup with hot sauce and crusty bread, if desired.

Variation
Try subbing your favorite dark leafy green for the kale. Chard or collards work beautifully in this soup, too. Or try mustard greens, for a uniquely piquant soup.

● ● ●

FOR THE LOVE OF CORN: AREPAS, PUPUSAS, TORTILLAS, AND MORE

*M*aybe the words in this chapter sound like names you should have remembered from your Early American history books. Be relieved that *arepas* and *pupusas* are memorable and filling foods that you'll look forward to working into your regular recipe rotation. But you're right on the history part. Whenever you're enjoying one of these dishes, you're eating a truly Old World food that is as terrific and enjoyable now as it was to ancient folks in Central and South America thousands of years ago. Latin Americans really know how to eat their native corn: roasted, grilled, fried, or in soups, as well as grinding it for a flour. This chapter contains a sampling of two of my favorite ways to enjoy specially prepared corn flours of Central America and South America.

Arepas are a very thick tortilla or can also be a fat little cake made from a differ-

ent style of masa harina (more about that in the Pantry section, page 13) than what is used in Central America. They are usually only eaten in Colombia and Venezuela, with slight variations between regions. *Arepas* feature a crisp and chewy outer crust with a dense and moist interior and are sometimes sliced and stuffed to the gills with fillings, to form a hefty sandwich.

Pupusas are a wonderful Central American treat with roots deep in Salvadorian culture. Using Mexican-style masa, the dough is stuffed and patted into a thick tortilla, grilled, and served with a light tomato sauce and a generous helping of the cool, crunchy marinated slaw *curdito*. Personally, they've become something of an obsession, and since each *pupusa* needs only a few tablespoons of filling, it's fun to experiment with leftovers for unique *pupusas* every time you make them.

Last but never least are a few other essentials. Homemade corn (and whole wheat, too) tortillas are a revelation if you've never bothered with them: just a few minutes of your time and any meal can be pumped up with soft, fresh tortillas. *Sopes* are adorable tortilla coasters built for heaping on the toppings. And *cachapas* are not to be missed by fresh corn fans! Tasty, sweet, fresh corn pancakes are a rockin' way to enjoy summer corn at the height of the season.

PUPUSAS STUFFED WITH BLACK BEANS AND PLANTAINS

- Makes eight 5- to 6-inch *pupusas*, serves 4 generously
- Time: About 45 minutes, not including making the *curdito* or tomato sauce
- Gluten Free, Soy Free

Pupusas are fat, stuffed, grilled tortillas with a cute name that hail from El Salvador. The fun of *pupusas* is in the combination of hot grilled masa harina, tasty fillings, tangy tomato sauce, and cool Salvadorian-style coleslaw known as *curdito*. *Pupusa* cravings are likely to strike once you get in the habit of making these!

Tip: Shaping *pupusas* (as with tortillas, arepas, and handmade flatbreads), takes practice. The perfectly formed *pupusa* should be thicker in the center and tapered at the edges, with no holes or cracks to expose the filling. No matter what shape your *pupusas* may be, they will still be tasty, so don't despair if they're not perfect looking. Keep *pupusas* on the small side, about 5 inches or less in diameter, for easy shaping and cooking.

Make-ahead Tips: Up to two days ahead, prepare the tomato sauce and fillings. To shorten your filling preparation time, use leftover beans (refried is fine) and fried plantains. Use 2 tablespoons total of leftover beans, veggies, tofu, seitan, or faux cheese per *pupusa*.

The night before, prepare the *curdito* and let it marinate in the fridge. When it's time to eat, heat the sauce, fluff the chilled slaw, and serve immediately with the hot *pupusas*.

Filling

2 cloves garlic, chopped

1 tablespoon olive oil

1 fresh green chile (mild or hot, your choice), seeded and diced

1 cup cooked black beans (if using canned, drain and rinse)

1/4 cup water

1/2 teaspoon ground cumin

1/2 teaspoon dried oregano

Salt and pepper

1 ripe, cooked plantain, baked or fried (see page 117 for how to bake ripe plantains)

1 tablespoon lime juice

1 cup shredded mozzarella-style vegan
cheese (optional)

Masa Dough
2 cups instant Mexican-style masa harina
1³/4 cups or more warm water
¹/4 teaspoon salt

Salvadorian Marinated Slaw (page 79)
Simple Latin Tomato Sauce (page 46)

1. Prepare the filling first: In a heavy skillet, combine the garlic and olive oil and fry over medium heat until sizzling and fragrant, about 30 seconds. Add the chiles, black beans, water, cumin, and oregano, and bring to a simmer. Cook for 6 to 8 minutes, or until the water has been absorbed but the beans are still moist. Turn off the heat, season with salt and pepper, if desired, and let the beans cool enough to be handled. Meanwhile, dice the cooked plantain into ¹/4-inch chunks and toss with the lime juice. Set the fillings (and shredded vegan cheese, if using) aside in small bowls near your work surface.

2. Prepare the masa: In a large bowl, stir together the masa harina, warm water, and salt. The dough should be moist and firm but not too sticky; if too dry, drizzle in a little more warm water; if too wet, sprinkle with a tablespoon or two of additional masa harina. I like my dough to be a little on the moist side, as it may dry somewhat while forming the *pupusas*. Divide the dough into eight equal portions and

roll into balls. Cover with a damp, clean kitchen towel to keep moist while shaping the *pupusas*.

3. To form a *pupusa*, cup a ball of dough in your palm and use the fingers of your other hand to form it into a little bowl, taking care to pat the sides and bottom to more or less the same thickness. It's a little like making those little ashtray pot things out of clay when you were in first grade. You want to create a hole about the size of a large walnut. Firmly press 1¹/2 to 2 tablespoons of filling into the indentation, plus about a heaping tablespoon of beans and a few chunks of plantain. Fold over the sides of your "bowl" on top of the filling and firmly press down.

4. Now comes the shaping part. Moisten your hands a little. With gentle yet firm patting motions, begin pressing your *pupusa* down and out. Use your palms to occasionally flatten the entire *pupusa* a little, then use the pads of your fingers to shape and press outward the edges of your *pupusa*. The traditional way of forming it is to do a little of this motion all at once, while incrementally turning the *pupusa* in your palms a little bit at a time to work on the edges.

5. At this point the *pupusa* masa may crack, or some of the filling may poke out here or there. Two ways remedy this: Moisten up your fingers just a little and smear a bit of dough over the offending crack. Or, locate the former bottom of your masa "pot"; the dough tends to

Pupusa Filling Explosion!

Pupusas are ready and waiting to take on any filling you challenge them with, so let the filling fiesta begin! You don't need a lot; about 1¹/₂ cups of filling total should be plenty for this recipe. Part of the fun of learning to make good *pupusas* is playing with any number of fillings . . . so be sure to have a steady supply of leftovers (and *curdito*) on hand!

Bean and Tofu Chicharrones: Use about half a recipe each of Home-style Refried Beans (page 86) and Tofu Chicharrones (page 101) for a batch of *pupusas*. This is a vegan adaptation of a very popular Salvadorean *pupusa* filling.

Bean and Chorizo: Use equal parts Home-style Refried Beans (page 86) and two links of Seitan Chorizo Sausages (page 36), chopped finely.

Roasted Zucchini and Vegan Cheese: Slice ¹/₂ pound of zucchini or yellow summer squash into ¹/₂-inch-thick pieces, toss with 1 tablespoon of olive oil, and sprinkle with salt and chile powder to taste. Roast at 350°F for 25 to 30 minutes, stirring frequently, until the squash is browned and tender. Stuff each *pupusa* with zucchini and a tablespoon of shredded meltable mozzarella-style vegan cheese.

Zucchini Blossom and Vegan Cheese: A traditional Salvadorian filling is an edible jungle flower called *loroco*. Maybe wild loroco isn't growing in your backyard, but always-abundant zucchini blossoms from the garden are possibly threatening a takeover. Lightly sauté 6 to 8 fresh blossoms with 1 tablespoon of olive oil until wilted and sprinkle with salt to taste; chop into bite-size pieces. Pair up with shredded vegan cheese, as directed for the Roasted Zucchini filling. Also look for canned Mexican-style zucchini blossoms, or if the *pupusa* gods smile upon you, perhaps your local Central American market carries pickled loroco flowers.

Squash and Bean: Steam or bake less than ¹/₂ pound of winter squash (pumpkin, calabaza, butternut, etc.) until tender. Mash and season with salt, cracked pepper, and lime juice. Use equal parts mashed squash and refried beans.

Shredded Seitan and Bean: Use less than half a recipe of Latin Shredded Seitan (page 106, original recipe or Mexican chile) plus refried beans. Good with a bit of vegan cheese, too.

Veggie Suprema: Sauté with 1 tablespoon of olive oil, plus ¹/₃ cup each of two or more of the following: fresh corn kernels, minced red onion, seeded and chopped red bell pepper, seeded and roasted red peppers, green onions, cremini mushrooms, and/or sliced green olives. Add some chopped garlic, too, and a touch of shredded vegan cheese, if you like. Season to taste with salt and lime juice.

Pizza Pupusa: A scandalous untraditional twist. Fill *pupusas* with shredded mozzarella-style vegan cheese, a little bit of store-bought chopped veggie pepperoni, and sliced olives or pepperoncini peppers. Absolutely serve this one with Simple Latin Tomato Sauce seasoned with plenty of dried oregano!

be thicker on this end. Carefully pinch off a small piece of this excess dough and smooth the area you took it from. Use this dough to patch up any cracks. Ultimately, you may still have some thin spots and cracks, but as long as your *pupusa* is holding its shape, no worries. You're on your way to *pupusa* mastery.

6. Cover the shaped *pupusas* with a damp, clean kitchen towel or waxed paper. Lightly oil and heat a cast-iron skillet or heavy-bottomed pan over medium heat. The skillet is ready when a few drops of water sizzle on contact. I like to brush *pupusas* with a little peanut or olive oil right before cooking, for a crisper crust.

7. Grill a few *pupusas* at a time, 4 to 6 minutes, flip, and repeat on the other side. Occasionally press down the center and edges gently with your spatula. Cooked *pupusa* masa should be firm and golden; a few dark spots on the surface is fine, even desirable. If serving all of the *pupusas*, you may want to keep them warm in an oven, wrapped in foil, while preparing the rest.

8. Always serve piping hot *pupusas* with a side of warm Simple Latin Tomato Sauce and a generous heap of Salvadorian Marinated Slaw. Slices of avocado and your favorite hot sauce will just make you even more popular with your new *pupusa* fans.

HOMEMADE SOFT CORN TORTILLAS

- **Makes one dozen 5- to 6-inch tortillas**
- **Time: Less than 15 minutes (if using a tortilla press; a little longer if using a rolling pin)**
- **Gluten Free, Soy Free**

If you can lift a bag of masa harina, you can make homemade corn tortillas and enjoy soft, toasty, corny goodness tonight! Homemade tortillas are best kept simple with basic toppings such as a strip of grilled tempeh or a spoonful of guacamole. Or serve with beans or a hearty Mexican posole. The key is to keep fresh off-the-grill tortillas well covered, to keep them warm and pliable until it's time to eat. This recipe isn't really too different from what's on the bag of masa, but I see it as a way to inspire making homemade tortillas in the event you've never tried!

Tip: An aluminum tortilla press makes tortillas so easy that maybe it's tempting to skip toast at breakfast in favor of these. A quick Internet search can reveal quality tortilla presses for under ten dollars. A rolling pin and some waxed paper are fine substitutes for a press, but once you're hooked on corn tortillas, it's an investment that will pay for itself in endless moments of fresh tortilla joy.

1½ cups Mexican masa harina, such as
   MASECA brand
1¼ cups warm water
½ teaspoon salt

1. In a mixing bowl, combine the harina, water, and salt well to form a firm but pliable dough. If it's too crumbly, stream in a little more water; if too moist, sift in a tiny bit more harina. Knead the dough for 2 to 3 minutes, until smooth. Divide the dough into twelve equal portions and roll into balls. Cover with a damp, clean kitchen towel to keep moist. Heat a cast-iron skillet or griddle (avoid using nonstick) over medium-high heat. Do not oil the skillet. The pan is ready when a few drops of water flicked onto its surface sizzle rapidly.

2. If you're using a tortilla press: Line the press with a single long piece of plastic wrap or waxed paper folded in half. Place a ball of dough in the center of the plastic wrap, squish down the dough, and bring down the lever to lock it in place. Alternatively, if you do not have a press, you can use two pieces of plastic wrap or waxed paper and a rolling pin. Place a ball of tortilla dough between the plastic and roll very thinly, less than ⅛ inch, turning the tortilla around a few times to get an even thickness.

3. Now that your tortilla dough is flat, gently peel off the top layer of plastic. Flip the tortilla onto your hand, remove the second sheet of plastic, and place the tortilla in the pan. Cook on each side for 30 to 40 seconds, or until the surface of tortilla looks dry and feels mostly firm, not too doughy, when pressed. Take care not to overcook, to avoid hard, dry tortillas. Flip the hot, freshly cooked tortilla into a folded clean kitchen towel and cover completely with the towel to keep in the heat and steam. Continue to cook the rest of the dough and to stack and cover the tortillas.

4. Serve the hot tortillas immediately. As the tortillas start to cool, they will stiffen and become more likely to crack if folded, so keep them wrapped in a clean cloth napkin or in a covered container, taking out only as many tortillas as you're going to eat.

5. Store tightly wrapped or covered in the fridge. Tortillas reheat perfectly in a microwave; just wrap in a damp paper towel and heat on high for 15 to 20 seconds, until hot and pliable.

WHOLE WHEAT FLOUR TORTILLAS WITH CHIA

- **Makes eight 7- to 8-inch tortillas**
- **Time: Less that 30 minutes**

Makin' flour tortillas at home is a little more work than mixing up a batch of corn tortillas. Homemade wheat tortillas may not be as uniformly perfect looking as store-bought ones, but their excellent flavor and chewy texture are well worth the effort. These whole-grain tortillas get an extra nutritional boost from nutty little chia seeds (of Chia Pet fame), an ancient food from Central America that's loaded with omega 3s, fiber, protein, and a mild poppy seed–like crunch. My flour of choice is white whole wheat flour, lighter than standard whole wheat flour. Pair fresh tortillas with beans or grilled protein and any salsa.

Leave out the chia seeds, if you wish, and opt for using all-purpose flour if you prefer a traditional wheat tortilla (but you may want to reduce the water initially to ½ cup and add more as needed). For lighter-tasting whole-grain tortillas, use up to half or two-thirds all-purpose flour in place of the whole wheat.

Tip: Not just for growing green hair on weird pottery anymore, chia seeds are definitely a health food store find, but are becoming increasingly available due to their awesome nutritional value.

- **2 cups white whole wheat flour, plus extra flour for rolling**
- **2 tablespoons chia seeds**
- **½ rounded teaspoon salt**
- **¼ teaspoon baking powder**
- **¼ cup nonhydrogenated vegetable shortening, at room temperature**
- **2/3 cup warm water**

1. In a large mixing bowl, combine the flour, chia seeds, salt, and baking powder. Stir together with your fingers then, with a pastry cut-ter or fork, cut in the shortening until the flour has a sandy texture. Alternatively, you may use a food processor to blend the flour mixture with the shortening. Pour in the water and stir (fingers are best) to form a stiff dough; knead for about a minute to form a smooth but firm ball. If the dough appears dry, drizzle in a tiny bit of water and knead into the dough.

2. Divide the dough into eight pieces and roll into balls. Cover with a damp, clean kitchen towel and let the dough rest for 10 to 12 minutes. Prepare a work surface for rolling the dough—lightly dust with a little flour and have ready a rolling pin. If desired, you can roll between waxed paper, but I found it works just as well without. In addition, line a large, shallow bowl with a few large, clean kitchen towels for wrapping the hot tortillas (or use a tortilla warmer, page 26).

3. Just before you are ready to make the tortillas, heat a large cast-iron skillet or *comal* (the original tortilla grill, page 27) over medium heat. Take a ball of dough and press it down slightly onto your floured board. Use the rolling pin to roll the ball into a very thin (less than 1/8 inch or thinner) circle 7 to 8 inches in diameter. To help form a nice-looking circle of dough, roll the dough once or twice with long strokes of the rolling pin, then turn the circle around 45 degrees and repeat; continue to rotate and roll to keep the circle from turning lopsided. Flip occasionally to help shape the tortilla. It's okay if it's not perfect . . . each tortilla has its own distinctive personality!

4. Place the rolled dough on the preheated skillet and cook until bubbles start to form and the edges look a little dry, 1 1/2 to 2 minutes. Flip the tortilla with tongs or your fingers (careful!) and grill for another 1 to 1 1/2 minutes; do not overcook or it will get hard and dry, but a few puffy browned spots are fine. Place the hot tortilla in the lined bowl and immediately wrap with kitchen towels. Roll out another tortilla, place on the griddle, and while it's cooking, roll out another one. Cook the remaining dough into tortillas in this way, stacking the hot tortillas on top of one another and making sure to cover tightly with the towels. Serve the hot tortillas immediately or reheat by wrapping in moistened paper towels and microwaving on medium power or by heating on a preheated skillet until soft.

TAQUITOS WITH CHORIZO AND POTATOES

....
● Makes 12 to 14 *taquitos*, serving 4 or 5 as an entrée
....

Here's a recipe for those tasty stuffed tortilla cylinders always a hit on Mexican menus and much requested from my recipe testers. Seitan chorizo and cilantro enliven its classic potato filling. Typically, *taquitos* are deep-fried, but I prefer to strategically pan-fry them (like a spring roll) with less oil. Serve *taquitos* with any salsa, Red Chile Sauce (page 45), and Home-style Refried Beans (page 86) for a fun weeknight dinner or hearty weekend brunch.

Tip: I just insisted you make some homemade corn tortillas, but for best results with *taquitos*, use store-bought tortillas. Being so thin and wide, they roll easily into a *taquito* tube shape.

1 pound potatoes
4 cloves garlic, chopped
1 tablespoon peanut or vegetable oil
1 small yellow onion, diced
2 teaspoons dried Mexican or ordinary oregano
1/2 teaspoon ground cumin
2 links Seitan Chorizo Sausages (page 36), chopped finely
2 tablespoons lime juice
1/2 teaspoon salt, or to taste
Freshly ground black pepper
2 tablespoons finely chopped fresh cilantro
12 to 14 corn tortillas
Vegetable oil, for pan-frying

1. Clean and scrape any eyes or discoloration from skin of the potatoes, then chop into bite-size chunks. In a large soup pot, combine the chopped potatoes and enough cold water to cover by 3 inches. Cover and bring to a boil over high heat, lower the heat to low, and simmer for 25 to 30 minutes, until the potatoes are extremely tender and easy to mash when pressed with a fork. Turn off the heat, reserve about ¼ cup of the potato-cooking liquid, and drain the potatoes.

2. Meanwhile, in a large skillet over medium heat, fry the garlic in the peanut oil until the garlic starts to sizzle, about 30 seconds. Stir in the onion and cook for 6 to 8 minutes, until tender and translucent; stir in the oregano, cumin, and chorizo, and fry for 5 minutes. Add the drained potatoes, lime juice, salt, and ground pepper, and use a potato masher to mash the potatoes with the vegetables and chorizo to completely mix them together. Turn off the heat and stir in 2 tablespoons of the potato-cooking water and the cilantro. Stir the ingredients well and taste the mixture; adjust the seasonings with more lime juice and salt, if necessary. The potatoes should be very firm but a little moist; if too dry, stir in additional potato-cooking water to moisten. Let the potato filling cool just enough to handle but use while still warm.

3. Create a *taquito* assembly line by first heating a corn tortilla, then filling and rolling it, and finally frying it. First, preheat a cast-iron skillet over medium heat. Take a corn tortilla, place it on the heated griddle for 30 seconds, then flip it over and heat until the tortilla is hot, soft, and pliable. It's important to keep the tortillas warm and moist, as they may crack if cooled while rolling the taquitos.

4. To shape a *taquito*, place about 2 heaping tablespoons of filling in a line down the center of the hot tortilla, patting the filling all the way to the edges. Over medium heat, fry the taquito in 2 tablespoons of vegetable oil in a large preheated cast-iron skillet. Place the *taquito* seam side down in the hot pan; it's important to fry the seam side first, as this will help hold the *taquito* together as it cooks. Cook on the seam side for about 2 minutes, or until golden and firm, then gently roll over the *taquito* and cook on the other sides for 1 to 2 minutes each, or until golden. Assemble and repeat with all of the *taquitos*, frying up to four at a time. Add another tablespoon of oil to the pan whenever the *taquitos* need more browning. Transfer the *taquitos* to serving plates and eat immediately or to a pan in a 300ºF oven and keep warm until ready to serve.

Variations

Replace the corn tortillas with flour ones and you have yourself a *flauta*, if that's what you really *quiero*.

Omit the seitan chorizo and substitute 1 cup shredded mozzarella- or Jack-style vegan cheese.

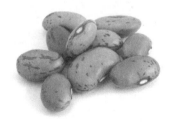

There are no burrito recipes in this book. No, *señor*, not a one. The reason is, if you're looking for a burrito recipe, probably you eat too many anyway! But, seeing that there are some out there who really feel they need a burrito recipe, here's a guide (okay, it's a recipe!) for a deluxe burrito with all the works. For simpler fare, leave out the addition of tofu, seitan, or tempeh or the garnishy vegetables such as the lettuce or onions. For best results make sure your beans, rice, and tofu, seitan, or tempeh are warm prior to filling.

> 1 (8- to 10-inch, or larger) store-bought
>   wheat tortilla (see Tip)
> 1/4 to 1/3 cup any bean recipe or refried beans
> 1/4 to 1/3 cup any rice (Cilantro-Lime Rice [page 95] always works,
>   or just long-grain brown with a twist of lime juice)
> 1/4 to 1/3 cup any tofu, seitan, or grilled tempeh, diced finely
> 2 to 3 tablespoons any salsa (it's fine to use store-bought salsa)
> A handful of shredded cabbage or finely chopped lettuce

Toppings
> Diced avocado
> Tomato
> Thinly sliced onion
> Thinly sliced, pickled jalapeño peppers

1. First reheat the wheat tortillas to soften them. Preheat a cast-iron skillet over medium heat and lay a tortilla in the center of the pan. Heat for 30 to 44 seconds, then flip and heat for another 30 seconds, until the tortilla is soft and flexible. Place the hot tortilla on your work surface.

2. To fill and fold, place your fillings in an oblong mound slightly off-center (a little closer to you than true center) of the tortilla. Don't go too crazy with the total amount of filling as it will be difficult to roll the burrito tightly if it is too full (about a cup of filling is fine for an 8-inch tortilla). Fold the right and left sides of the tortilla toward the filling, covering the filling only partially. Then lift and fold over the edge closest to you, so that it partially covers the filling and overlaps the two previously folded edges. Now, firmly holding the tortilla along its right and left sides to keep those first two flaps folded in, carefully and firmly roll the filling end away from you, toward the last unfolded edge of the tortilla. Roll it tightly, as this will greatly help the burrito to hold together while eating. You should now have a neat little burrito!

3. Add an extra dimension of delicious by grilling this baby burrito. Lay the burrito seam side down onto that skillet you've previously heated and grill for 2 to 3 minutes, until it is nicely toasted and the seam has firmed up. Very carefully turn the burrito onto the other side and

grill until toasted as desired. Every now and then, you might want to press down gently on the burrito with a wide spatula to speed up the toasting process.

Tip: For burritos, use store-bought tortillas over homemade ones, unless you're skilled at rolling them very, very thinly. You'll need the tortilla to be very flexible to fold it right. Also, plenty of interesting varieties are now available, such as spinach, tomato, garlic, and that old workhorse, the whole wheat tortilla. Or even try using tortillas labeled for use with the dreaded "wrap" sandwich and making what they should be called anyway . . . a burrito.

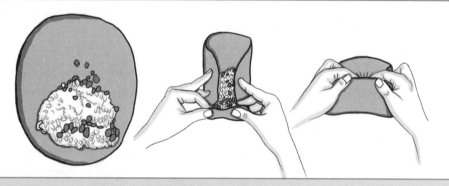

1. Fill only lower third of tortilla
2. Fold tortilla sides, then bottom edge over filling
3. Roll while firmly holding sides of burrito

CHORIZO-SPINACH SOPES

- **Makes 8 *sopes*, 2 per serving**
- **Time: About 45 minutes**

Adorable Mexican *sopes* (SO-pehs) are fat little tortillas with a raised edge, served open faced and designed to hold more of whatever you "smother" them with. Here, we pile them with garlicky sautéed spinach and seitan chorizo, but they could be stacked in-stead with taco fillings such as beans, vegetables, or shredded vegan cheese.

Sopes are made by a two-step process: First, they're cooked like regular tortillas on a dry, hot grill; then they're lightly sautéed, to crisp the edges. Brushing with oil and finishing in the oven is a nice alternative to frying, for a lightly chewy crust. This filling can be made while baking the *sopes*, for a manageable and exciting weeknight dinner.

Sopes

1 recipe of dough from Homemade
  Soft Corn Tortillas (page 165)
Canola or peanut oil, for oven "frying"
  or pan-frying

Chorizo-Spinach Topping

2 tablespoons olive oil
4 cloves garlic, minced
4 links Seitan Chorizo Sausages (page 36),
  diced small
2 bunches fresh spinach (about 2 pounds),
  well washed, thick stems removed,
  chopped coarsely
2 tablespoons lime juice
Salt and freshly ground pepper

Toppings

Cashew Crema (page 51)
Shredded green or red cabbage
Sliced avocado
Sliced radish
Pickled Red Onions (page 43)
Any salsa

1. Preheat a cast-iron skillet over medium heat. If baking the sopes, preheat the oven to 375°F.

2. Make the sopes first: Divide the tortilla dough into eight equal portions and roll into balls. Cover with a damp, clean kitchen towel to keep moist

3. To form a sope: Pat the dough into a circle 1/4 to 3/8 inch thick and about 3 1/2 inches wide.

Now place the thick tortilla in your palm. Using your other hand, pinch it with your finger and thumb to form a small raised ridge around the edge of the tortilla; it should be 1/4 to 3/8 inch high. Your sope will look like a tiny tart. Place the sope flat side down on the preheated skillet and cook for 2 to 3 minutes, until the dough has firmed and the bottom has a few toasted spots. Continue to shape the sopes and place them flat side down onto the skillet.

4. Once the sopes are grilled, you can either bake or fry them. If baking, transfer the hot sopes to a lightly oiled baking sheet and generously brush with oil, making sure to brush the sides and the raised edge. Bake the sopes at 375°F for 12 to 14 minutes, until firm. Keep warm in a 250°F oven until ready to serve, but if the sopes are to remain in the oven for longer than 15 minutes, cover with foil to prevent their drying out. Alternatively, to fry the sopes, pour 1/2 to 3/4 inch of oil into a cast-iron skillet and heat over medium-high heat. The oil is ready when a small piece of dough dropped into the hot oil sizzles immediately and vigorously. Some recipes call for measuring the temperature of the oil at a specific 350°F, but your sopes will be just fine as long as your oil passes the sizzle test. Sauté one or two sopes at a time for 4 to 6 minutes, until their surfaces are golden. Drain on paper towels or crumpled brown paper and keep warm in a 250°F oven until ready to serve.

5. Make the spinach filling while the sopes are cooking: In a large nonstick skillet over

medium heat, heat half the olive oil and fry half of the garlic, stirring, for 30 seconds. Add the diced chorizo and cook, stirring occasionally, for 5 minutes, or until the edges of the chorizo are slightly browned. Remove the chorizo from the pan and add the remaining oil and garlic. When the garlic starts to sizzle, add the spinach by the handful and sauté, stirring occasionally, adding more spinach until all of the spinach has wilted and is tender, 6 to 8 minutes. Sprinkle with lime juice, salt, and pepper to taste.

6. To serve: mound a generous portion of spinach in the center of a *sope*. Top with some of the fried chorizo, then shredded cabbage, avocado, any other goodies, and lastly some Cashew Crema. I like to dilute the *crema* so that it's pourable rather than sour cream–like, but that's up to you. *Sopes* can be messy eating, so it's okay to grab and eat these using both hands!

BLACK-EYED–BUTTERNUT TOSTADAS

- Serves 8 as an appetizer or 4 as a hearty main entrée
- Time: About 45 minutes
- Gluten Free, Soy Free

Tostadas (popular crispy fried tortillas stacked with toppings) can be piled with most anything, such as succulent squash and hearty black-eyed peas. They're ideal for New Year's Day (as a twist on the Amer-

ican Southern tradition of that lucky black-eyed pea meal) but try pintos, black beans, or your favorite bean the during the rest of the year. Ready-to-use tostadas (common in Mexican markets) are convenient, but frying up your own tortillas is a surprisingly snappy and satisfying business.

Serve with Fresh Tomato Salsa (page 50), Classic Roasted Tomatillo or Classic Roasted Tomato Salsa (page 47), or purchase a prepared salsa—a chipotle-based salsa goes especially well with the sweet winter squash.

8 corn tortillas

Peanut or vegetable oil, for shallow frying

1/2 pound butternut squash, peeled, seeded, and diced into 1-inch cubes

4 cloves garlic, chopped

3 tablespoons olive oil

1/2 pound red onion, minced

1 to 2 jalapeño or serrano chiles, seeded and minced

1/2 teaspoon ground cumin

1 (15-ounce) can black-eyed peas, rinsed and drained, or 2 cups cooked

1 large tomato, diced small

Salt and freshly ground pepper

Toppings

2 cups thinly chopped romaine lettuce or thinly shredded cabbage, or a combination of both

1 ripe avocado, peeled, seeded, and sliced thinly

Pickled Red Onions (page 43) or thinly
    sliced rings of fresh red onion
Fresh Tomato Salsa (page 50), Classic
    Roasted Tomatillo Salsa (page 47), or
    any purchased salsa

1. Prepare the tortillas for the tostadas first. Preheat the oven to 300ºF. Heat about 1/2 inch of peanut oil over medium-high heat until a small piece of tortilla immersed in the oil sizzles and browns in less than 30 seconds. Fry one tortilla at a time, flipping once and frying for about 2 minutes on each side. Drain on crumpled brown paper bags or paper towels. Keep warm in a 250ºF oven until ready to serve.

2. Place the squash in a large pot. Cover with cold water and bring to a boil over high heat. Lower the heat and simmer until the squash is tender, 25 to 30 minutes. Drain and lightly mash the squash with a potato masher or large fork; cover and keep warm. In a large skillet over medium heat, fry the garlic in the oil until the garlic starts to sizzle, about 30 seconds. Add the onion and chile pepper and continue to sauté until the onion is soft and translucent, about 2 minutes. Sprinkle in the ground cumin and add the black-eyed peas and tomato, stirring occasionally and frying for 4 minutes. Remove from the heat and mash about one-third of the peas with the back of a spoon. Stir the mashed squash into the pea mixture and stir to combine. Season with salt and pepper and keep the mixture warm until serving time.

3. To assemble the tostadas: Spread about 4 tablespoons of the mixture on a warm, fried tortilla. Top with salsa, lettuce, onions, and avocado.

Homemade Tortilla Chips

If you fried tortillas for those tostadas, you passed the test to make tortilla chips at home. Use a knife or kitchen shears to slice corn tortillas like a pie, for triangles ready for frying. Fry and drain as directed for the tostadas, sprinkle with salt (or chile powder or a sprinkle of lime juice) and serve hot. Store the chips in a folded paper bag (plastic could make them soft) in a cool place. Reheat the chips in a preheated 300ºF oven for 8 to 10 minutes, until crisp and hot. Or get creative and cut the tortillas into long strips or freaky angles, for a classy garnish for any posole stew or salsa!

CHIPOTLE, SEITAN, AND POTATO TACOS

- **Makes about 6 large tacos**
- **Time: About 1 hour, including boiling, filling, and frying everything**

A hodgepodge of a taco—soft, grilled corn tortillas piled high with beer-marinated seitan and roasted potatoes (or sweet potatoes!)—a crazy and luscious mess to eat. But it's not a too-crazy thing to make on a weeknight with premade seitan ready to go or a purchased bag of shredded cabbage. There are several components to this dish, but most are simple and quick enough to prepare while other ingredients are marinating or cooking. Preroasting the potatoes in the oven will have you spending less time standing over the stovetop. You can also easily make the potatoes, Cashew Crema, and marinated seitan a day or two in advance.

Make the tacos with just one tortilla, or make monster-size ones by using two overlapping tortillas. It's helpful to have extra tortillas on hand, just in case!

1½ pounds white or sweet potatoes, scrubbed but unpeeled, diced into ½-inch chunks
3 tablespoons olive oil
Salt
½ recipe (two loaves) Steamed White Seitan (page 35), sliced into ⅛-inch strips no longer than 1 inch

Marinade
¾ cup beer, preferably Mexican
2 cloves garlic
1 to 2 chipotles in adobo, seeded and chopped finely
1 to 2 teaspoons chipotle adobo sauce
1 teaspoon dried oregano
1 teaspoon ground cumin
2 tablespoons lime juice
2 tablespoons olive oil
½ teaspoon salt

Optional Garnishes
Any salsa
Finely shredded cabbage
Chopped fresh cilantro
Chopped onions, thinly sliced radishes, or Pickled Red Onions (page 43)

For Assembly
Cashew Crema (page 51) or your favorite vegan sour cream, thinned with a little lime juice or water
6 corn tortillas, or 12 for double-tortilla extra-large tacos

1. Prepare the potatoes first: Preheat the oven to 400°F. Spread the diced potatoes on a large, rimmed baking sheet, sprinkle with the oil, and toss to completely coat in the oil. Sprinkle with a little bit of salt and roast for 18 to 20 minutes, flipping the potatoes halfway through, until browned and tender. Set aside.

2. While the potatoes are roasting, marinate the seitan. Whisk together all the marinade ingredients in a large bowl. Add the seitan strips, using tongs to coat the slices. Marinate for 15 minutes, stirring the strips occasionally. While all that roasting and marinating action is going on, chop, shred, and arrange for serving the other taco toppings. The shredded cabbage is highly recommended, as it adds wonderful crunch. Chill until ready to use.

3. When the seitan is ready to cook, set aside the marinade. Heat a cast-iron pan or grill pan

over medium-high heat. Generously oil the pan with a cooking oil that has a high smoking point (such as peanut) and place one-quarter of the seitan in the pan (don't crowd). Cook the seitan for 3 to 4 minutes per side, flipping once, until the seitan is browned, crisped on some of the edges, but not overly dry. Stack the seitan on a small plate near the stove to help keep it warm.

4. When the seitan is done, fry a portion of the potatoes at a time. Add a little extra oil to the pan if it seems dry and pour a tablespoon or a little more of the remaining marinade over the potatoes as you're reheating them. Cook the potatoes enough to make them hot but still juicy with the marinade. Repeat with the remaining potatoes, stacking them on the dish with the seitan. Wipe down the cast-iron skillet, oil very lightly if necessary, then place a tortilla on the hot surface. Heat the tortillas just enough to soften and heat them, flipping once, the whole process taking about a minute.

5. To assemble a taco: Place a hot tortilla on a serving dish. (For extra-large tacos, use two tortillas, overlapping them to make one large

 ## Taco Toppings!

Tu casa (a.k.a. your kitchen, the best vegan "taco truck" in town) is a popular place when your friends figure out that your tacos are awesome. Tacos are limitless in what you can top them with, so go with your gut (of course) when it comes to what sounds *delicioso*. Along with your favorite salsa, avocado slices, or guacamole (page 48), try one of the following combos, or a combo of combos, or make up something new!

- Refried pinto beans (page 86) + Salvadorian Marinated Slaw (page 79) + Pickled Red Onions (page 43)
- Chimichurri Baked Tofu (page 100) + refried cannellini beans (page 86) + roasted garlic (rub whole heads of garlic with olive oil and roast until tender)
- Sautéed spinach with raisins and capers (see Swiss Chard recipe, page 123) + Tofu Chicharrones (page 101)
- Sautéed potatoes as above, with beer marinade. Stir in one small jar of drained pickled nopales (Mexican "cactus" paddles, page 125) and fry until hot. Top with Cashew Crema (51), shredded green cabbage, and thinly sliced radishes
- Refried black beans (page 86), fried Chorizo Seitan Sausages (page 36) and shredded crisp Romaine lettuce
- Latin Shredded Seitan, either regular or Mexican chile style (page 106), Salvadorian Marinated Slaw (page 79), chopped pickled jalapeño, and a drizzle of Fresh Gazpacho Salsa Dressing (page 70)
- Tempeh Asado (page 110), shredded green cabbage, sliced radishes, Creamy Ancho Chile Dressing (page 70), and diced ripe tomato, sprinkled with lime juice

tortilla.) Arrange equal parts seitan and potatoes down the center of the tortilla(s). Top with salsa, if using; then shredded cabbage and other veggies, if using; drizzle with Cashew Crema, and finally a few radish slices. Fold up and expect stuff to drip out the other end you're not eating, but no worries since everyone else will be doing the same. It's all *bueno*.

AREPAS (VENEZUELAN- AND COLOMBIAN-STYLE "TORTILLAS")

- Makes 6
- Time: About 40 minutes for Venezuelan arepas, 20 minutes for Colombian
- Gluten Free, Soy Free

Arepas are often described as "corn bread," though, unlike American cornmeal products, they more resemble very thick tortillas with a crunchy-chewy crust and moist interior. They're almost exclusively eaten in Venezuela and Colombia and must be made with the regional *masarepa* precooked corn flour. The best arepas have dark char marks on their crust; the easiest way to get this effect is to first grill the arepas on a cast-iron griddle, for a perfect toasted aroma and texture.

Arepas are served piping hot, usually split and filled with any savory thing your masa-filled heart desires. For luxuriantly stuffed arepas, try the Sexy Avocado-Tempeh Filling (page 181) or Oyster Mushrooms and Pimiento Peppers (page 180).

Tip: The most common brands of Venezuelan or Colombian *masarepa* are Harina PAN, Venezuelana, or Goya. (Many say Harina PAN when referring to this kind of masa in general.) Check the package; if your *masarepa* is either manufactured or imported from Colombia or Venezuela, you're in the clear. Yellow and white Harina PAN can be used interchangeably, as they taste the same. Never substitute Mexican-style masa harina.

2 cups white or yellow Venezuelan- or Colombian-style masa harina flour
1/2 teaspoon salt
2 1/4 cups warm water, or more
A small amount of vegetable oil (use a high-smoking-point oil, such as refined canola), for grilling

1. Preheat a well-seasoned cast-iron griddle or other thick-bottomed skillet over medium high heat. Lightly brush with vegetable oil. If you're making Venezuelan style arepas, also preheat the oven to 350ºF and have ready a baking sheet. The griddle is ready to use when a drop of water dropped onto its surface sizzles loudly.

2. In a large bowl, combine the *masarepa* flour and salt. Form a well in the center of the flour and pour in the warm water. Use your

hands to mix the water into the *masarepa* to form a soft mass, then knead with your fingers, eliminating any lumps and creating a smooth, moist dough. The dough should have the consistency of very firm, moist, and heavy mashed potatoes. If the dough seems too stiff, drizzle in a little extra water.

3. Divide the dough into six equal portions and roll into balls. Place a ball in your palm and, with gentle yet firm patting motions, begin pressing down your arepa. Use your palms to occasionally press the disk just a little flatter, then use your fingers to shape and press the edges outward. Do a little of this motion all at once while incrementally turning the arepa in your palms to work on the edges. Shape each arepa into a disk 3 1/2 to 4 inches wide by 1 1/4 inches thick.

4. Gently place two to three arepas in the preheated, lightly oiled pan, leaving enough room that they can be easily flipped. While the other arepas cook, place the remaining shapely new arepas on a cutting board and cover with either a damp, clean kitchen towel or plastic wrap. Cook each arepa for 8 to 10 minutes on each side to form a crust, flipping just once. Some dark, browned spots are ideal. If desired, try cooking the arepas on a well-greased preheated grill pan, grilling each side for 10 to 12 minutes or until nice browned grill marks are created. Then place the grilled arepas on the baking sheet and bake for another 14 to 16 minutes, flipping halfway through. The arepas are ready when they have a firm crust and sound slightly hollow when tapped underneath.

5. To fill an arepa: Slice horizontally about three-quarters of the way to form a "pocket" not unlike filling a biscuit or pita bread. Add plenty of your desired filling(s) and eat piping hot. Remove a little of the doughy interior if you want to pack in even more filling . . . ridiculously overstuffed arepas are popular in Venezuela and make messy and fun eating.

6. Serve hot arepas immediately or keep warm by loosely wrapping in foil. Arepas should be eaten hot, as they tend to toughen up when they get cool. Reheat arepas by grilling again, or by warming in a microwave for 30 seconds and then slapping on the grill if you want the interior very hot and the crust recrisped.

Variation

Colombian-style Arepas: These are made from the same masa harina but are usually shaped much thinner and considerably wider than the Venezuelan type, yet still considerably thicker than Mexican tortillas. For Colombian-style arepas, shape each ball of dough into a disk, but make it ½ to ⅜ inch thick and 5 to 6 inches wide. Cook as directed, 8 to 10 minutes per side, to develop a firm crust with a few dark spots. There's no need for the second baking step, just eat 'em hot off the griddle, once a nice crust has formed.

Colombian arepas sometimes have extra goodies kneaded into the dough and are eaten as snacks or sometimes made a little smaller to accompany rice, beans, and the works for a hearty meal. For really delicious arepas, make Colombian Grilled Arepas with Corn and Vegan Cheese (below).

COLOMBIAN GRILLED AREPAS WITH CORN AND VEGAN CHEESE

- Makes 6 large, thin arepas
- Time: About 30 minutes

Cheesy arepas like these have been slowly invading NYC street fairs. Colombian-style arepas—thin, griddle-baked with corn and/or vegan cheese kneaded into the dough—are comforting, lip-smacking as an entrée (with salad or with soup) or sliced into quarters for finger-food-tastic appetizers. Once you get into the arepa habit, you may think twice about making same-old quesadillas. Fortunately new meltable mozzarella-style vegan cheese (vastly superior to vegan cheeses of the past) is now available to make Latin recipes like this a dream come true! Serve with So Good, So Green Dipping Sauce (page 43), Colombian Green Onion Salsa (page 44), Creamy Avocado-Tomato Salsa (page 39), or your favorite hot sauce.

2 cups fresh or frozen corn kernels (thawed and drained, if frozen)
1½ cups finely shredded mozzarella-style vegan cheese, preferably one that melts (optional)
2 tablespoons melted nonhydrogenated vegan margarine, cooled
1 recipe basic arepa dough (page 177)
Vegetable oil, for grilling

1. Knead the corn, cheese, and melted margarine into the arepa dough until everything is distributed evenly throughout the dough. Preheat a cast-iron griddle or other thick-bottomed skillet over medium-high heat. Lightly brush with vegetable oil.

2. Divide the dough into six equal portions and roll into balls. Place a ball in your palm and with gentle yet firm patting motions, press the dough down to form your arepa. Aim to shape the arepas into thin disks 1/2 to 3/8 inch thick and 5 to 6 inches wide. Use your palms to occasionally press the disks flat just a little as you turn the arepas in your hands while using the pads of your fingers to press and shape their edges.

3. Gently place one or two arepas into the preheated, oiled pan, leaving enough room that they can be easily flipped. While the other arepas cook, place the remaining shapely new arepas on a cutting board and cover with either a damp, clean kitchen towel or plastic wrap. Fry

each arepa for 12 to 14 minutes, flipping once or twice, until the surface is golden, the cheese has softened or melted, and a few dark, toasted spots have formed. Oil the pan as needed to cook the remaining arepas. Transfer the hot arepas to a cutting board, slice in half or into quarters, and serve immediately.

Variation

Colombian Arepa con Chicharron: Mix 1 cup of Tofu Chicharrones (page 101) into the arepa dough for an extra-smoky, "meaty" treat.

AREPAS STUFFED WITH OYSTER MUSHROOMS AND PIMIENTO PEPPERS

- Makes 6 generously stuffed arepas
- Time: About 1 hour
- Gluten Free, Soy Free

Stuffed Venezuelan-style arepas with mushrooms and roasted red peppers are marvelously messy and delicious *bocadillos.* You can use any mushroom you like in this dish, but light-colored mushrooms are best as they contrast nicely with the pimientos. You could even get sneaky and make tapas-size mini-arepas for totally "wow!" appetizers. Either way, these arepas go great with chilled white wine, Sangria (page 219), or your favorite Caribbean beer.

Make-ahead Tip: Arepas taste best if eaten after being freshly made, so cook and fill them within 30 minutes of serving. Make the filling an hour in advance and gently warm on the stovetop or microwave, but don't overcook.

1 recipe Venezuelan-style Arepas
   (page 177), kept warm in a 250ºF oven

Mushroom-Pimiento Filling

1 pound oyster mushrooms or other
   delicately flavored, light-colored
   mushrooms
3 tablespoons olive oil
4 cloves garlic, minced
1 small yellow onion, diced
1 (6-ounce) jar red pimiento peppers,
   drained and chopped finely
1 cup finely chopped ripe red tomatoes
1 tablespoon finely chopped fresh cilantro
   or flat-leaf (Italian) parsley
1/2 teaspoon ground cumin
1/4 cup white wine
3/4 teaspoon salt, or to taste
Freshly ground black pepper
Your favorite bottled hot sauce
   (Tabasco is fine)

1. Use a paper towel or clean kitchen towel to brush off any debris from the mushrooms. Cut off any tough stems and slice the mushrooms into thin strips. In a large nonstick skillet, heat 1 tablespoon of the oil over medium heat and add the mushrooms. Cook for 8 to 10

minutes, stirring occasionally, until the mushrooms have reduced in bulk by about half and are tender. Transfer the cooked mushrooms to a dish and set aside.

2. Add the remaining 2 tablespoons of oil to the skillet and stir in the garlic; cook until the garlic starts to sizzle, about 30 seconds. Stir in the onions and pimientos and fry until the onions are soft and translucent, 6 to 8 minutes. Stir in the tomatoes, cilantro, and cumin and cook until the tomatoes are soft and most of their juices have evaporated, about 10 minutes. Add the white wine, stir, and cook until bubbling, then stir in the cooked mushrooms and salt and season with ground pepper to taste. Cook the mixture for 6 to 8 more minutes, until the wine has been mostly absorbed but mixture is still moist. Taste the mushrooms and adjust the seasoning with more salt, pepper, and hot sauce, if desired. Use this filling hot or warm to stuff the arepas.

3. To fill the arepas, place a hot arepa on a cutting board. Firmly secure it to the board with your fingers (you may want to wear an oven mitt if the arepa is very hot) and use a sharp knife to slice the arepa three-quarters of the way through horizontally. It's important to not completely slice the arepa in half as you want to have a "pocket" (a little like a very thick pita bread) to fill. Stuff a generous amount of the mushroom filling into the arepa and serve immediately. If you're serving the arepas all at once, keep a baking sheet in the warm oven so

that you can place the filled arepas on it and keep them warm until everything is ready to serve. Serve with more hot sauce, if desired.

AREPAS WITH SEXY AVOCADO-TEMPEH FILLING (AVOCADO PEPIADA AREPA)

....

- **Makes 6 generously stuffed arepas**
- **Time: About 45 minutes including making arepas, not including chilling time**

....

The literal queen of stuffed Venezuelan arepas, *reina pepiada* sandwiches (*pepiada* being an old Venezuelan term for "sexy," in a fully loaded sort of way) are packed with a mild chicken and avocado salad. Here, tempeh is our stunt *pollo*. This version is also updated with chopped green onions and the surprise ingredient of Mexican jicama (not Venezuelan at all, but neither is the tempeh!). Cool, creamy salad in a hot, crisp arepa is an unforgettable and undeniably sexy combination.

Make-ahead Tip: The filling can also be made a day in advance, which could be a good idea, considering the flavors need a little bit of chilling to properly meld.

1 (8-ounce) package tempeh, cut into
   1/2-inch cubes
1 tablespoon soy sauce
1/2 cup vegan mayonnaise

2 tablespoons lime juice

1/4 teaspoon freshly ground black pepper,
or more to taste

2 green onions, green parts only, sliced
finely

1 cup shredded jicama (slice first, peel,
then shred)

1 to 2 ripe avocados

6 hot Venezuelan-style arepas
(page 177)

1. In a large saucepan with a lid, bring to a boil 1½ quarts of water. Add the tempeh and cook for 10 minutes, stirring occasionally. Drain the tempeh completely, sprinkle with the soy sauce, and set aside until it's cool enough to handle. In a large bowl, whisk together the mayonnaise, lime juice, and ground pepper until smooth. Fold in the green onions, jicama, and cooled tempeh and turn to coat completely with the mayonnaise mixture. Cover the bowl and chill for 30 minutes so that flavors blend.

2. Peel the avocado, remove the pit, and slice the flesh into ¼-inch slices. To assemble, slice the hot arepas three-quarters of the way through horizontally, leaving one end intact, so that you create a pocket (a little bit like a pita bread). If you prefer, you may scoop out a little bit of the doughy insides to create more room for the fillings. Layer some avocado slices into the arepa, then generously pack in as much of the tempeh filling as possible.

3. Serve immediately. Stuffed arepas are completely messy eating, but that's part of the fun! If desired, serve with your favorite hot sauce.

Variation

Traditional Petits Pois: The traditional filling contains peas, the tiny and sweet *petits pois* variety. If you can't get fresh, then frozen *petits pois* are the only way to go (do not use canned). Add ½ cup lightly cooked (tender but still bright green) *petits pois* along with the green onions.

SAVORY FRESH CORN PANCAKES (CACHAPAS)

- Makes about eight 6-inch pancakes
- Time: About 45 minutes

My favorite Venezuelan food might be *cachapas*, sweet and savory fresh corn pancakes. *Cachapas* are served with soft cheese and eaten as a hearty breakfast, light lunch, or snack . . . if it's possible to stop oneself from eating the whole batch.

Making a great *cachapa* had long bedeviled my family because fresh corn grown in the United States is rather watery compared to the corn in South America and difficult to form into a sturdy pancake. That and constructing a vegan version without eggs took some practice. With the help of some nontraditional ingredients, at last I arrived at a vegan *cachapa* that tastes as good as I remember. *Cachapas* are made quite big in Venezuela but petite pancakes cook faster and withstand flipping better. Fresh corn is vastly preferable to frozen.

Serve with your favorite nonhydrogenated vegan margarine. While it's not traditional, I also love slices of avocado and tomato on *cachapas*. Or even a healthy dab of Creamy Avocado-Tomato Salsa (page 39).

3 generous cups fresh or frozen
   corn kernels (thawed and drained,
   if frozen)
1/2 cup soy or other nondairy milk
1/3 cup Venezuelan- or Colombian-style
   masarepa (don't use Mexican
   masa harina)
3 tablespoons all-purpose flour
2 tablespoons ground flaxseed,
   preferably golden
3 tablespoons sugar
1/2 teaspoon baking powder
1/2 teaspoon salt
Peanut or corn oil, or
   high-smoking-point nonstick
   cooking spray, for frying
Shredded, meltable mozzarella-style
   vegan cheese (optional)

1. In a blender jar, combine the corn, soy milk, *masarepa*, flour, flaxseed, sugar, baking powder, and salt. Pulse everything until a thick chunky batter is formed with a consistency similar to that of creamed corn. If necessary, stir the in-gredients with a rubber spatula (not while the blender is running, of course) to make sure everything is blended together. Let the batter sit for 10 minutes and stir a few times before using.

2. While the batter is resting, heat a large, well-seasoned cast-iron pan or griddle over medium heat. It's ready to use when a few drops of water flicked on its surface sizzle immediately. Generously oil the surface of pan with the oil or cooking spray.

3. Scoop 1/3 cup of batter and spread on the cooking surface, using a circular motion to evenly distribute the batter. Keep your *cachapa* less than 3/8 inch thick. Cook for 3 to 4 minutes, until most of the pancake's surface is no longer shiny wet and the edges appear solid. Slide a wide, thin spatula underneath the pancake and carefully flip it over. The cooked side of the *cachapa* should be golden brown. Cook on the other side for another 2 to 3 minutes and lift it off the pan with a spatula.

4. To serve with vegan cheese, sprinkle the shredded cheese over the cooked top of the *cachapa* after you've flipped it the first time. After the bottom has cooked for 2 minutes, fold the pancake over the cheese like an omelet. Cook for another minute or so to allow cheese to melt, flip one more time, and serve.

5. Serve immediately or stack on a serving plate.

Tips for the Cachapa Chef

- If your *cachapas* fall apart when flipping, try making them slightly smaller. Use ¼ cup of batter.

- An evenly heated cooking surface is key for well-browned *cachapas*. If your kitchen range isn't the most even surface in the world, occasionally move your pan around to help distribute the heat. It's easy to tell things are a little lopsided if your pancakes are scorched on one side and pale on the other.

- Dark brown scorch marks are completely acceptable, even desired on a cachapa's surface.

- Cast iron is superior for *cachapa* cooking, as it conducts high heat ideally. Nonstick surfaces may lead to pale, anemic-looking pancakes.

11

YOU, TOO, CAN TAMALE

*F*or the uninitiated, *tamale* is the name for a wide group of foods based on masa harina, wrapped in a corn husk or banana leaf and either steamed or boiled. Almost any filling or sauce, savory or sweet, can find its way into tamales. Tamales have many different names and ingredients in Central America, the Caribbean, and many parts of South America . . . the combination of softly steamed masa surrounding yummy fillings makes for substantial street food or a festive meal when dressed up with side dishes. They have the advantage of often being portable and tasty (tamales were the "fast food" of Aztec warriors, after all!). The following recipes are Mexican-ish in flavor and style.

TAMALE TIPS FOR EVERYBODY

Tamales freeze beautifully and are so easy to reheat on the stove or in a microwave.

Many a frozen (months old, even) tamale has kept me going when the cupboards were bare. But I cannot tell a lie . . . if you're hungry right now, you should just make a salad or microwave a frozen burrito and not attempt a few dozen tamales. Even if you dropped everything and poured your undivided attention into tamale making, you probably wouldn't see a ready-to-eat morsel for two hours. So before you're starving and up to your elbows in tamale masa, please carefully go over the following tips!

That said, I promise, with a little advance planning, you'll soon be more stuffed with tamale goodness than a chile relleno. The tamale recipes in this book make a lot. It takes almost the same amount of energy (both human and kitchen appliance) to make a dozen as it does three dozen tamales, so if you've set aside the time, it's always better to make as many as you can stand (just freeze 'em!). And if you have help, the assembly stage goes fast.

With some time, the right ingredients, and a little technique, a big batch of the tamales of your dreams can be yours. You do dream of tamales as much as I do, right?

Tamales wrappers are easily tied with shreds of corn husk. However, if you suspect you'll be short on husks, use cotton kitchen string to tie the ends of the tamales.

Shopping and Ingredients

Buy more corn husks than you think you may need: I usually pick up at least two packs of husks. Corn husks are natural products and therefore can vary widely in shape, consistency, quality, and quantity from brand to brand, even package to package. Buy the largest, cleanest-looking husks packed in thick, neat bundles. Store any leftover dry corn husks in a large, loosely sealed plastic or paper bag.

Unless specifically stated, most of the tamales in this book require Mexican-style masa harina. Nothing else will do. For the easiest tamale making, look for instant masa harina. This harina (which simply means "flour" in Spanish) is made from corn treated with lime water and ground into a fine, silky, off-white flour. The most common brand I find in the Northeast is MASECA, which is sold in 5-pound white paper sacks. When in doubt, check to see where your masa harina is made or imported from: it should be from Mexico (or perhaps Central America), but for Mexican tamale-making avoid *masarepa* from Colombia or Venezuela, as it is an entirely different kind of corn flour product. Do not confuse *maicena* with masa harina, either . . . it's Spanish for "cornstarch"!

Preparing the Corn Husks

Dried corn husks must be soaked prior to using, to make them soft and bendable. To get them tamale ready, carefully separate the husks. Don't bother peeling each and every one apart. Just pull apart in bunches of two or four at a time, whatever easily separates without too much effort. For the savory tamales in this book, you'll need, minimum, two dozen long husks at least 4 inches wide; extra husks are always a good idea. Since dried husks are often not uniform in size, you'll want to pull out a few more, perhaps compensating with two smaller husks for one great big husk. Once you start making tamales, you'll soon see size does matter.

To soak the dried husks, fill a large, deep pan with at least 3 inches of warm water. A large lasagne pan works great for this. Press the husks down into the pan to immerse them in the water and let soak for 15 to 20 minutes, occasionally swishing the water around to help loosen up any husks that may be sticking to one another. The husks are ready to use when soft and easily pliable.

If using corn husks for tying tamales, take two to three long husks and tear into ½-inch-thick ribbons with your fingers.

Leave them in the water to remain pliable while you are assembling the tamales.

Setting up a tamale assembly line will take you far, especially if you're stuck making the whole batch by yourself (oh well, more tamales for you). I prepare for assembly and set up my workspace in the following order:

1. Prepare and soak the corn husks: at least 24 for the savory tamales, 2 to 3 for tearing into strips to tie them with, plus 6 or more for lining the steamer basket.

2. Prepare the filling, as it will cool enough to handle while you're making the masa and doing other things.

3. Set up the actual tamale assembly space, such as a large, clean cutting board and extra-large plates for stacking the finished tamales.

4. Set up steaming basket including filling steaming pot with 3 to 4 inches of water and lining the steaming basket with a few extra soaked corn husks.

5. Make the tamale dough. I like to make it right before I'm ready to start the filling, and use it warm. If you can't use your tamale dough right away, place in a mixing bowl, cover the top very tightly with plastic wrap, and chill. Use within a day and allow the dough to warm to room temperature before using.

6. Assemble the tamales by spreading the dough onto the soaked husks, then filling, wrapping, and tying. About halfway through making the batch of tamales, I like to put a lid on the steaming pot and try to get the water boiling over high heat by the time I finish the last tamale.

7. Place the tamales in the steamer basket. The easiest way to do this is by leaning the tamales against the sides of the basket, overlapping them slightly in a spiraling pattern. If you have too much space in the center (enough that tamales are falling over), fill the space with a crumpled ball of foil or a small cup or bowl. Don't pack the tamales too snugly; leave a little room to allow them to expand while cooking. Place the basket into the preheated pot, cover, and steam the tamales for at least 50 minutes, up to 1 hour 15 minutes.

8. Test the tamales for doneness: carefully remove a single tamale, let it cool for a few minutes, and peel back the wrapper from one end. The tamales are done when the husk wrapper pulls away easily. Cooked masa feels solid and has a somewhat firm yet tender texture. Maybe you could say it's like firm, sliced polenta, but way better. Sometimes cooked tamales may still be a little sticky. Slightly sticky tamales sometimes just need a little more cooling, about 20 minutes, to firm up and no longer be tacky.

Steaming

Lining your basket with a few corn husks can make cleanup faster. That way, on the chance occasion tamale dough pops out of its husk a little when cooking, it's just spilling out onto more corn husk rather than all over the steaming basket.

Keep a careful eye on the water in the steaming pot. You want just enough to reach about ½ inch from the bottom of the steamer basket; no water should touch the cooking tamales. However, don't let the water evaporate completely, as you may end up scorching both your pot and your tamales. Yes, you can literally find yourself burning water . . . even famous cookbook authors do it sometimes. Pour a few cups of water into the pot if it looks as if it needs it, by taking out the steamer basket first rather than pouring the water all over your precious little bundles.

Eating Tamales

Don't eat the corn husk! A friend requested I add this last bit just in case someone isn't aware that tamales need to be disrobed first before eating. Depending on how macho your guests are, two to three 4-inch tamales make a meal when paired with the works: rice, beans, and salad. If tamales are all you require, then four-plus tamales per guest are a hearty meal, plus plenty of hot sauce, salsa, and beer to wash it all down.

Freezing and Reheating Tamales

I promised you a freezer of homemade tamales and I'm hoping I've now done you right. To freeze tamales, just leave them in their corn-husk jackets and pack firmly into plastic bags; I usually double-bag them in gallon-sized resealable plastic bags, maybe write the date on them, and then forget about them. Like Buck Rogers in some distant future, when I need tamales the most, I pull them out of suspended animation and back into the world.

The easiest way to reheat frozen tamales is to generously moisten a clean kitchen towel or several paper towels, then wrap two or three frozen tamales and microwave on high for 4 to 5 minutes. Check to see if they are thawed and hot in the center, heated up just enough to make the tamales hot and moist throughout. You can also resteam the tamales just the way you cooked them in the first place. Frozen tamales take about 20 minutes to completely reheat this way, enough time to make yourself a side salad and tell those non-tamale-helpers in your life to go get themselves a frozen burrito instead.

SAVORY VEGAN MASA DOUGH

- **Makes about two dozen tamales**
- **Time: About 30 minutes**

Vegan tamales start with vegan masa dough. This is a fluffy, very rich dough that makes sublime melt-in-your-mouth tamales. The steaming masa will fill your kitchen with a delectable tamale perfume. It's important to use the best-quality vegan non-hydrogenated margarine or shortening you can find; as of this writing, Earth Balance margarine and shortening is my go-to brand for tamales.

Tip: Tamale dough should be cooked as soon as it is made. For complete tamale-making guidance, read Tamale Tips for Everybody (page 185), the filling recipe, and this dough recipe completely before making tamales, to make sure you have your ingredients and equipment all set. Total tamale making time—from dough to steaming—can take about 2½ to 3 hours (if it's just one person shaping them, that is), so plan accordingly!

1/2 cup nonhydrogenated vegetable shortening
1/2 cup nonhydrogenated vegan margarine
3 1/2 cups Mexican masa harina
2 teaspoons baking powder
1 teaspoon garlic powder
1/2 teaspoon salt
3 cups warm light-colored vegetable stock or "chicken"-flavored vegetable stock

1. In a large bowl, use a handheld mixer to cream together the shortening and margarine until creamy and light. If using a stand mixer, be sure to frequently scrape the sides of the bowl with a rubber spatula. Sift in the masa harina, baking powder, garlic powder, and salt then continue to beat for about 3 minutes, until a sandy-looking mixture forms. Pour the vegetable stock into the masa mixture and continue to beat until all of the liquid is absorbed and a fluffy dough forms, about 5 minutes.

2. The tamale dough should have a moist but not overly wet consistency—similar to mashed potatoes—and be easily spread with a rubber spatula. If the mixture seems too wet, sprinkle in another tablespoon or two of masa harina. If too dry, drizzle in a tablespoon of vegetable broth until the desired consistency is reached. Use this dough right away for making tamales.

BLACK BEAN–SWEET POTATO TAMALES

- Makes about two dozen tamales
- Time: 1 1/2 to 1 hour 45 minutes

My favorite all-vegetable filling for tamales! Soothing sweet potatoes and earthy black beans spiked with chipotles in adobo sauce are amazing already. Hugged in tamale dough, it's an achievement in food perfection worth throwing a real fiesta for. If I ever had a Thanksgiving tamale party, this would be the main attraction.

24 large dried corn husks, plus 6 to 8 more
for tying the tamales and lining the
steamer basket
1 pound sweet potatoes (2 small to
medium-size are better than a large one)
1/2 teaspoon ground cumin
1/4 teaspoon salt
Freshly ground pepper
2 tablespoons olive or peanut oil
4 cloves garlic, minced
1/2 pound yellow onion, diced
2 chipotle peppers in adobo sauce,
minced, plus 2 tablespoons sauce, or
more to taste
1/4 cup vegetable broth or white wine
2 cups cooked black beans
1 recipe Savory Vegan Masa Dough
(page 188)

Tip: For complete tamale-making guidance,
go to Tamale Tips for Everybody (page 185)
for every step, including steaming.

1. Soak the corn husks in warm water. When
you're ready to assemble the tamales, tear two
or three long husks into 1/4-inch-wide strips.
Keep the strips in water until ready to use.

2. Preheat the oven to 375ºF. Pierce the
sweet potatoes several times with a fork, wrap
in foil, and place on a baking sheet. Bake for 35
to 40 minutes, until the sweet potatoes are
soft enough to be easily pierced with a knife.
Remove from the oven, unwrap, slice the
sweet potatoes in half lengthwise, and let cool.

When cool enough to handle, remove the
skins, place the sweet potatoes in a bowl, add
the ground cumin, and season to taste with
salt and pepper. Use a fork or potato masher
to mash the potatoes to a chunky puree.

3. Prepare the black beans: In a large nonstick skillet over medium heat, combine the
olive oil and garlic. Allow the garlic to sizzle for
30 seconds, stirring occasionally. Add the
onion and fry until the onion is translucent,
about 5 minutes. Add the chipotles and their
sauce and the vegetable broth, stir, and simmer for 1 minute. Add the black beans, bring
the mixture to a simmer, and cook until most of
the liquid is absorbed but beans are still moist,
about 4 minutes. Turn off the heat and allow
beans to cool.

4. For each tamale: Spread a generous 1/4
cup of dough down the center of a pliable
soaked corn husk, leaving at least 11/2 inches
on either end. This will form an oblong shape 4
to 5 inches wide and 3/8 to 1/2 inch thick.
Spoon 1 generous tablespoon of sweet potato
down the center of the tamale dough, then top
with 1 tablespoon of black beans.

5. Now grab both edges of the corn husk that
are not covered with dough. Bring the edges toward each other and push the sides of the masa
dough together to encase the filling. Gently
press the tamale to form a firm, solid tube shape.
Tightly twist each end of the tamale wrapper (so
it looks a little like a wrapped piece of candy)

and tightly tie each end with a soaked corn-husk strip. Some sauce may leak out of the dough into the interior of the corn husk wrap, but it will not have any effect on the steamed tamales. Repeat with the remaining dough, filling, and husks. When you're finally tired of making tamales, it's time to get the steamer basket ready.

6. To steam the tamales: Remove the steamer basket from the pot. Fill the pot with 2 to 3 inches of water, or whatever level will stay below the steamer basket. Cover and bring to a boil. Meanwhile, line the bottom of the steamer basket with some soaked corn husks. Set the tamales, unwrapped end upright, into the steamer basket, first layering them around the sides of the basket and working inward. Top the tamales with any leftover soaked husks, if you have them, place the steamer basket in the pot, and cover.

7. Steam the tamales for at least 55 minutes, up to 1 hour 5 minutes. Check the pot occasionally to make sure the water has not evaporated; add more hot water as needed. Test to see if the tamales are ready by removing a tamale and peeling back some corn husk. Fully cooked tamale dough will be tender but solid, not wet. Remove the entire basket from the pot, place on a dinner plate, and let stand, covered, for at least 15 minutes to cool. Handle the tamales carefully (tongs are handy) as they will still be hot and steaming.

Serve these tamales hot with any chile sauce plus beans, rice, or salad, if desired. To serve tamales, you can unwrap them for your guests or let them do the honors.

RED CHILE–SEITAN TAMALES

- Makes about two dozen tamales
- Time: About 1½ hours, not including Red Chile Sauce or Red Steamed Seitan

These saucy tamales bear a striking resemblance toward their meatier classic red chile tamale cousins. Seitan and red chile sauce together don't mess around when it comes to making a luscious, full-flavored, "meaty" tamale. Make double the recipe for Red Chile Sauce if you plan on serving the entire batch of tamales in one serving . . . especially if your tamale eaters are a saucy bunch.

> 24 large dried corn husks, plus 6 to 8 more for tying the tamales and lining the steamer basket
>
> 2 loaves Steamed Red Seitan (page 34, or about ¾ pound purchased or homemade seitan, sliced into ¼-inch pieces
>
> 5 tablespoons peanut or other vegetable oil
>
> ½ pound yellow onion, cut in half and sliced into thin strips
>
> ¼ pound red bell pepper (half a large pepper), seeded and sliced into thin strips
>
> 1 recipe Red Chile Sauce (page 45)
>
> 1 recipe Savory Vegan Masa Dough (page 188)

Tip: For complete tamale-making guidance, go to Tamale Tips for Everybody (page 185) for every step, including steaming.

1. Soak the corn husks in warm water and, when you're ready to assemble the tamales, tear two or three long husks into 1/4-inch-wide strips. Keep the strips in water until ready to use.

2. In a large cast-iron skillet, heat 3 tablespoons of the peanut oil over medium heat. When a piece of seitan sizzles when placed in the pan, add the rest of the seitan and stir to coat in the hot oil. Using a metal spatula to stir, fry the seitan until the edges are starting to turn crisp and brown, about 10 minutes. Transfer the seitan to a large mixing bowl.

3. Pour in the remaining 2 tablespoons of oil, heat over medium heat, and add the onion and pepper. Fry in the same manner as the seitan until the onion turns translucent and soft, 10 to 12 minutes. Turn off the heat and pour the onion and peppers into same bowl as the seitan. Add 1 1/2 cups of the chile sauce to the seitan mixture, and stir to coat. Set aside the remaining sauce to serve with the cooked tamales. Allow the mixture to cool enough to be handled.

4. I like to shape these tamales the "open-ended" method. In the center of a large corn-husk, spoon 2 to 3 tablespoons of masa dough. Using your fingers, spread or pat the dough toward the wide end of the husk, while also spreading the dough outward. Properly formed dough should be about 1/4 inch thick, about 1/4 inch from the wide end (what will be the open end) of the husk and 3 1/2 to 4 inches wide. You will want at least 2 inches of uncovered corn husk on either side of the spread dough, plus at least 3 inches of uncovered space at the tapered end of the husk.

5. For each tamale, spoon about 2 generous tablespoons of filling onto the dough slightly closer to the wide edge; use about 3 chunks of seitan, a few strands each of onions and peppers, and 2 teaspoons or more of sauce.

6. Now grab both edges of the corn husk that are not covered with dough. Bring the edges toward each other and push the sides of the masa dough together to encase the filling. Gently press the tamale to form a solid shape and carefully tuck one of the edges of the corn-husk under the other. Tightly wrap the free end of the corn husk around the tamale and then fold over the tapered "tail" end of the husk on top of the tamale. (Don't worry if any sauce leaks out of the folded tamale dough.) Take a long strip of corn husk and tie around the base of the tamale, about 1/2 inch from the end. Tie a tight knot to keep the wrapper from unraveling. Repeat with remaining dough, filling, and husks. When you're tired of making tamales, it's time to get the steamer basket ready.

7. Steam as directed for Black Bean–Sweet Potato Tamales, page 189.

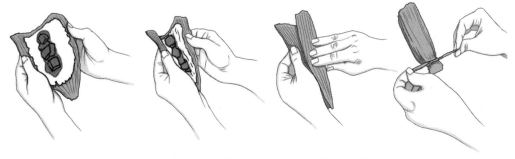

1. Hold filled tamale dough by corn-husk sides
2. Bring sides together, pressing dough over filling
3. Fold corn-husk sides over dough
4. Tuck tail end of corn husk and tie tightly

CHOCOLATE MOLE VEGGIE TAMALES

Makes about two dozen tamales
Time: 1¹/2 to 1 hour 45 minutes

Tamale + potatoes + chile chocolate mole sauce equals *sí, señor*, I'll have another! Serve with more mole sauce or warm tomatillo sauce or roasted tomato salsa. Sweet spicy chocolate mole works wonders inside and on top of tamales.

Tip: Look for the special MASECA for Tamales brand of masa harina (the kind that comes in a tan paper bag [see Pantry section, page 14]); its rustic grainy texture and unique corn flavor are fantastic with this mole filling. The dough may require less liquid than usual, so reduce the total

liquid to about ½ cup. In the unlikely event you'll need more broth, you can slowly add it back into the dough.

24 large dried corn husks, plus 6 to 8
    more for tying the tamales and lining
    the steamer basket
1 pound potato, peeled and diced into
    ¹/2-inch cubes
¹/2 pound carrots or pumpkin, peeled
    and diced
1 loaf White Steamed Seitan, finely diced,
    or 1 generous cup cooked pinto beans,
    rinsed
¹/2 cup fresh or frozen green peas
    (rinsed with warm water, if frozen)
1¹/2 cups prepared Chocolate-Chile Mole
    Sauce (page 51)
1 recipe Savory Vegan Masa Dough
    (page 188)

Tip: For complete tamale-making guidance, go to Tamale Tips for Everybody (page 185) for every step, including steaming.

1. Soak the corn husks in warm water and, when you're ready to assemble the tamales, tear two or three long husks into 1/4-inch-wide strips. Keep the strips in water until ready to use.

2. Prepare the filling: Boil the potatoes for 14 to 16 minutes, until tender. During the last 5 minutes of cooking, stir in the carrot, then drain and rinse with cold water. In a large mixing bowl, combine the cooked vegetables, seitan, peas, and Chocolate-Chile Mole Sauce, and stir to coat the vegetables completely with the sauce. Have ready the prepared dough and corn husks.

3. For each tamale, spread a generous 1/4 cup of dough down the center of a pliable soaked corn husk, leaving at least 1 1/2 inches on either end. Form an oblong shape 4 to 5 inches wide and 3/8 to 1/2 inch thick. Spoon about 2 generous tablespoons of mole filling onto the dough down the middle.

4. Now grab both edges of the corn husk that are not covered with dough. Bring the edges toward each other and push the sides of the masa dough together to encase the filling. Gently press the tamale to form a firm, solid tube shape. Tightly twist each end of the tamale wrapper (so it looks a little like a wrapped piece of candy) and tightly tie each end with a soaked corn-husk strip. Repeat with the remaining dough, filling, and husks.

5. Steam as directed for Black Bean–Sweet Potato Tamales (page 189).

6. Serve these tamales hot with extra Chocolate-Chile Mole Sauce plus beans, rice, or salad, if desired. To serve the tamales, you can unwrap them for your guests or let them do the honors.

FARMERS' MARKET TAMALES

- **Makes about two dozen tamales**
- **Time: 1 1/2 to 1 hour 45 minutes**

A delicate tamale filled with fresh vegetables worked right into the dough, inspired by the tamales from the Sinaloa region of Mexico. There's no "filling" each one, so these are just a little easier on your inner tamale-making-grandmother.

These are a great all-purpose veggie tamale. You can really vary these with whatever you score at the farmers' market; from zucchini and tomatoes to butternut squash and potatoes. A little bit of capers adds a tangy surprise to every other bite.

Green Tomatillo Sauce (page 40) complements the fresh flavors of these tamales perfectly. For a complete feast, serve these up with Home-style Refried Beans (page

86, using pintos or a white bean, perhaps) and Cilantro-Lime Rice (page 95).

24 large dried corn husks, plus 6 to 8 more for tying the tamales and lining the steamer basket

1 pound zucchini or other summer or winter squash, peeled, seeded, and cut into 1/4-inch cubes

1/2 teaspoon salt (for summer squash only)

4 cloves garlic, minced finely

4 green onions, trimmed and chopped finely

1 tablespoon olive oil

1 cup fresh or frozen corn kernels (thawed and drained, if frozen)

1 cup fresh or frozen green beans, cut into 1/2-inch pieces

1/2 cup fresh or frozen green peas

1/2 cup finely diced seeded tomato, or 1/4 cup finely chopped sun-dried tomato

1 large carrot, diced into 1/4-inch cubes or grated

1/4 pound waxy potato (one smallish potato), diced into 1/4-inch cubes

2 teaspoons dried oregano or dried epazote

1/2 teaspoon ground cumin

1 tablespoon lime juice

1/2 cup capers, drained

1 recipe Savory Vegan Masa Dough (page 188)

Tip: For complete tamale-making guidance, go to Tamale Tips for Everybody (page 185) for every step, including steaming.

1. Soak the corn husks in warm water and, when you're ready to assemble the tamales, tear two or three long husks into 1/4-inch-wide strips. Keep the strips in water until ready to use.

2. For the filling: Place the zucchini in a bowl, sprinkle with the 1/2 teaspoon salt, and let sit for 15 minutes. The squash will release excess water; when ready to use, rinse well and drain. Winter squash, however, does not need to be salted.

3. While the squash is draining, sauté the garlic and green onions with the olive oil in a large, deep, nonstick skillet over medium heat until the onion is softened, 4 to 5 minutes. Add the squash, corn, green beans, peas, tomato, carrot, and potato. Cook and stir occasionally until the squash is slightly tender, 6 to 8 minutes. Remove from the heat, let cool enough to touch, and drain any excess liquid from the vegetables. Season with the oregano, cumin, and lime juice. Add the vegetables and capers to the tamale dough and gently knead the dough to distribute everything.

4. For each tamale: Scoop 1/3 cup of dough and pat into an oblong shape about 2 1/2 inches wide and about 2 inches thick down the center of a corn husk, leaving at least 1 1/2 inches on either end. Grab both edges of the corn husk that are not covered with dough. Bring the edges toward each other and push the sides of the masa dough together to encase the filling.

Gently press the tamale to form a firm, solid, tube-like shape. Tightly twist each end of the tamale wrapper (so it looks a little like a wrapped piece of candy) and tightly tie each end with a soaked corn-husk strip. Repeat with the remaining dough, filling, and husks.

5. Steam as directed for Black Bean–Sweet Potato Tamales (page 189).

PINEAPPLE-RAISIN SWEET TAMALES

....

- ● **Makes about 16**
- ● **Time: About 1 1/2 hours**

....

Pineapple, raisins, and sweet spices are popular blend of flavors for dessert tamales. Try them with hot Mexican-style chocolate for a cozy cool-weather treat or perhaps even vegan vanilla ice cream for an all-new kind of à la mode. Since all the ingredients are blended right into the masa, there's no filling and folding. Just shape the dough, wrap 'em, and steam them up.

Tip: Using MASECA for Tamales? You may want to increase the masa harina up to 2 2/3 cups to compensate for this moister corn flour.

> **16 large dried corn husks, plus 6 to 8 more for tying the tamales and lining the steamer basket**

> **2/3 cup nonhydrogenated vegan margarine, softened**
> **2/3 cup light brown sugar**
> **2 1/3 cups Mexican masa harina**
> **1 1/2 teaspoons baking powder**
> **1 1/2 teaspoons whole aniseed**
> **1 1/4 teaspoons ground cinnamon**
> **1/4 teaspoon salt**
> **1 (20-ounce can) crushed canned pineapple with juice**
> **2/3 cup golden raisins**

Tip: For complete tamale-making guidance, go to Tamale Tips for Everybody (page 185) for every step, including steaming.

1. Soak corn husks in warm water and, when you're ready to assemble the tamales, tear two or three long husks into 1/4-inch-wide strips. Keep the strips in water until ready to use.

2. In a large mixing bowl, use a hand mixer to cream together the margarine and brown sugar until light and fluffy, about 4 minutes, frequently scraping the sides of the bowl with a rubber spatula. Add the masa harina, baking powder, aniseed, ground cinnamon, and salt, and continue to beat until a crumbly mixture forms, about 3 minutes. Pour in the crushed pineapple with its juices and beat for 3 to 5 more minutes, scraping frequently, to form a soft dough. The dough will be a little moister than savory tamale dough; if it seems too wet, stir in a few tablespoons of masa harina at a time until a desired consistency is reached.

Add the raisins and knead into the dough to distribute them evenly.

3. For each tamale: Scoop 1/4 to 1/3 cup of dough and spread in the center of a pliable soaked corn husk, leaving at least 1 1/2 inches on either end. Form a square or rectangular shape about 3 inches wide and no more than 1/2 inch thick.

4. Grab both edges of the corn husk that are not covered with dough, bring edges toward each other, and gently fold the edges so that they overlap. Fold the long top and bottom ends of the tamale on top to form a square or squat rectangular package. Use a corn-husk strip to tie the package together in the middle, keeping the long ends of the corn husks down.

Try keeping these tamales on the small side to help create this square package–like shape, but if it doesn't work out, use the long candy wrapper–like shape with the ties at both ends (as in the Farmers' Market Tamales, page 194). Repeat with the remaining dough, filling, and husks. When you're almost done making them it's time to get the steamer basket ready.

5. Steam as directed for Black Bean–Sweet Potato Tamales (page 189).

Variation

Coconut-Pineapple Tamales: A tropical paradise in a corn husk. Fold 1 cup of grated unsweetened coconut into the dough, along with the raisins.

12

EMPANADAS!

*B*reakfast, lunch, dinner . . . what do these have in common in Español? They're all times to eat empanadas, the original handheld savory or sweet pie! A whole world of tasty seitan, beans, and vegetables wrapped up in a tender wheat crust is just waiting for you, worthy of your precious cooking time. If that wasn't enough reason to dust off the old rolling pin, there is an entire school of delicate corn-crusted empanadas, fried to perfection and without a trace of gluten. Empanadas keep well in the refrigerator and are the best there is for a light meal or hearty snack. A Sunday afternoon of empanada making can keep you in delicious and convenient handheld meals until the middle of the week (unless you really do eat empanadas all day long).

WHEAT EMPANADA DOUGH

- Makes about a dozen 6-inch dough rounds
- Time: About 35 minutes, not including the chilling time

This produces a pastry crust that can be baked or fried and filled with just about anything for delightful empanadas. Although you put it together like a piecrust, this dough is less fussy, more forgiving. The result is a tender crust that's not overly flaky or greasy and is up to the task of holding even the juiciest fillings in place.

There is no denying that making empanadas—especially mixing, rolling, and cutting out the dough—can be time consuming. Make time work for you by putting together some (or even all) of the components a day in advance. I highly recommend mixing, chilling, and cutting the dough the night before, so that when it's empanada time, you can focus on making the filling and baking them.

Tip: Drop a few ice cubes in the water for colder water that helps keep the gluten strands in the dough shorter. Shorter gluten equals a more tender pastry. And tender pastry equals tender, more loving empanadas.

3 cups all-purpose flour

1 1/2 teaspoons salt

1/4 teaspoon baking powder

6 tablespoons chilled nonhydrogenated vegan shortening

2 tablespoons chilled nonhydrogenated vegan margarine

3/4 cup cold water, or more as needed

1. In a food processor bowl, pulse together the flour, salt, and baking powder for a few seconds. Slice the shortening and margarine into 1/2-inch chunks, add to the food processor, and pulse until everything resembles fine, sandlike crumbs. If your food processor bowl is small, prepare everything in two batches. If you prefer, you can also use a large fork or pastry cutter to blend the fats into the flour.

2. Pour the flour mixture into a large bowl and stream in the cold water while mixing the dough with your fingers. Continue adding just enough cold water that you can press the mixture together to form a soft and stretchy dough. Briefly knead a few times, divide into two balls,

flatten each into a round about an inch thick, and wrap tightly with plastic wrap. Handle the dough minimally to keep it from getting tough. Chill it overnight or for at least 4 hours.

3. Tear about ten pieces of waxed paper to about 7 inches square and keep them near your workspace. Lightly dust a large, stable rolling surface and a rolling pin with all-purpose flour. Roll one of the dough rounds about 3/8 inch thick, stretching and pulling the dough a little if necessary. To keep the dough from getting tough, use long rolling motions, occasionally lifting the dough by the edges and turning it a little to ensure an even thickness throughout.

4. Using a 6-inch-diameter bowl pressed into the dough as a guide, take a small, sharp paring knife and run it around the edge of the bowl to cut out circles. Or, use a huge round cookie or biscuit cutter. Stack the circles of dough on top of one another, separating them with the waxed paper pieces to keep them from sticking. Chill the dough scraps, while you roll and cut the remaining unworked dough

Frozen Empanada Dough

Don't want to get acquainted with a rolling pin? Look for premade frozen empanada dough circles in the freezer section of your local Latin grocery. It's also a good idea to have some on hand if you know you're making a double batch of empanadas and want to be certain you'll won't run out of dough. These "wrappers" often require thawing for at least an hour before using, so plan accordingly. But first, be sure to read the ingredients very carefully! Some brands may contain animal fat. Unfortunately, the pretty orange ones (tinted with annatto) usually contain lard, but you may be able to find dough circles that are made with just vegetable shortening.

into rounds. Gather up all the remaining dough scraps, reroll them only one more time, and cut out as many circles as possible.

5. Chill the finished dough circles, the entire stack well wrapped in plastic wrap while preparing the filling, or store in the refrigerator for up to a week. Keep the empanada dough chilled until you're ready to fill and bake 'em.

Richer Wheat Dough

Use this slightly richer version of the empanada dough for Bolivian-style *salteñas* (page 204) or for wrapping sweet fillings.

> 3 cups all-purpose flour
> 1/3 cup sugar
> 1 1/4 teaspoons salt
> 1/2 teaspoon baking powder
> 6 tablespoons chilled nonhydrogenated vegan shortening
> 4 tablespoons chilled nonhydrogenated vegan margarine
> 3/4 cup cold water, or more as needed

CREAMY CORN-FILLED EMPANADAS (EMPANADAS HUMITAS)

....

- Makes about a dozen 6-inch empanadas
- Time: About 1 hour, not including making the dough

....

Empanadas are a real treat stuffed with a creamy corn filling, a favorite filling in Argentina and Chile. *Humitas* is the name for a whole family of baked or steamed foods made with pureed fresh corn that are found all over South America, and they're so good you'll feel as if you're getting away with something with every delicious bite. As with most regional recipes, there are many variations on how chefs like to season their *humitas*; I like adding chives, green onion, or even spring garlic scapes for zesty pungent zing in the sweet corn filling.

> 1 recipe Wheat Empanada Dough (page 199), cut into 6-inch rounds
> 3 tablespoons nonhydrogenated vegan margarine
> 3 tablespoons finely chopped chives, garlic scapes, or green onions
> 1 teaspoon dried basil, crumbled
> 5 cups fresh or frozen corn kernels (thawed and drained, if frozen; removed from 6 to 8 ears of corn if fresh)
> 3 cloves garlic, chopped
> 1/4 cup cornstarch
> 2/3 cup soy creamer or other heavy cream substitute, or any nondairy milk
> 1 tablespoon lemon juice
> 1 teaspoon salt, or more to taste
> A big pinch of cayenne
> Freshly ground black pepper
> 1/3 cup soy creamer or nondairy milk, for brushing

1. Keep the prepared dough rounds chilled while preparing the filling. In a heavy-bottomed pot, melt the margarine over medium heat, add the chives and dried basil, and sauté for 2 minutes. In a blender jar, pulse the corn kernels, garlic, cornstarch, soy creamer, lemon juice, salt, cayenne, and pepper into a thick batter. Pour the corn mixture into the pot containing the chive mixture and cook for 8 to 10 minutes, stirring occasionally with a silicone spatula or a wooden spoon, until the filling thickens to the consistency of thick porridge. Remove from the heat, taste, and adjust the seasonings, if desired, with salt, ground pepper, or even little more lemon juice.

2. When ready to assemble the empanadas, preheat the oven to 400ºF. Line baking sheets with parchment paper.

3. Take a dough round, gently stretch it slightly outward by its edges, and brush lightly with soy creamer. Scoop a generous 1/3 cup of corn filling into the center of the round and spread it over half of the round; leave about 1/2 inch of space along the edge of the dough. It's especially important to make sure this filling doesn't spill over the edge; the wet filling can make crimping the edges a little tricky. Fold the unfilled dough over the filling, stretching and pulling it just enough to completely encase everything. (You will now have a semicircular patty.) With your fingers, firmly press down the edges of the dough, then seal by firmly pressing the tines of a fork into the edges of the em-

panada. Carefully lift and place the empanada on a prepared baking sheet, and brush with more soy creamer. Repeat with the remaining dough and filling, dividing the filling equally among the dough rounds.

4. Bake the empanadas for 24 to 26 minutes, or until their crust is golden and their edges begin to brown. A little of the filling may bubble out of the edges, but once you get the hang of crimping the edges it won't happen very often. Allow the empanadas to cool for about 5 minutes before serving, as the filling will be extremely hot right out of the oven. To reheat, either wrap in foil and bake at 350ºF for 8 to 10 minutes, or microwave on high for 30 to 35 seconds. Store leftovers chilled in a tightly covered container.

SHREDDED SEITAN AND MUSHROOM EMPANADAS WITH RAISINS AND OLIVES

....
- Makes about one dozen plump 6-inch empanadas
- Time: About 1 hour with baking, not including making the dough rounds
....

South American–style empanadas have gained a certain foothold in New York City. These pockets of baked wheat crust can encase most anything, and this seitan filling stands up to its meatier contemporary with salty black olives and sweet dark raisins.

Steamed Red Seitan is grated and enriched with a little finely minced mushroom to create a tender filling that's tempting even for those of the carnivorous persuasion.

Tip: This filling is extremely versatile and practically every Latin American country has a variation on the shredded or ground meat + olives + raisins idea. Use this filling for corn-crust empanadas, arepas, in tacos, or even as is with any rice. Or use it for filling *patacones* (page 65).

1 recipe Wheat Empanada Dough
   (page 199), rolled into 6-inch rounds
½ recipe (two loaves) Steamed Red
   Seitan (page 34), chilled (for easiest
   shredding)
½ pound cremini mushrooms (or any
   brown mushroom), cleaned, tough
   stems removed
3 tablespoons olive oil
4 cloves garlic, peeled and minced
½ pound yellow onion, minced finely
2 tablespoons red wine or vegetable broth
1½ teaspoons smoked paprika
1½ teaspoons dried oregano
½ teaspoon ground cumin
¼ teaspoon ground cinnamon (optional)
Salt and freshly ground black pepper
½ cup black olives (kalamata or oil-cured
   Greek olives), pitted and sliced in half
⅓ cup dark raisins
⅓ cup soy creamer or nondairy milk, for
   brushing

1. To prepare the seitan filling: use a large-holed grater and gently grate the Red Steamed Seitan. Use your fingers to tear apart any remaining nubs too small to grate. The grated seitan will be crumbly but moist and springy. Very finely mince the mushrooms, chopping them as small as the bits of shredded seitan (the idea is that they will blend into the seitan; these are not chunky vegetable empanadas).

2. In a 12-inch nonstick skillet, heat together the olive oil and garlic over medium heat, until the garlic starts to sizzle and becomes fragrant. Stir in the onion and fry until translucent, about 5 minutes. Stir in the mushrooms and cook until they darken and release their juices, another 5 to 6 minutes. Add the red wine, paprika, oregano, cumin, and cinnamon (if using), stirring occasionally, and bring to a simmer. Stir in the grated seitan and, stirring constantly so that seitan absorbs liquid but is still moist, cook for 6 to 8 more minutes. Use a silicone spatula to fold the seitan into the vegetable mixture and really press it into the liquid to help it absorb more seasonings. Remove from the heat, let cool for a few minutes, and taste the mixture. Add salt and ground black pepper to taste. Stir in the olives and raisins. Set aside until cool enough to comfortably handle.

3. When ready to assemble the empanadas, preheat the oven to 400ºF. Line baking sheets with parchment paper. Have handy the prepared dough rounds, soy creamer, and a pastry brush.

4. Take a dough round, gently stretch it slightly outward by its edges, and lightly brush with soy creamer. Scoop up a generous 1/3 cup of filling, making sure to get a few raisins and olive slices with each scoop. Place the filling into the center of the round and spread it over half of the round; leave about 1/2 inch of space along the edge of the dough. It's especially important to make sure this filling doesn't spill over the edge; the wet filling can make crimping the edges a little tricky.

5. Fold the dough over the filling, stretching and pulling it just enough to completely encase everything. (You will now have a semicircular patty.) With your fingers, firmly press down the edges of the dough, then seal by firmly pressing the tines of a fork into the edges of the empanada. Carefully lift and place on a prepared baking sheet and brush with soy creamer. Repeat with the remaining dough and filling, dividing the filling equally among the dough rounds.

6. Bake the empanadas for 24 to 26 minutes, or until the crust is golden and the edges begin to brown. A little of the filling may bubble out of the edges, but if you crimp it firmly enough it won't be much of an issue. Allow them to cool for 6 to 8 minutes before serving, as the filling will be extremely hot right out of the oven.

7. To reheat, either wrap in foil and bake at 350ºF for 8 to 10 minutes, or microwave on high for 30 to 35 seconds. Store leftovers chilled in a tightly covered container.

SWEET AND SPICY SEITAN-POTATO EMPANADAS (BOLIVIAN SALTEÑAS)

- Makes about a dozen 6-inch empanadas
- Time: About 1 1/2 hours with baking and cooling the filling, not including making pastry dough circles

In Bolivia the big, richly spicy and juicy empanada called *salteña* is king. It's a real handheld meal with a chunky saucy filling wrapped up in a sweeter wheat crust. *Salteñas* look different, too. Rather than having the typical half-moon shape, these look like plump little boats topped with a twisted braid of dough. This recipe may seem epic, but take heart that it's still simpler and faster than the animal-loaded original. Serve with you favorite hot sauce or So Good, So Green Dipping Sauce (page 43).

Tip: A pretty "braid" along its top seam is the *salteña*'s calling card and serves the practical function of holding in its juices. Dough braiding requires some practice to get just right, but the basic technique can be worked quickly once you get the hang of it. Press the side of your thumb into the raised edge of dough at a 45-degree angle. Now pinch the dough between your thumb and the knuckle of your index finger, while pressing the dough down slightly. Then place your thumb in the imprint made by your index finger and pinch again in the same manner, working from one end of the empanada to the other. The resulting crimp will have a wavy, braid-like appearance.

1 recipe Wheat Empanada Dough (richer variation, page 201), well chilled

1 pound waxy potatoes, peeled and diced into 1/2-inch cubes

1 large carrot, peeled and diced into 1/2-inch cubes (about 1 cup)

3 tablespoons olive or peanut oil

1/2 recipe (two loaves) Steamed Red or White Seitan (pages 34 and 35), diced into 1/2-inch cubes (about 2 generous cups of chopped seitan)

4 cloves garlic, chopped

1/2 pound yellow onion, diced into 1/2-inch cubes

1 1/2 teaspoons ground cumin

1 1/2 teaspoons dried oregano

2 teaspoons red hot chile sauce or paste, or more to taste (use fiery rocoto pepper for very hot salteñas)

A generous twist of freshly ground black pepper

1/2 cup fresh or frozen peas

1/2 cup dark raisins

2/3 cup sliced green olives

1 2/3 cups rich vegetable broth

4 teaspoons arrowroot powder or cornstarch

1 tablespoon sugar

1/2 teaspoon salt, or to taste

1. Place the potatoes and carrots in a heavy saucepan and cover with cold water. Bring to a boil over high heat, lower the heat to a simmer, and cook until the potatoes just start to turn tender but are not mushy, 10 to 12 minutes. Drain in a colander over the sink and rinse with cold water to stop the vegetables from cooking further. Leave the colander in the sink to drain any excess water.

2. Now make the seitan veggie filling. If desired, you can do this step in advance and keep the filling chilled until it's time to bake the empanadas. In a heavy-bottomed pot, heat 1 tablespoon of the oil over medium heat and add the diced seitan, sautéing for 5 minutes, or until the edges start to brown. Transfer to a plate. Heat the remaining 2 tablespoons of oil over medium heat and add the garlic and onion, frying until the onion becomes soft and translucent, 8 to 10 minutes. Stir in the cumin, oregano, and hot sauce and grind a few twists of pepper over everything. Add the seitan, drained potatoes and carrots, peas, raisins, and olives and fry for about 2 minutes.

3. While the seitan mixture cooks, use a wire whisk or a fork to beat the vegetable broth, arrowroot, sugar, and salt in a mixing cup until dissolved. Add to the seitan mixture and stir occasionally until the mixture starts to boil. The mixture will begin to thicken now, so switch to stirring constantly until a thin gravy has formed. Taste the gravy; it's fully cooked when no chalky texture remains. Adjust the seasoning, if needed, by adding more salt, pepper, or even hot sauce, if desired. Remove from the heat and allow the filling to cool for at least 25 minutes. It should be cooked enough to handle easily.

4. When ready to assemble the empanadas, preheat the oven to 400ºF. Line baking sheets with parchment paper. You may want to use baking sheets with a raised edge for these empanadas, as juices may bubble out.

5. Take a dough round, place it on a lightly floured surface, and gently stretch it slightly outward by its edges. Scoop up a generous 1/3 cup of filling (making sure to scoop up some of the gravy) into the center of the round, leaving at least 1/2 inch of space along the edge of the dough. Quickly grab two opposite ends of the dough and pinch together to form a "purse" to help prevent the gravy from spilling out. Continue to press the edges together and work toward the top to create a bottom-heavy, half-circular purselike shape. Now really press those edges of the dough together, enough to squish the dough out to create an edge 1/2 inch wide.

Carefully crimp the edges and tuck them under (see the tip about making a braided edge). It's an important step to make sure all of the filling is secured inside the crust.

6. Gently lift the empanada by hand (or use a thin spatula) and place on the prepared baking sheet. Brush the top and sides generously with soy creamer. Continue with the rest of dough and filling, dividing the filling equally among the dough rounds.

7. Bake the empanadas for 28 to 30 minutes, or until the crust is golden and the edges are browned. A little of the filling may bubble out of the edges, but as you get better at crimping the edges of the dough it won't be much of an issue. Allow them to cool for 6 to 8 minutes before serving, as the filling will be extremely hot right out of the oven.

8. To reheat: either wrap in foil and bake at 350ºF for 8 to 10 minutes, or microwave on high for 30 to 35 seconds. Store leftovers chilled in a tightly covered container.

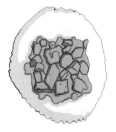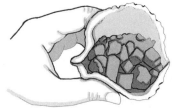

1. Place filling on dough
2. Pinch dough upright to seal

In Colombia and Venezuela, empanadas use a dough made from the same South American precooked corn flour that's used for making arepas. After working with homemade wheat dough, working with corn dough will be something of a revelation; thanks to the precooked *masarepa*, this dough comes together in mere minutes. And because there's no gluten, you can knead and rework the dough all night long without fearing the wrath of a tough empanada.

Corn-crusted empanadas are best deep-fried. Or they can be baked instead, if you prefer; the crust will be chewier instead of crisp, in that case. These empanadas are so easy to pull together, you'll want to experiment with different fillings and textures. Try making one or more of the following fillings for your next empanada-frying fiesta! Prepare the corn dough and fill and fry just like in the recipe for potato-pumpkin empanadas (page 205).

- Use the shredded seitan, olive, and raisin filling (page 202) for a "meaty" and very traditional-style filling. Serve with Green Onion Salsa (page 44) or any salsa.
- Fill with equal parts black bean Home-style Refried Beans (page 86) and finely shredded meltable mozzarella-style vegan cheese (one of the most typical and beloved of fillings for corn empanadas). Serve with any salsa or hot sauce.
- Stuff with the oyster mushroom and pimiento pepper arepa filling (page 180)
- Fill with leftover seitan ropa vieja (page 107) plus a little leftover rice.
- Colombian-style Red Beans (page 90), especially roja bola beans, are particularly outstanding and hearty inside empanadas. Great with a little bit of sweet roasted or fried plantains, too.

CORN-CRUSTED PUMPKIN-POTATO EMPANADAS

- Makes about 20 small empanadas
- Time: About 1 hour, including boiling, filling, and frying everything
- Gluten Free, Soy Free

Colombia and Venezuela empanada fillings vary widely and I like this vegetable-only medley of pumpkin and potato simmered in a *sofrito*. Colombian empanadas are always fried, which (of course) greatly enhances the corn's flavor. These smaller empanadas make deluxe appetizers, or present them three at a

time for an entrée. Always serve with tangy and fresh-tasting Colombian Green Onion Salsa (page 44) by spooning a little dab of salsa onto every empanada bite.

Make-ahead Tip: Use half a recipe of Sofrito con Tomate (page 33) in place of the oil, onion, pepper, and tomato.

Filling

3/4 pound pumpkin, calabaza, or winter squash, peeled, seeded, and diced into 1/2-inch cubes

3/4 pound white potato, peeled and diced into 1/2-inch cubes

3 tablespoons vegetable oil

3 cloves garlic, minced

1 large onion, diced

1/2 green bell pepper, seeded and
diced finely

1 large tomato, seeded and diced

1/4 cup chopped fresh cilantro

1 teaspoon ground cumin

1 teaspoon dried oregano

1 teaspoon salt, or to taste

Freshly ground pepper

Dough

2 1/2 cups Harina PAN, Colombian- or
Venezuelan-style precooked *masarepa*
corn flour (do not use Mexican
masa harina!)

2 cups warm water

1 teaspoon salt

Vegetable oil, for deep frying

1. Prepare the filling first. Place the pumpkin and potato pieces in a large stockpot. Add enough cold water to cover by 2 inches and bring to a boil over high heat. Lower the heat to a simmer, partially cover, and cook until the potatoes are tender, 20 to 24 minutes. Drain and set aside.

2. Heat the oil in a large skillet over medium heat, stir in the garlic, and fry until the garlic is fragrant and sizzling, about 30 seconds. Add the onions and green pepper and cook for 15 minutes, stirring occasionally, until the vegetables are soft. Stir in the tomato, cilantro, cumin,

oregano, salt, and pepper, and cook for another 10 minutes, until the tomatoes have released their juices and are very mushy. Stir the cooked pumpkin and potato into the sofrito, mashing it occasionally to form a chunky mixture. The filling should be moist but not overly juicy; if so, continue to cook and stir until excess liquid has evaporated. Remove from the heat and taste the filling, adjusting the seasoning with more salt and pepper, if necessary.

3. While the filling cools, prepare the corn dough. In a large mixing bowl, combine the *masarepa*, warm water, and salt. You can use a wooden spoon or your fingers to stir the ingredients together. Once the dough starts to thicken, use your fingers to knead the dough and eliminate any lumps. The dough should be soft, slightly moist, and dense. Keep covered with plastic wrap or a clean, damp kitchen towel when not using.

4. Line a large plate with paper towels or crumpled brown paper, for draining the oil from the empanadas. Preheat the vegetable oil for frying in a large heavy pot (cast iron is best) over medium-high heat. Make sure that there are at least 2 1/2 inches of oil in the pan, as the empanadas will need to be mostly covered in the oil to ensure even cooking. The oil is hot enough when a small piece of dough placed in the hot oil immediately starts to bubble rapidly and fry quickly. The idea is to use very hot (but never smoking) oil so that the outsides of the empanadas cook evenly without soaking up too much grease.

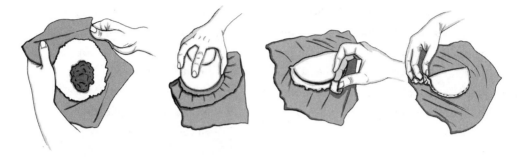

1. Holding plastic wrap, fold dough over empanada filling
2. Use a bowl or cup and firmly press on top of plastic wrap
3. Remove the bowl. Gather dough trimmings.
4. Empanada now has a sealed edge and half-moon shape

5. While the oil is heating, assemble the empanadas. Spread a large piece of plastic wrap on a work surface (do not use waxed paper; only plastic wrap will keep the dough from sticking) and have ready a rolling pin and a small bowl or large mug about 4 inches in diameter. Take a lump of dough a little less than 2 inches in diameter, roll into a ball, and place on the plastic wrap. Fold the plastic wrap on top of the dough (leaving about 5 inches free around the dough), flatten slightly, and proceed to roll the dough into a circle about 1/4 inch thick or slightly less.

6. Scoop a heaping tablespoon of filling into the center of the circle and, taking hold of the plastic underneath, fold the dough over to form a semicircle. Now for the fun part: turn your bowl upside down and line it up with the curve of the dough. Use it to firmly press down to cut through the dough. You've just sealed and trimmed the excess dough for a perfectly shaped empanada;

lift up the bowl and you'll see a cute half-moon pocket. Carefully lift off the plastic wrap, roll away the excess trimmed dough, and put the scraps back with the rest of the dough. (You can reroll corn dough scraps as much as you like, since there's no gluten to toughen.) Continue to fill, fold, and cut the empanadas.

7. To fry: Place the newly shaped empanada directly into the hot oil to fry. Depending on the size of the pot, fry two to three empanadas at a time; don't overcrowd the pan. (Keep extra unfried empanadas on a plastic-lined surface.) Fry for 6 to 8 minutes, turning each empanada occasionally with metal tongs or a slotted spoon. The empanadas are ready when their crust is golden, firm, and crisp on the edges. Remove from the oil, very carefully shake off any excess grease, and place on the paper-lined plate to drain for a minute or two. Serve immediately but be careful biting into a piping hot empanada. To bake: This is not at all traditional but an option if you'd rather not fry. Preheat the oven to 375°F. Oil a baking sheet or line it with parchment paper. Place the empanadas on the prepared sheet and lightly brush the tops with a little vegetable oil. Bake for 20 to 22 minutes, until their crust is firm and golden.

BEANS, RICE, AND SWEET PLANTAIN EMPANADAS

....

- Makes about 20 small empanadas
- Time: About 1 hour, including baking the plantains and frying everything
- Gluten Free, Soy Free (if the seitan is omitted)

....

These plump little empanadas are styled after the Venezuela national dish *pabellón criollo* and a bite of everything you require in a meal—beans, plantains, and rice (and perhaps a little shredded seitan, too). The filling for these guys entirely could also be crafted from leftovers of last night's vegan Latin feast. Any rice is welcome in the filling, any kind of seitan or tofu, and even a few bits of vegetables can be worked in for maximum tastiness: use leftover Fried Sweet Plantains (page 115) and black bean Home-style Refried Beans (page 86) instead of making the bean filling below. Serve with Colombian Green Onion Salsa (page 44), Creamy Avocado-Tomato Salsa (page 39), or your favorite hot sauce.

2 ripe plantains (yellow with black spots, soft when squeezed)

Black Bean Filling

2 tablespoons olive oil
2 cloves garlic, chopped
1 small yellow onion, diced
1/2 green bell pepper, seeded and diced
1 plum tomato, diced finely
1 teaspoon ground cumin
1/2 teaspoon dried oregano
1 (15-ounce) can black beans, drained and rinsed, or 2 cups cooked
1/4 cup vegetable broth or water
1/2 teaspoon salt, or to taste
Freshly ground black pepper

1 cup cooked rice, either plain white or any leftover flavored rice
1 recipe corn dough from Corn-Crusted Pumpkin-Potato Empanadas (page 207)

1. Preheat the oven to 350°F and tear off a 12-inch-long piece of aluminum foil. Peel the ripe plantains as directed for Fried Sweet Plantains (page 115), wrap in the foil, and bake for 18 to 20 minutes, until soft. Unwrap, let cool enough to handle, and dice into 1/2-inch-thick pieces.

2. While the plantains are baking, make the black beans. In a large, heavy cast-iron skillet, combine the oil and garlic over medium heat. Allow the garlic to sizzle for 30 seconds, then add the onion, bell pepper, and tomato. Using

VIVA VEGAN!

a wooden spoon to stir it occasionally, fry until the onion begins to turn translucent, 8 to 10 minutes. Sprinkle in the cumin and oregano and fry for another 30 seconds. Stir in the beans and vegetable broth and increase the heat to medium-high. Bring to a boil, then lower the heat to medium. Simmer for 15 to 20 minutes, until most of the liquid is absorbed and the beans are softened. Using a spoon, lightly mash the beans until the mixture is chunky. Remove from the heat and let cool enough to handle.

3. While the filling is cooling, prepare the corn dough according to the directions on page 208. Keep covered with plastic wrap or a clean, damp kitchen towel while not using.

4. Line a large plate with paper towels or crumpled brown paper for draining the oil from the empanadas. Preheat the vegetable oil for frying in a large, heavy pot (cast iron is best) over medium-high heat. Make sure that there are at least 2 inches of oil in the pan, as the empanadas will need to be mostly covered in the oil to ensure even cooking. The oil is hot enough when a small piece of dough placed in the hot oil immediately starts to bubble rapidly and fry quickly. The idea is to use very hot (but never smoking) oil so that the outsides of the empanadas cook evenly without soaking up too much grease.

5. While the oil is heating, assemble the empanadas: Spread a large piece of plastic wrap on a work surface (do not use waxed paper; only plastic wrap will keep the dough from sticking) and have ready a rolling pin and a small bowl or large mug about 4 inches in diameter. Take a lump of dough a little less than 2 inches in diameter, roll into a ball, and place on the plastic wrap. Fold the plastic wrap on top of dough (leaving about 5 inches free around the dough), flatten slightly, and proceed to roll the dough into a round about 1/4 inch or slightly less.

6. Scoop a heaping teaspoon *each* of plantains, beans, and rice into the center of the round. Taking hold of the plastic underneath, fold over the dough to form a semicircle. Turn your bowl upside down and line it up with the curve of the dough. Use it to firmly press down to cut through the dough. You've just sealed and trimmed the excess dough for a perfectly shaped empanada; lift up the bowl and you'll see a cute half-moon pocket. Carefully lift off the plastic wrap, roll away the excess trimmed dough, and put the scraps back with the rest of the dough. (You can reroll corn dough scraps as much as you like, since there's no gluten to toughen.) Continue to fill, fold, and cut the empanadas.

7. Either place the newly shaped empanada directly into the hot oil and start frying or set it down on a plastic-lined surface. When you're ready to fry, slide two or three empanadas into the preheated oil at a time, taking care not to overcrowd the pan. Fry for 6 to 8 minutes, turning each piece occasionally with metal tongs or a slotted spoon. The empanadas are ready when their crust is golden and firm and crisp on the edges.

8. Remove from the oil, very carefully shake off any excess grease, and place on the paper-lined plate to drain. Serve immediately, but be careful biting into a piping hot empanada. To bake: This is not at all traditional but an option if you'd rather not fry. Preheat the oven to 375ºF. Oil a baking sheet or line it with parch-ment paper. Place the empanadas on the pre-pared sheet and lightly brush the tops with a little vegetable oil. Bake for 20 to 22 minutes, until their crust is firm and golden. Serve hot.

Variation

Shredded Seitan: Use about half a recipe of Latin Shredded Seitan (or less, you don't need too much) and add a little bit (about a teaspoonful) to the other ingredients. Or re-place the rice entirely with shredded seitan.

Sweet Rice Pudding Empanadas

Empanadas can be sweeties, too. For a classy dessert-style empanada, fill small rounds (cut about 4 inches in diameter) of Wheat Dough (richer variation page 201) with 1/4 cup apiece of cooled Simply Arroz con Leche rice pudding (page 234). Assemble as directed for baked em-panadas, brush well with soy creamer, and sprinkle with cinnamon sugar (2 tablespoons of sugar plus 1/2 teaspoon of ground cinnamon) before baking. Bake in a preheated 350ºF oven for 20 to 24 minutes, or until golden brown. Serve warm and à la mode with a scoop of vegan vanilla ice cream!

13

DRINKS

Latin-style drinks are among the most memorable Latin food experiences. You never forget your first sip of fruity sangria, cup of thick spiced hot chocolate, or minty *mojito*. There are so many great Latin drinks out there I feel like it would take a lifetime to cover (or gulp) them all; with these recipes, you'll be on your way to getting a *refresco* in your hand faster than you can say *horchata!*

CREAMY HORCHATA

- Makes about 6 cups
- Time: About 30 minutes, not including overnight chilling
- Gluten Free, Soy Free

Horchata is the Mexican version of the rice-based beverages popular all over Latin America and the one that most North Americans have likely experienced. This recipe has a hint of lime and almonds, with a rich, smooth, and creamy finish. If you already enjoy rice milk, you'll love a frosty glass of *horchata* on a hot day or paired with spicy, salty foods. Top with grated cinnamon or chocolate for a flavorful garnish.

2 cups almond milk, preferably
    unsweetened, plus 2 additional cups
    almond milk or rice milk
2 cups water
2 (3-inch) sticks cinnamon
1/2 cup sugar
Zest from 1 lime, sliced into 1/2-inch strips
6 cloves
1/2 cup long-grain white rice
1/3 cup sliced almonds, lightly toasted and
    ground finely
Ground cinnamon or finely ground
    Mexican sweet drinking chocolate
    (Ibarra, for example), for garnish

1. In a large pot, combine 2 cups of the almond milk, and the water, cinnamon sticks, sugar, lime zest, cloves, rice, and ground toasted almonds. Cover and bring to boil, then lower the heat to a simmer; stir and cover. Cook for 20 minutes, stir,

and turn off the heat. Remove the lime zest, cover, and let the mixture cool to room temperature before transferring to the refrigerator to chill for at least 2 hours or overnight.

2. When the mixture is completely cool, stir in the additional almond milk and remove the cinnamon sticks. Strain by using one of these methods: layer cheesecloth on top of a small bowl, pour the mixture through, and then twist and squeeze the cheesecloth to extract as much liquid as possible. Or, pour the mixture through a fine metal sieve positioned over a bowl and gently press out any remaining liquid with a spoon. Many testers liked to save the drained rice and serve as a chunky cool rice pudding (just to be sure to remove the lime zest and cloves!)

3. Stir the *horchata* and chill; serve it very cold over ice cubes. Sprinkle each serving with ground cinnamon or finely grated sweet Mexican drinking chocolate.

Variation

Agavelicious Horchata: Substitute 1/3 cup of agave syrup for the sugar.

REAL BROWN SUGAR LIMEADE (AGUA DE PAPELÓN)

- ● **Makes about 1 1/2 quarts**
- ● **Time: Less than 15 minutes, not including chilling time**
- ● **Gluten Free, Soy Free**

This intensely flavored, amber-hued limeade is made with minimally refined sugar cane juice (*panela*) instead of run-of-the-mill brown sugar. Limeade like this is an old-fashioned pick-me-up beverage in Colombia and Venezuela, valued for being chock-full of minerals from the unprocessed *caña* and loved because, who doesn't like limeade? Serve it chilled with plenty of ice cubes and a slice of lime or mint sprig.

Papelón or *panela* (as it's called in Venezuela and Colombia) is perhaps the simplest cane sugar there is, produced by cooking the juice of freshly squeezed sugar cane down to a solid, crystallized mass. Look for it in Latin groceries, sold in heavy, dark round or rectangular cakes. The old-fashioned way to make *agua de papelón* is to soak the *panela* in water overnight until it dissolves. My dad does this, but impatient types like me prefer to cook the *panela* to a simple syrup for faster *agua* drinking pleasures. This recipe easily doubles and the undiluted syrup keeps well in a tightly covered container in the fridge.

$1/2$ pound *panela* (also called *papelón*
or *piloncillo*)
1 cup water
$1/2$ cup freshly squeezed lime juice
3 cups cold water
Thin slices lime or mint leaves,
for garnish

1. Using a sharp, heavy knife, coarsely chop the *panela* into $1/2$-inch pieces. Place in a large saucepan, cover with the water, and bring to a boil over medium heat. Reduce and stir occasionally until the sugar has melted, about 5 minutes, then remove from the heat and let cool. Stir in the lime juice. Then, either store the syrup in a glass or plastic, covered container in the refrigerator or, if serving immediately, pour into a large pitcher.

2. To serve limeade, add the cold water to the pitcher, stir well, and pour into chilled glasses filled with ice cubes. Garnish with lime slices or mint. This syrup is slightly concentrated to compensate for melting ice cubes but, if desired, dilute more or use less water for very sweet *agua de papelón*.

TROPICAL FRUIT SHAKE (BATIDO)

- Makes 1 drink, about 12 ounces
- Time: Less than 10 minutes
- Gluten Free, can be made Soy Free

The original fruit smoothies, *batidos* made with local tropical fruits have been keeping Latin Americans cool for generations. And healthy, too, as tropical fruits are loaded with vitamins, antioxidants, and in the case of papayas and pineapples, plenty of digestive enzymes, too. Unfortunately, most fresh tropical fruits travel terribly, becoming flavorless by the time they've arrived north to our supermarkets.

But there's a superconvenient solution! Most any Latin American market will have packets of great-tasting frozen tropical fruit pulp in the freezer section. There's no washing, peeling, or seed-picking, either.

Water-based *batidos* are light and refreshing enough to drink every day; add richer vegan milks or even vegan ice cream for a more luxurious treat.

Mixing Your Batido

When you're blending, try different (or multiple) frozen fruit purees! Sweet purees such as *mamay*, *piña* (pineapple), or papaya may not need much sugar or any. Other sour purees such as passion fruit (sometimes called *maracuyá*), *lulo* or *naranjilla* (a sour orange consumed in Colombia), or *tamarindo* (tamarind) will need considerably more. Some fruits fall somewhere in between like *mora* (Andean blackberry) or my favorite, *guanábana* (also called soursop), so when adding sugar to fruit shakes, go easy at first, then add more after everything has been blended. Keep a selection of purees in reasealable plastic bags in the freezer for a quick *batido* anytime.

4 to 5 ounces frozen tropical
   fruit puree, such as papaya,
   guanábana, *mamay*, *mora* (Andean
   blackberry), *tamarillo*, *lulo*, passion
   fruit, or coconut
1 cup ice cold water or almond milk,
   rice milk, or favorite nondairy milk
Agave syrup or sugar to taste,
   anywhere from 1 to 3 tablespoons
A handful of ice cubes (optional)

1. Break the frozen fruit puree into chunks and place in a blender jar. Add the remaining ingredients and pulse on the "ice crushing" setting, blending until the fruit and ice are blended and the *batido* is frothy. Pour into a tall glass and serve immediately.

Variations

Merengada: Use rich soy milk and add 3 tablespoons cold nondairy soy creamer for a smoother, richer Latin-style fruit "milkshake." Sneaking in a little vegan vanilla ice cream is great for an extra-special treat.

Truly Tropical Banana Smoothie: Add 1 frozen banana, chopped, along with the rest of the ingredients, and blend for a thick tropical smoothie. You can get away with using less sugar to compensate for the banana's natural sweetness.

REAL HOT CHOCOLATE AND VARIATIONS

- Serves 4
- Time: Less than 15 minutes
- Gluten Free, can be made Soy Free

Chocolate: we all love it and want it the world over. In chocolate's hometown, Central and South America, the traditional way to get your daily allowance is via a warm, soothing "real" cup of creamy hot chocolate made with Latin-style drinking chocolate bars—never cocoa powder mixes!—and your favorite nondairy milk of choice.

Drinking chocolate is typically flavored with spices, vanilla, or nuts and varies from country of origin: the Mexican brand Ibarra features almonds and cinnamon; the Colombian brand Lukar is spiked with ground cloves. My new favorite brand, Taza, is actually made in Massachusetts; go figure. Most Latin drinking chocolate is vegan. Although I've yet to see one that had any sneaky dairy products added, just to be sure to always read the ingredients.

Tip: Most directions on drinking chocolate packages call for about an ounce of chocolate per serving. I've increased it a little for smoother, richer flavor with more foam. A low-calorie drink this is not, but what else is better on a chilly autumn evening?

6 ounces any Latin-style drinking
   chocolate bars, chopped coarsely
1/3 cup water
3 1/2 cups soy, almond, rice, hemp, or other
   nondairy milk, or a combination

1. In a 2-quart saucepan with a lid, combine the chocolate and water. Bring to a simmer over medium heat, stirring to melt the chocolate. Stir in the nondairy milk and continue to heat until steaming, but take care not to boil, 6 to 8 minutes.

> Latin-style hot chocolate is often whisked or beaten to produce a creamy foam topping. Most famous of these special instruments is the Mexican *molinillo* which looks like the funky lovechild of a rattle and a scepter and is briskly rolled between one's palms. If you don't have one, don't worry—a wire whisk or a handheld immersion blender fitted with a whisk attachment is just as effective.

2. Turn off the heat and use a *molinillo*, wire whisk, or a handheld immersion blender to beat the chocolate until a thick layer of foam forms on top, anywhere from 2 to 6 minutes. Alternatively, try pouring the hot chocolate into a blender jar and pulse for 45 seconds or more to create the foam. Ladle the chocolate into serving cups, making sure to include a serving of foam on top of each.

Variations

For richer chocolate: replace 1 cup of the nondairy milk with soy creamer or coconut milk.

Toddy Caliente: Simmer the nondairy milk with a cinnamon stick or piece of orange zest. Remove before beating either by hand or with a blender. Spike each hot chocolate with a tablespoon of rum, Kahlúa, or brandy.

Quiero Vegan Café con Leche!

Before there was a big national coffee chain on every corner, Americans in the know could satisfy that craving for a creamy coffee at any decent Latin bakery (especially a Cuban or Puerto Rican one). *Café con leche* is what we've come to know as a latte, perhaps milkier and less foamy that the stuff served at the corporate coffee joint. For a homemade *café con leche* experience, anything from a basic stovetop espresso pot to a full-service espresso machine works just fine.

   Cuban-style Coffee: Sweet Cuban-style coffee is fun to make at home. For authentic flavor, look for deep, dark, Cuban-style espresso roast coffee; Bustelo brand is plentiful and cheap in New York City supermarkets, for example.

   Place 2 tablespoons (or more!) of sugar into the base of your espresso pot, brew the coffee as directed, and as the coffee drips into the pot, it will dissolve the sugar. Be sure to remove

continues

your espresso maker pot just prior to when the brewing stops to prevent the coffee from spilling over. Stir the espresso slightly, then pour into demitasse cups and serve.

Alternative method: If you don't feel like sugaring up your stovetop espresso pot or machine, an easy alternative is to brew your espresso as usual and pour the sugar into a small (less than 6-ounce) coffee cup or a small milk pitcher. This cup should be just large enough to contain your entire serving of brewed espresso when finished. Drizzle in a teaspoon of hot espresso and stir vigorously with a small spoon to form a creamy paste with no sugary grit. If the sugar doesn't completely dissolve, drizzle in a little more espresso and continue stirring until smooth. Now slowly pour the remaining hot espresso into the paste while constantly stirring. A well-made *cafécito* will have a thin layer of light brown foam, the *espumita*, on top, but if it doesn't, you'll still have one high-powered shot of espresso.

Café con Leche: Consumed everywhere in Latin America, if *café con leche* is your ultimate destination, stir a steamed (or microwaved until hot) cup of your favorite nondairy milk into your sweet little shot of espresso. Thick creamy hemp or coconut-based (not actual coconut) milk is *fabuloso*!

For a complete Cubano café experience, serve with a slice of crusty bread, well buttered with your favorite vegan margarine and pressed until browned and crunchy in a panini grill (or use the technique for Cubano Vegano Sandwiches on page 66) and enjoy bites of buttery toast along with sips of sweet creamy coffee. Ahhhh, *sabroso*!

SIMPLE SYRUP

- Makes 1 cup
- Time: Less than 10 minutes
- Gluten Free, Soy Free

Simple syrup is the basis of lots of easy-to-make cocktails and even frozen desserts such as Fresh Papaya-Lime Sorbet (page 239). Make a batch and keep it chilled, and you'll always be prepared for impromptu parties. This recipe is easily halved or doubled.

1 cup sugar
1 cup water

1. Combine the water and sugar in a small saucepan and bring to a boil over high heat. Lower the heat to a simmer, stir, and cook for another 5 minutes, until all the sugar has been dissolved. Remove from the heat and let cool to room temperature. To speed up the cooling process, fill a large metal mixing bowl with ice, cover with cold water, and carefully settle the saucepan into the bowl, making sure the ice water doesn't spill over into the syrup. Let sit for 15 to 20 minutes until cold.

Make-ahead Tip: If you're in no rush, you can make the syrup up to a week in advance and store it in the refrigerator in a tightly covered container until ready to use.

SANGRIA

- Makes 2 liters
- Time: 30 minutes
- Gluten Free, Soy Free

It's not a Spanish meal without this timeless blend of wine, brandy, and fruit juice. Although sangria is often associated with the Old World, it's enjoyed all over the Americas. Oranges, lemons, or apples are classic additions, but I gravitate toward tropical fare such as papaya, mango, or pineapple. It is strong, but you can go easy on the brandy, if you like, or toss in an ice cube for a gentler sangria.

A good sangria can be—or even *should* be—crafted out of inexpensive dry red wine and brandy. Rigging up wine with fruit and liquor would ruin that spendy twenty-year-old vintage. But say you do want special-occasion sangria. Then it's time to invest in a good brandy such as apple-scented Calvados, stir in a few shots of Grand Marnier, and power-boost that sangria with a crushed (and vegan) port wine.

1 orange (preferably a Valencia or "juice" orange)
1 lemon
1/2 cup simple syrup (page 218)
2/3 cup brandy
1/2 cup freshly squeezed orange juice
2 tablespoons freshly squeezed lemon juice
3 cups mixed fresh fruit, such as apple, papaya, pineapple, mango, any melon, strawberries, or raspberries, chopped into bite-size pieces
1 (750 ml) bottle dry red wine, chilled
Ice cubes (optional)

1. Wash the orange and lemon well. Use a heavy, sharp chef's knife to quarter the fruit and slice each piece into paper-thin slices, discarding any seeds. In a large glass pitcher, combine the simple syrup, brandy, orange juice, lemon juice, sliced orange, lemon, and chopped fruit. Stir and set aside for 30 minutes for the fruit to absorb the brandy flavors.

2. Before serving, pour the chilled red wine into the pitcher and stir into the brandy mixture. To serve, pour the sangria into 16-ounce glasses and use a large spoon to ladle in plenty of fruit. Serve immediately. If desired, add a few ice cubes to help temper the alcohol.

Make-ahead Tip: Prepare the fruit and soak in the brandy mixture up to a day in advance of stirring into the wine.

Variations
Use a good-quality fruity brandy, such as Calvados.

Add 2 tablespoons of the following: A sweet crushed port wine, Grand Marnier or Cointreau, or a good cherry brandy.

For a sweeter sangria, stir in more simple syrup.

MOJITO

- Serves 1
- Time: Less than 10 minutes
- Gluten Free, Soy Free

Simple syrup makes this effortless. A mojito in hand, and that next sweltering summer evening in your apartment could be considered just "tropical."

> ¼ cup loosely packed whole mint leaves
>   (remove stems)
> 1 tablespoon lime juice
> 2 tablespoons simple syrup (page 218)
> 2 tablespoons light rum
> Ice cubes
> Chilled club soda
> Mint sprigs or thin lime slice, for garnish

1. Place the mint leaves in a tall, narrow glass and add the lime juice and simple syrup. With either a muddler (special bar tool for these things) or the opposite end of a long wooden spoon, gently crush the mint while stirring the juice and syrup into the leaves. Do this for about a minute, then add rum. Pile in ice cubes and pour in enough chilled club soda to almost reach the top of the glass. Top off with a mint spring or lime slice and a swizzle stick. Stir and sip and contemplate the joys of drinking your greens (minty greens, that is).

MICHELADA
(SPICY, SALTY, ICE-COLD BEER)

- Serves 1
- Time: Less than 10 minutes
- Gluten Free

Need a break from margaritas and mojitos? It's the enigmatic Michelada or *cerveza preparado* to the rescue, a fascinating marriage of ice-spiked beer, lime, salt, and savory hot sauce. Before you toss this book aside and grab a pitcher of mango daiquiris, hear me out! Micheladas are especially suited for fans of beer, Bloody Marys, or salted margaritas. Experiment with your favorite hot sauce and Mexican beer for a different kind of Michelada for every day in the summer.

Tip: The salt and chile powder mixture makes enough for two or more Micheladas, and it's easy enough to store in a tightly covered container for when the next heat wave strikes. The sharp, bright flavors of pequín and costeño chiles contrast perfectly with beer; follow the chile toasting and grinding instructions on page 264 to make your own for truly memorable Micheladas.

> 1 tablespoon coarse margarita salt or
>   kosher salt
> ¼ teaspoon ground Mexican chile powder
>   or ground dried chile, such as pequín or
>   costeño chiles

Lime wedge, plus another for garnish

1 tablespoon freshly squeezed lime juice

1 to 2 teaspoons Mexican hot sauce, or more to taste

1 dash vegan Worcestershire sauce

Ice cubes

1 (12-ounce) bottle Mexican beer, chilled

1. If desired, chill a tall 16-ounce beer glass in the freezer for an hour before serving, so that it gets frosty. Stir together the coarse salt and chile powder in a small saucer. Take a lime wedge and rub it along the rim of the beer glass, then dip the wet rim into the salt mixture, twisting the glass to coat the rim evenly. At the bottom of the glass, stir together the tablespoon of lime juice, hot sauce, and Worcestershire sauce. Fill the glass with ice cubes and pour in the chilled beer to the top, stir a few times, and garnish with the remaining lime wedge. Serve immediately.

14

DESSERTS AND SWEETS

*B*reakfast, or really any time, is a good time for a *postre* or *dulce*. European-style cakes and pastries are popular all over Latin America, but I suspect you came here to indulge in crunchy churros, billowy sopaipillas, creamy caramel flan, or sweet treats filled with tropical flavor.

Latin desserts are typically very sweet, more so than American or European palates might be used to. Also, a few old-fashioned Latin American desserts are made with ingredients that may surprise you: corn, sweet potatoes, and pumpkin. Fans of puddings have come to the right place—puddings of all kinds have a special place in Latin kitchens. Often made with grains and fruits, these desserts are substantial enough for a breakfast treat. For something more decadent, try the caramel-sweet *dulce de leche* that transforms any standard dessert—or crepes or shortbread rounds—into dessert *en Español*. It can even be enjoyed straight up with a spoon (as many testers can attest to, and maybe you, too!).

CHURROS

- **Makes about two dozen 4-inch churros**

Churros are fingers or loops of sugar-coated fried pastry that, not to be outdone, are served with cups of thick hot chocolate. Churros are sometimes considered doughnuts, but may I be brash and say they're better: they have a light crunch, come in fun-to-eat shapes, and most important, are so easy (maybe too easy) to make at home. Churros can vary from country to country in shape and size: in Venezuela, they're shaped into dainty loops, whereas Mexican churros are quite long and spiked with cinnamon, for example. You may already be familiar with the Mexican-style cinnamon-sugared churro, but many Latin countries like their churros with just a dusting of granulated sugar.

For general deep-frying tips, see Deep-frying on page 261. Making churros is one of those special occasions worth pouring cups of oil into a pan. Share them with friends or family as a weekend treat to spread the goodness around.

Tip: A *churrera* is special tool that sort of looks like a cookie press and is specially made for making churros. If you are in the habit of churros, it might be wise to invest in one of these, but for the rest of us there's good old pastry bags and pastry tips. Look for a star-shaped tip in a large but not huge size . . . one with a tip around ³⁄₈ inch wide at the opening should work just fine. For home frying, simple 4- to 5-inch sticks of dough at this thickness are easy to press out with a pastry bag and fry up nicely.

Speaking of a cookie press, that could work, too, if you have a tip or plate that's around the same dimensions of a large star-shaped pastry tip.

1 cup all-purpose flour
1 tablespoon tapioca flour or
   cornstarch
1/8 teaspoon baking soda
1/4 teaspoon salt
11/4 cups water
1 rounded tablespoon dark brown sugar
1 tablespoon nonhydrogenated vegan
   margarine
1/4 teaspoon vanilla extract
Mild-flavored vegetable oil (canola, corn,
   sunflower, or a blend) for deep-frying,
   enough for at least a 2-inch depth

Sugar for Rolling the Churros
1/4 cup granulated sugar
1/4 teaspoon ground cinnamon for
   Mexican-style churros (optional)

1. In a mixing bowl, combine the flour, tapioca flour, baking soda, and salt. In a large saucepan, combine the water and brown sugar and bring to a boil, then add the margarine and heat until melted. Lower the heat to low, stir in the vanilla, and pour in a little of the flour mixture at a time, mixing constantly with a silicone spatula or large fork. The mixture will look lumpy at first, but continue to add flour and stir; it will be very thick but don't let it stop you, just keep stirring! After all of the flour has been added, remove from the heat and continue to stir for about a minute, to form a thick, smooth dough. For this last step, you may find it easier to scoop the dough into a mixing bowl, but if your pan is large enough you can continue mixing it there. Let the dough cool for 10 minutes.

2. While the dough cools, pour the frying oil into a 3-quart heavy pot (cast iron is best) and preheat over medium-high heat. Make sure that there are at least 2 inches of oil as, to cook properly, churros should be able to float in the oil. Cover a large plate with paper towels or crumpled brown paper for draining the hot churros. The oil will need anywhere from 10 to 14 minutes to get hot enough (but not smoking); when at the correct temperature, the hot oil will have a gently rippling surface. The idea is that the oil will be sufficiently hot for the

churros to cook evenly without soaking up too much grease.

3. Fit a large pastry bag with a large star-tip nozzle. Use a rubber spatula to scoop the dough into the bag; grab the ends of the bag and shake several times so that the dough drops farther down toward the nozzle. Gather the top ends of the bag and firmly twist toward the dough so that it will press out of the nozzle when you're ready to fry. If you're using a *churrero* or cookie press, follow the manufacturer's directions for assembling and loading with the dough.

4. Spread the sugar on a dinner plate, stirring in the cinnamon, if using.

5. Test the oil to see if it's ready by pinching off about 1/4 teaspoon of dough and dropping it into the hot oil. Immediately, it should start to bubble rapidly and to fry quickly. To make the churros: twist down the top of your pastry bag, squeeze the top, and press a length of dough about 4 inches long directly into the hot oil. Use your fingers or sharp kitchen scissors to pinch the churros free from the pastry tip. *While you're at it, please be careful around hot oil and never, ever drop water into hot oil.* You can fry up to five churros at a time in a 10-inch pot without crowding them; just take care not to squeeze dough directly onto another frying churro. Use either metal tongs or a metal slotted spoon to gently turn the churros occasionally. Fry for 4 to 6 minutes, or until the churros are firm and slightly golden. Remove from the oil, very carefully shake off any excess oil, and place on the paper-lined plate to drain.

6. I like to let churros cool for 2 to 3 minutes (rather than dumping piping hot into the sugar, where it can create an oily mess), before placing them in the sugar and gently rolling to coat. Serve warm with hot chocolate.

CHOCOLATE PARA CHURROS

- Makes four 1/2-cup servings of thick chocolate
- Gluten Free, can be made Soy Free

Compared to Real Hot Chocolate (page 216), this recipe is much thicker, like a smooth, thin pudding, and is designed for dipping your freshly made churros. If you prefer frothy chocolate, prepare Real Hot Chocolate instead. Make *chocolate para churros* while the dough is cooling, keep it covered in a pan on the stovetop, and give it a brisk whisk right before serving.

4 ounces sweetened Latin drinking
    chocolate (any brand, such as
    Ibarra, Lukar, or Sol), chopped
    coarsely
1/3 cup water
1²/3 cups nondairy milk, such as almond,
    soy, hemp, or a combination
2 teaspoons cornstarch

1. In a 2-quart saucepan with a lid, combine the chocolate and water. Bring to a simmer over medium heat, stirring to melt the chocolate. Whisk in 1⅓ cups of the nondairy milk and continue to heat until steaming (take care not to boil), about 8 minutes. In a measuring cup, stir together the remaining ⅓ cup milk and the cornstarch until dissolved. Pour into the steaming milk and stir constantly until the mixture thickens slightly, 4 to 5 minutes. This can happen suddenly, so keep stirring for an accurate measure of the consistency. Taste: the cornstarch is cooked when the chocolate does not taste chalky but instead has a smooth texture. Turn off the heat and cover the pan. When ready to serve, whisk the chocolate and pour into four cups. Serve with warm churros.

SOPAIPILLAS WITH ORANGE FLOWER–AGAVE "HONEY"

....

● **Makes 2 dozen or more fried pastries**

....

This recipe for little puffy fried pillows of dough is derived from my mom's Mexican friend Rosa Maria's other Mexican friend Elva from her travels in New Mexico, for a cross the border and back again experience. I've replaced the traditional honey accompaniment with agave syrup; its consistency is similar to that of a light honey, plus a gentle simmer with cinnamon and citrus further deepens this vegan alternative. The not-so-secret ingredient of orange flower water adds a special floral aroma to the agave syrup, for additional honeylike flavor.

Tip: Orange flower water is made by a distillation of orange flowers in water and is usually imported from France. It doesn't taste like oranges at all, but instead has a spicy floral perfume and flavor. Look for it in the baking aisle or baking extracts section in fancy gourmet stores. If you can't find it, just leave it out of the recipe.

> 2 cups all-purpose flour
> 2¼ teaspoons baking powder
> ¼ teaspoon salt
> 1 tablespoon light brown sugar
> ¼ teaspoon vanilla extract
> ⅔ cup soy, almond, or other nondairy milk
> 2 tablespoons nonhydrogenated margarine, slightly softened
> Peanut oil or vegetable oil, for deep-frying

Agave "Honey"
> ½ cup agave syrup, preferably dark
> 1 tablespoon water
> 1 (3-inch) stick cinnamon
> Thin 1-inch sliver lime or lemon zest
> ⅛ teaspoon orange flower water (optional)

1. In a large mixing bowl, stir together the flour, baking powder, and salt. In a mixing cup,

stir the brown sugar and vanilla extract into the soy milk until mostly dissolved. Add softened margarine to the flour mixture and use a pastry cutter or a fork to blend it into flour to form a sandy mixture. Make a well in the center of the mixture.

2. Gradually stir in the soy milk mixture and mix until a soft dough forms. Lightly knead for about 2 minutes, then divide the dough into two portions and flatten each piece into a rough square shape. Wrap in plastic wrap or waxed paper. Let the dough rest for half an hour at room temperature (this will help the gluten relax and make rolling easier). While the dough is resting, prepare the agave honey.

3. In a large cast-iron Dutch oven or similar large heavy pot, heat about 2¹/2 inches of oil over medium-high heat. The oil will need about 10 minutes to get hot enough (around 350ºF; see Churros [page 223] for additional deep-frying information); while the oil is heating, lightly flour a large work surface and rolling pin. Roll a piece of dough into a very thin rectangle, 1/8 of an inch thick or slightly less. Use a sharp knife to cut squares or diamonds 3 to 3¹/2 inches long. Trim any ragged edges from the dough. Repeat with the remaining dough.

4. Test the oil by dropping a scrap of dough into the hot oil. It should fry very rapidly and puff up within 30 seconds. Fry three or four sopaipillas at a time, until golden on each side and puffed, 1 to 1¹/2 minutes per side. Do not crowd the pan; overcrowding may cool the oil and prevent the dough from puffing properly. Use a mesh skimmer or tongs to carefully transfer the sopaipillas onto layered paper towels or crumpled brown paper to drain. Serve warm, either drizzled with agave syrup or serving it on the side as a dip.

5. Prepare the Agave "Honey": Combine all of the ingredients except for the orange flower water in a small saucepan. Bring the mixture to a gentle boil over medium heat, lower the heat to low, and simmer for 10 minutes . Turn off the heat, stir in the orange flower water, and set aside to cool for 10 minutes. Remove the cinnamon stick and lime zest and serve.

UN-DULCE DE LECHE

- **Makes about 1¹/2 cups**
- **Time: 45 minutes**

This Latin confection has really broken though to the American public, showing up recently in all kinds of things from ice cream to yogurt. For good reason: the sticky caramel-like sauce can be drizzled onto any cake, pudding, or ice cream, wherever a blast of Latin sweetness is required. It's ridiculously indulgent served with warm churros (instead of dusting with sugar) or sopaipillas. Or play innocent and use it as a fondue to dip fresh tropical fruit (or cookies).

Tip: Brown rice syrup's consistency and flavor plays a big part in this sauce; there's no substitute for it!

1 cup soy creamer or rich soy milk

4 teaspoons tapioca flour or arrowroot powder

1/2 cup brown rice syrup

1/2 cup light brown sugar

2 tablespoons nonhydrogenated vegan margarine

1 1/2 teaspoons vanilla extract

1. In a measuring cup, whisk together 1/4 cup of the soy creamer and the tapioca flour and set aside. In a large saucepan, combine the remaining 3/4 cup of soy creamer, and the brown rice syrup and brown sugar, and bring to a slow boil over medium heat. Stir in the margarine and lower the heat to low. Simmer the sauce for 30 minutes, stirring occasionally. The mixture should resemble a thick caramel sauce and easily coat the back of a wooden spoon.

2. Whisk the tapioca flour mixture again and stir it slowly into the simmering sauce. Continue stirring until the sauce thickens even more, simmering for another 10 minutes. Remove from the heat and stir in the vanilla. The sauce is now ready to use, yay!

3. Store extra *dulce* in a tightly covered container in the fridge; it lasts for weeks if not forever.

CREPES WITH UN-DULCE DE LECHE AND SWEET PLANTAINS

● Serves 4, two crepes each

● Time: About 45 minutes, not including making the sauce

Nothing says "Hey, I freakin' love you!" like serving your friends or *familia* or future special someone (no pressure!) some gorgeous Latin dessert crepes with sautéed sweet plantains and drizzled with buttery Un-Dulce de Leche sauce (page 227). Escalate the richness with a scoop of vanilla ice cream (especially a fantastic coconut-based nondairy ice cream).

Tip: For an epic discussion on how to identify and handle really sweet ripe plantains, see page 116.

Make-ahead Tips: There are several components to this recipe, so don't mess around, especially if you plan on serving these crepes for dessert after a more elaborate meal. Make the crepes up to three days ahead: stack them on a dinner plate, cover with plastic wrap, and chill. Reheat briefly on a preheated oiled griddle, for about 1 minute or until hot, flipping once. You can also make the *dulce* sauce up to a week in advance; just keep chilled and heat on the stovetop or in a microwave for 40 to 50 seconds, stirring occasionally, until warm. You could even fry the plantains that day, chill, and either microwave or briefly heat on the stovetop.

Crepe-making Tip: A few items that will make your crepe-making experience all the easier: a silicone basting brush (which can withstand contact with a hot pan), non-stick cooking spray, a crumpled paper towel for wiping the crepe pan or skillet, and a long, thin spatula (like the kind used to frost cakes) for turning the crepes.

Crepes

- 1½ cups soy or almond milk
- ⅓ cup cold water
- ¾ cup all-purpose or whole wheat pastry flour
- ⅓ cup chickpea (garbanzo) flour
- 2 tablespoons sugar
- ½ teaspoon salt
- Nonstick cooking spray and/or softened nonhydrogenated vegan margarine

Brown-Sugared Sweet Plantains

- 4 very ripe plantains (most black with dark yellow–streaked skin, should feel soft when gently squeezed)
- 4 tablespoons nonhydrogenated vegan margarine
- 4 tablespoons brown sugar
- 4 teaspoons lime juice
- 4 tablespoons dark or spiced rum
- Nonstick cooking spray

For Assembly

- 1 recipe Un-Dulce de Leche (page 227), gently warmed on the stove or microwave

1. For the crepes: In a blender jar, combine the soy milk, water, flour, chickpea flour, sugar, and salt. Pulse until you have a smooth, thin batter. Pour into a container, cover, and chill for at least an hour or overnight. When ready to cook, stir the batter briefly if the ingredients have separated. Heat a 10- to 12-inch crepe pan or skillet over medium-high heat; the skillet is ready when a few drops of water flicked onto the pan sizzle. Spray with nonstick cooking spray. For additional buttery flavor, dab a silicone brush into softened nonhydrogenated margarine and brush along the bottom and sides of pan, but you can skip this if you use plenty of nonstick spray for each crepe.

2. Ladle ⅓ to ½ cup (use the larger quantity for a bigger pan) of batter into the center of the pan. As the batter starts to sizzle, immediately begin to tilt the pan (use your wrist) in a circular motion to spread a thin layer of batter to the edges of the pan. Continue to tilt the pan as the batter spreads and then sets. If you're new to crepes, you'll find you get better the more you make them; often your first crepe isn't nearly as nice as the last one in the batch.

3. Cook the crepe until the top looks dry and the edges appear firm, 1 to 1½ minutes. Gently run the spatula (a long, thin one works

ideally here) under the crepe to loosen it, carefully flip the crepe, and cook it on the other side for 30 seconds. Slide the crepe onto a dinner plate. Spray more oil or brush more margarine onto the crepe pan before starting the next crepe; if the crepes start to stick, give the pan another hit of nonstick cooking spray. If bits of batter collect on the pan or the pan seems too oily, quickly swirl the crumpled paper towel across the surface of the pan to remove the crumbs. Cook the rest of the crepes, stacking them one on top of another. If not serving immediately, cover the entire batch with plastic wrap and store in the refrigerator.

4. For the fried sweet plantains: Preheat a cast-iron or nonstick skillet over medium heat. On a cutting board, use a very sharp paring knife to slice both ends off a plantain and run a shallow cut—only deep enough to slice the skin but not the flesh—from one end of the plantain to the other. Peel off the skin and slice on a bias into 1/2-inch-thick slices.

5. Spray the preheated pan with nonstick cooking spray and melt a tablespoon of margarine on its surface. Slide one-third of the plantain slices into the pan and fry for 4 to 6 minutes, flipping a few times until the plantains are soft and turning golden. Sprinkle with one-third of the brown sugar, lime juice, and rum and sauté for another 2 to 4 minutes to gently caramelize the surface of the plantains. Remove from the pan and repeat with the re-

maining plantains. If the surface of your pan gets too sticky, wipe with a paper towel before frying more plantains. Cover the cooked plantains with foil, or warm them in the oven or microwave (remove foil first if microwaving) if they start to get too cold.

6. To assemble: Lay a crepe on a serving plate, drizzle half of the crepe (a semicircle) with some Un-Dulce de Leche, and layer that part with three or more slices of plantain. Fold the crepe in half, drizzle half that surface with more sauce, add three or more slices of plantain, and fold again so that now you have a curvy triangle. Top with another plantain slice and more *dulce*. Repeat on the same plate if you're serving two at a time.

Variation

Crepes à la Mode: Top a crepe with a scoop of favorite vegan vanilla ice cream and, you guessed it, drizzle with more dulce sauce!

COCONUT TRES LECHES CAKE

- **Serves 9**
- **Time: About 1 1/2 hours including baking time, not including overnight chilling**

Literally "milk cake," Tres Leches Cake may sound a little ambiguous but it's just a sweet spongy cake moistened in milky syrup, covered with a creamy topping and garnished with fresh fruit. The thing about nonvegan Tres Leches Cake is that it's really only *una leche*—it's like saying, "cow, cow, cow." This sublime vegan adaptation makes it real with three totally different milks: coconut milk, silky almond milk or rice milk, and versatile soy milk.

What likely originated in Nicaragua has found a home across the cuisines of Latin America. This vegan incarnation of this cake leans heavily (and heavenly) with coconut for a tropical Caribbean vibe. Make this cake a day in advance, as it really benefits from a long rest in the refrigerator.

Tip: The easiest way to obtain coconut cream is to open a full-fat (don't use lite) can of coconut milk and skim it off the top. Or look for little cans of coconut cream (usually sold for mixing up piña coladas) or semisolid bars of creamed coconut. Either of these work great for the topping (but be sure to read the ingredients list to make sure they're vegan).

Cake

- 1 cup soy milk
- 1 tablespoon lemon juice
- 1/3 cup canola oil
- 3/4 cup sugar
- 2 teaspoons vanilla extract
- 1/2 teaspoon coconut, lemon, or orange extract
- 1 1/4 cups all-purpose flour
- 3 tablespoons cornstarch
- 1 teaspoon baking powder
- 1/4 teaspoon baking soda
- 1/4 teaspoon salt

Soaking Syrup

- 1 cup regular or lite coconut milk
- 2/3 cup almond milk
- 1/3 cup granulated sugar
- 1/3 cup light brown sugar
- A big pinch of ground cinnamon
- 2 tablespoons light or spiced rum

Topping

- 6 ounces soft silken tofu (half of an aseptic water-packed tofu block)
- 3 tablespoons coconut cream
- 1/3 cup water
- 1/2 teaspoon agar flakes, or 1/4 teaspoon agar powder
- 1/2 cup granulated sugar
- 1/4 cup rice milk or additional almond milk
- 2 tablespoons tapioca flour or arrowroot
- 1/2 teaspoon vanilla or orange extract

For Assembly

- 1/3 cup grated coconut
- Fresh strawberries or blackberries or chunks of mango or pineapple, for garnish

1. Make the cake first. Preheat the oven to 350°F and oil an 8-inch square baking pan. In a mixing bowl, stir together the soy milk and lemon juice; the mixture will appear to curdle. Stir in the oil, sugar, vanilla, and coconut extract

and whisk until smooth. Sift in the flour, cornstarch, baking powder, baking soda, and salt. Gently fold in the dry ingredients just enough to moisten; do not overmix, a few small lumps are okay. Pour into the prepared baking pan, spreading it evenly and using a rubber spatula to completely scrape all of the batter out of the bowl. Bake for 30 to 32 minutes, or until a toothpick inserted into the center of the cake comes out clean. Remove the cake from the oven, let cool for a minute or two, then use a toothpick to poke holes into the cake at about 1/2-inch intervals.

2. While the cake is baking, make the soaking syrup. Mix all the syrup ingredients except the rum in a small saucepan and bring to a slow boil over medium-high heat, stirring the mixture constantly with a wire whisk. After the mixture has boiled for about 1 minute, lower the heat to low. Simmer the syrup for 30 minutes, stirring occasionally, until the mixture has a syrupy consistency and coats the back of a spoon. Remove from the heat and let cool for 10 minutes. Stir in the rum and drizzle over the warm cake . . . it's important that the cake be warm so that the syrup can be better absorbed. Cover the cake with plastic wrap and chill for at least 4 hours or, even better, overnight. Some extra syrup may not be completely absorbed by the cake but no worries—everything will still taste great.

3. To prepare the topping: Blend the silken tofu with the coconut cream in a food proces-

sor until smooth. In a small saucepan, combine the water and agar flakes and bring to a boil over medium-high heat, stirring constantly. Lower the heat and simmer for 4 to 5 minute to melt the agar flakes. A few tiny specks of agar remaining is fine, but most of it should be dissolved. Add the sugar and stir to dissolve. In a mixing cup, use a fork or wire whisk to whisk together the rice milk and tapioca flour. Pour this mixture into the agar mixture and cook, stirring constantly, until thickened, 3 to 5 minutes. The mixture should taste smooth and not chalky. Use a rubber spatula to scrape the mixture into a food processor and add the silken tofu. Blend until very smooth. Add the vanilla and pulse one more time to incorporate it.

4. Remove the plastic from the top of the cake and spread the tofu mixture evenly over the top. Sprinkle with the grated coconut, cover the cake, and chill for about 11/2 hours or until the topping is completely cooled and has firmed up slightly. Cut into nine squares and serve chilled, topped with sliced fresh fruit.

FRESH MANGO AND GUAVA BREAD PUDÍN

- Serves 6 to 8
- Time: About 1 hour

Bread pudding gets a lot of love in Latin America. Latin bread pudding is dense and firm enough to hold its own shape like a slice of cake, while being as sweet as a smile. This Caribbean-inspired version has strips of aromatic guava paste and slices of fresh mango baked into the top crust. I love *pudín* served warm with a scoop of ice cream, but if you find yourself eating spoonfuls straight from the fridge, that's just as well, too.

Tip: Guava paste is a chewy, ultrasweet fruity confection made from guavas and sugar cooked down forever. It comes in round tins or blocks, sometimes wrapped in dried banana leaf (look for *bocadillos* of paste). Guava paste sometimes includes milk caramel (you'll see tan layers in the paste), so read the ingredients to make sure it's completely cowless. For easier slicing, try chilling guava paste first.

1 pound day-old good-quality vegan white
    bread, cut or torn into small chunks
2/3 cup granulated sugar
1/4 cup light brown sugar
1/2 cup dark raisins
1/2 teaspoon ground cinnamon
3 1/2 cups soy milk or favorite rich
    nondairy milk
1 (3 by 1-inch) strip lemon or orange zest

How to Slice Mango

Slicing a fresh mango is best done with a thin, slightly flexible but very sharp, serrated knife. Place the knife about 3/4 inch from the nubby "stem" and balance the other end of the mango on a cutting board. The idea is to cut alongside the flat, wide seed of the mango (that runs almost the whole length of the fruit) to remove as large a slab of mango as possible while staying only just clear of the seed.

Using a gentle sawing motion, cut through the mango flesh. If you encounter resistance, you're probably cutting into the seed. No worries, just shift your knife slightly and continue cutting along until you've removed one side of the mango. Continue with the other side for the other mango half. Then trim around the exposed seed to remove any remaining flesh and skin from it (do not peel the halves). If you spot some mango seed bits on the flesh, just remove them, too.

Holding a mango half flesh side up, use that thin knife to gently slice 1/4-inch strips, side by side, end to end, into the flesh, taking care not to slice through the skin but slicing as deeply as possible. When you're done slicing, firmly grab the ends of the mango half and, pushing from the bottom, press the whole thing inside out. You'll have a bunch of mango slices sticking out and up that can be either cut off or gently removed with your fingers. Repeat with the other half and slice up any remaining bits of the mango you'd separately removed from the seed. Now for my favorite part . . . place the pit in your mouth and slurp off any remaining juicy mango bits. It's your delicious (and messy, best eaten over the sink) reward for showing that mango who's boss, so enjoy.

3 tablespoons nonhydrogenated
   vegan margarine
2 tablespoons cornstarch
2 tablespoons dark or spiced rum
2 teaspoons vanilla extract
5 ounces guava paste, sliced into
   thin strips
1 large ripe mango

1. Lightly grease a 9 by 11 by 2-inch baking pan. Place the bread pieces in a large mixing bowl. Add the granulated and light brown sugar, raisins, and cinnamon, and toss together. Set aside 1/2 cup of the soy milk in a measuring cup and pour the remaining 3 cups of soy milk into a large saucepan. Add the orange zest and, over medium heat, simmer the milk for 10 minutes, stirring occasionally. Add the margarine and stir to melt. Remove the orange zest and pour the hot soy milk over the bread mixture. Using a wooden spoon or rubber spatula, fold the ingredients to completely moisten the bread. Set the mixture aside and let it cool for 15 minutes, stirring occasionally. The bread will fall completely apart and will be very mushy and wet. While the bread mixture is cooling, preheat the oven to 375°F.

2. Into the remaining 1/2 cup of soy milk in the measuring cup, whisk the cornstarch, rum, and vanilla until smooth. Pour onto bread mixture and mix thoroughly. Pour into the prepared baking pan and top with strips of guava paste and strips of mango, poking them partially into the pudding. Bake for 40 to 45 minutes, or until the

top is lightly browned; the guava paste will melt and bubble and the mango will brown. A knife inserted into the center of the pudding should come out mostly clean (a few sticky crumbs are okay). The pudding will be like molten lava right out of the oven, so let it cool for at least 15 minutes before cutting and serving.

SIMPLY ARROZ CON LECHE

- Makes about 4 cups, or 8 half-cup servings
- Time: About 45 minutes
- Gluten Free, can be made Soy Free

Homemade Latin rice pudding is about as elemental and comforting as a dessert (or breakfast treat) can get, irresistibly warm and soothing. Practically every country has a home-style version of it. The name itself—it means literally "rice with milk"—aptly conveys its simplicity: rice is simmered on the stovetop with milk (rice or almond, please), generously sweetened and spiked with spices.

Tip: This pudding can be as thick or thin as you like; just cook longer if you are adding more nondairy milk. Just keep in mind that the pudding will continue to thicken after it has been removed from the heat. Arroz con Leche is best served warm the day it's made, but can be reheated easily enough on a stovetop or microwave. Just add a little extra nondairy milk or water to help loosen it up enough to stir easily.

6 whole cloves

2 strips citrus zest, such as orange, lemon, or lime (about 1 by 2 inches each)

1½ cups almond or rice milk, plus 1⅔ cups additional almond, rice, or soy milk, preferably vanilla flavored

⅔ cup uncooked long-grain white rice

⅔ cup sugar

1 (3-inch) cinnamon stick

A big pinch of ground allspice

½ cup dark or golden raisins

1 tablespoon dark rum (optional)

1 teaspoon vanilla extract

¼ teaspoon salt

1. Stick three cloves into each of the pieces of citrus zest. In a large, heavy-bottomed saucepan, combine the 1½ cups of almond milk, and the rice, sugar, cinnamon stick, allspice, and clove-studded zest. Bring to a boil over medium-high heat, stirring occasionally when the milk begins to foam. Lower the heat to low, cover, and simmer for 15 minutes, until the rice is very soft and mushy.

2. Pour in the additional 1⅔ cups of non-dairy milk, add the raisins, rum, vanilla, and salt, and stir. Bring the mixture to a boil again, lower the heat, and simmer for another 20 to 25 minutes, stirring occasionally, until very creamy and thickened. Remove from the heat

and allow to cool for 10 minutes. Remove the citrus zest, cloves, and cinnamon stick and pour into individual serving cups or a large serving bowl. Garnish with a sprinkle of ground cinnamon, if desired.

Variations

Arroz con Leche with Saffron: Set aside ¼ cup of warm nondairy milk in a small cup and combine with a pinch of saffron threads. Let soak for 8 minutes, strain out the threads, and stir into the rice pudding when you add the additional nondairy milk.

Arroz con Leche de Coco: Replace the additional 1⅔ cups of nondairy milk with one 15-ounce can of coconut milk. If desired, garnish the pudding with ½ cup of grated coconut that has been lightly toasted in a skillet over medium heat until golden, 3 to 5 minutes.

SWEET COCONUT CORN PUDDING (MAJARETE)

- Makes five or six ½-cup servings
- Gluten Free, can be made Soy Free

Majarete is a light sweet pudding from the Caribbean island nations and some South American countries. This recipe is based on *majarete* found in the Dominican Republic, which, corn-based, is made creamy with coconut scented with vanilla and cinnamon. *Majarete* is soothing and nourishing and it's not uncommon to find it served as a breakfast snack. It's best served slightly warm, after it's been allowed to cool just enough to firm up the texture.

Tip: Depending on how watery or juicy your fresh corn is, your *majarete* may have a thicker or thinner consistency every time. Just cook your pudding longer and keep stirring for a thicker pudding.

> 3 cups fresh corn kernels
> (from 4 to 5 ears of corn)
> 1 (14-ounce) can regular or lite
> coconut milk
> 2/3 cup sugar
> 2 (3-inch) cinnamon sticks
> 1/2 teaspoon salt
> 1/2 cup almond, rice, or soy milk
> 2 tablespoons cornstarch
> 1/4 cup yellow cornmeal
> Grated zest of 1/2 lemon
> 1 1/2 teaspoons vanilla extract
> 1/2 teaspoon coconut extract
> Ground cinnamon, for sprinkling

1. In a blender jar, pulse together the corn kernels, coconut milk, and sugar until smooth; some corn texture will remain. Empty into a large saucepan, add the cinnamon sticks and salt and bring to a boil over medium heat. Lower the heat to low, partially cover the pan, and simmer for 20 minutes, stirring occasionally.

2. In a measuring cup, whisk together the almond milk and cornstarch and then stir in the cornmeal. Pour this mixture into the simmering corn mixture and whisk rapidly until smooth. Add the lemon zest and cook for 10 to 12 minutes, stirring constantly until the pudding resembles a thin polenta, or continue cooking until the desired consistency is reached. Remove from the heat, stir in the vanilla and coconut extracts, and remove the cinnamon sticks.

3. Pour into individual 1/2-cup serving cups or ramekins or one large glass serving dish, sprinkle with ground cinnamon, and let cool for 15 minutes. Either serve slightly warm or chill for a firmer pudding.

DULCE DE BATATA (SWEET POTATO SWEET MASH)

....

- Makes about 2 1/2 cups
- Time: 1 to 1 1/2 hours, most time spent simmering on stove
- Gluten Free, Soy Free

....

This jamlike paste of fruit cooked down with sugar is such a traditional and old-school Latin sweet. Sweet potato is a popular choice for all kinds of *dulces* from the Caribbean all the way down to Uruguay, from fudgelike candies to spreadable preserves. This brilliant orange mash has a fresh flavor and thick, creamy texture. And it's less sweet than commercially sold dulces, for less of a culture shock to unaccustomed palates.

Sweet potato dulce is irresistible eaten by the spoonful warm out of the pot, or dolloped on toast, nondairy ice cream, vanilla yogurt, or Arroz con Leche. For an exciting twist on chocolate cake, use *dulce de batata* as a fat-free filling in Spiced Chocolate Cake and serve with a drizzle of Un-Dulce de Leche (page 227)

Tip: This recipe requires a long cooking time on the stove but it doesn't require constant attention. Just make sure to use a heavy pot and keep the heat low. I'm not saying go to the gym or pick up the dry cleaning in the meantime, but you don't have to hover near, watching it constantly!

2 pounds orange-flesh sweet potatoes, peeled and chopped into 1/2-inch chunks
2 (3-inch) cinnamon sticks
1 cup sugar
1 cup water
2 tablespoons lemon juice
A pinch of salt
1 1/2 teaspoons vanilla extract

1. Place the sweet potato chunks in a medium-size pot with a lid, add enough cold water to cover by about 3 inches, and add the cinnamon sticks. Cover and bring to a boil over high heat, then lower the heat to low and simmer for 30 to 35 minutes, until the potatoes are very tender. Remove the cinnamon stick, drain, and mash very well until creamy.

2. In a large pot, combine the sugar, water, lemon juice, and salt and bring to a boil over medium heat. Stir until the sugar is dissolved, then stir in the mashed sweet potatoes until completely incorporated. Lower the heat to medium-low and cook, stirring occasionally, until the mixture has reduced in size by about half and is very thick, like a jam, 1 to 1 1/2 hours. Remove from the heat and stir in the vanilla. Let cool to room temperature before eating or store in a tightly covered container in the refrigerator until ready to use.

Variations

Replace the granulated sugar with brown sugar for a rich, caramel-like flavor. The paste won't be quite as bright orange, however.

Stir in 2 tablespoons of rum or brandy into the paste during the last 20 minutes of cooking.

Stir in 1 cup of toasted grated coconut for a nutty-tasting treat.

CHOCOLATE ORANGE SPICE CAKE WITH DULCE DE BATATA

....

- Serves 8 to 10
- Time: 45 minutes, not including preparation of Dulce de Batata

....

Layers of spiced dark chocolate and bright orange *dulce de batata* filling make this cake a dramatic presentation with an appropriately autumn feel. If you're ready for a break from heavy buttercream frostings (and, hey, sweet potatoes are good for you!), this cake could even be a revelation. It's also a good choice for warm-weather dining, when greasy frostings would just melt away.

1 3/4 cups almond or rice milk

1/4 cup freshly squeezed orange juice

1 1/2 cups sugar

Grated zest of 1 orange, or 3/4 teaspoon orange extract

2/3 cup canola oil

2 teaspoons vanilla extract

2 cups all-purpose flour

2/3 cup unsweetened cocoa powder, plus more for dusting (optional)

1 1/2 teaspoons ground cinnamon, plus more for dusting (optional)

1/2 teaspoon ground allspice

1/2 teaspoon ground nutmeg or mace

2 teaspoons baking powder

1/4 teaspoon baking soda

1/2 teaspoon salt

1 recipe Dulce de Batata (page 236)
Confectioners' sugar (optional)

1. Preheat the oven to 350ºF. Spray with non-stick cooking spray two 9-inch round cake pans and line the bottoms of the pans with circles of parchment paper. An easy way to cut the parchment is to place a large sheet on a cutting board, firmly press the pan on top and run a very sharp paring knife around the bottom edge of the pan. Pull away the excess paper and you'll have a perfectly sized parchment paper lining.

2. In a mixing bowl or 4-cup measuring cup, whisk together the almond milk, orange juice, sugar, grated orange rind, canola oil, and vanilla extract. In a separate large bowl, sift together the flour, cocoa powder, ground cinnamon, allspice, nutmeg, baking powder, baking soda, and salt, stir well, and form a well in the center of the dry ingredients. Pour the wet ingredients into the well and gently stir everything together, occasionally scraping the sides of the bowl. Stir just enough to completely moisten the ingredients; some small lumps are okay. Do not overmix.

3. Divide the batter equally between the prepared baking pans and bake for 30 to 32 minutes, or until a toothpick inserted into the center of the cakes comes out clean. Remove the pans from the oven and let cool on a wire rack for 20 minutes. After 20 minutes, flip the pans over onto the racks, peel off the parchment paper from the tops of the cakes, and let the cakes cool completely, about an hour.

4. To assemble: Use a very sharp, long, serrated knife (a bread knife is ideal) to carefully slice each cake into two equally thick layers. Gently warm the *dulce de batata* either on the stovetop in a saucepan or in a microwave at 60 percent power. Stir the *dulce* to a spreadable consistency. Spread the softened *dulce* on a layer of cake, top with another layer, and repeat until all the cake is used. Leave the top of the cake plain as is, or decorate with a swirl of any remaining *dulce* or sift with confectioners' sugar, then cocoa powder mixed with a little bit of ground cinnamon. Slice and serve immediately, or store in the refrigerator in a tightly covered container.

FRESH PAPAYA-LIME SORBET

....

- ● **Makes about 1¹/2 quarts**
- ● **Time: Less than 20 minutes, not including freezing time**

....

Mmmmm, papaya! This creamy sorbet will turn heads and taste buds with its gorgeous orange-pink color and luscious tropical flavor. A teeny bit of vodka helps keep this sorbet from turning completely rock hard in the freezer (but leave it on a countertop for 10 minutes for easier scooping after the deep freeze). Seek out those huge "red" papayas from Mexico and Central America for best results. Served after a rich meal, it's cool and refreshing, plus the papaya has enzymes that aid digestion.

Tip: A papaya is ripe when it feels soft when gently pressed and has a tropical fruity aroma.

1 cup water
1 cup sugar
1 large red papaya (about 2 pounds)
3 tablespoons lime juice
1 tablespoon vodka

1. Make a simple syrup by combining the water and sugar in a small saucepan and bringing to a boil over high heat. Lower the heat to a simmer, stir, and cook for another 5 minutes, until all of the sugar has been dissolved. Remove from the heat and let the syrup cool to lukewarm.

2. Cut the papaya in half and use a large spoon to remove and discard the seeds. Peel the papaya and cut into chunks that can be pureed easily in your blender (do not use a food processor). Puree about 2 cups of chunks; you may need to stir the chunks of the first batch a few times to chop things up, but once these pieces of papaya are pureed it will be easy to liquefy the rest. Keep adding and pureeing handfuls of papaya chunks until you have 4 cups of very smooth puree.

3. In a mixing bowl, combine the papaya puree, lime juice, and vodka. Stir the cooled simple syrup into the puree until the mixture is smooth. Pour into a container, cover, and chill. Place the cold papaya mixture in your ice-cream maker and freeze according to the manufacturer's instructions. Keep any leftover sorbet in a tightly covered container in the freezer.

SWEET CORN ICE CREAM

- Makes about 1 1/2 quarts
- Time: 30 minutes, not including freezing time

You already love corn, but get ready to bring your love to a new level in a creamy ice cream form. Inspired by Brazilian *sorvete de milho*, sweet corn ice cream has a buttery yellow hue and an irresistible flavor that screams summertime! A touch of rum tastes great and helps keep the ice cream soft enough for easier scooping (but can be left out if to be served immediately). For best results, use juicy local farmers' market sweet corn in the peak of summer.

1 (14-ounce) can coconut milk (don't use lite coconut milk)
1/2 cup soy milk, soy creamer, or other nondairy milk
2 cups fresh corn kernels
1 (3-inch) cinnamon stick
1 tablespoon cornstarch
6 ounces silken tofu (half of an aseptic water-packed tofu block)
2/3 cup sugar
2 tablespoons rum
2 teaspoons vanilla extract

1. Open the can of coconut milk and spoon off as much of the solid coconut cream from the top as possible; place the coconut cream in a blender jar. Place about half of the remaining coconut water, and the soy milk, corn kernels, and cinnamon stick in a small saucepan and bring to a boil over medium heat. Lower the heat to low and simmer for 10 minutes. Meanwhile, whisk the cornstarch into the remaining coconut milk until smooth. After the corn mixture has cooked for 10 minutes, whisk in the cornstarch mixture and simmer for another 2 to 4 minutes, until the mixture has thickened and the cornstarch has cooked (the mixture should taste smooth, not chalky). Turn off the heat and let the mixture cool for 15 minutes.

2. Remove the cinnamon stick and add to the blender jar containing the remaining coconut cream, along with the silken tofu, sugar, rum, and vanilla extract. Blend until very smooth, pour into a container, and cover tightly.

3. Chill the mixture completely, then freeze in ice-cream maker according to manufacturer's instructions. For best texture, you may want to chill the corn ice cream for 20 minutes right after it's made, to firm it up, especially if the weather is very warm.

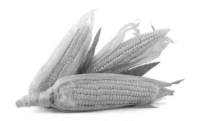

BUTTERY COOKIES WITH THICK DULCE DE LECHE FILLING (ALFAJORES)

● **Makes about two dozen 2-inch-diameter sandwich cookies**

Alfajores are the South American answer to Oreos: thick shortbread rounds hug buttery *dulce de leche* filling. The edges can be rolled in toasted coconut or almonds, or left unadorned. This recipe is something in between: a not-too-sweet cookie with a lightly crumbly texture and soft filling.

Tip: Since the vegan filling is somewhat more delicate than the cow stuff, I recommend either assembling these cookies right before serving (for crisper cookies with gooey centers), or chilling preassembled sandwiches in a tightly covered container. The cookies won't be quite as crisp but will fuse into a tender, melt-in-your-mouth wonder.

Tip: Do not substitute cornstarch for the tapioca flour in the filling recipe; cornstarch won't work right and you'll probably have a sauce instead of a thick spreadable filling. The thick *dulce de leche* filling has the consistency of a spreadable caramel and should not be overly oozy or runny.

Thick Dulce de Leche Filling
  (recipe follows)
3/4 cup nonhydrogenated vegan margarine, slightly softened (should
  not be melted or greasy looking)
2/3 cup confectioners' sugar
1 1/2 teaspoons vanilla extract
1/2 teaspoon finely grated lemon zest
1 1/2 cups all-purpose flour
2/3 cup cornstarch
1/4 teaspoon baking powder
A pinch of salt
1 tablespoon nondairy milk
1 tablespoon rum, brandy, or cognac
1/3 cup grated coconut or finely chopped
  almonds (optional)

1. Prepare the Thick Dulce de Leche Filling first, as directed. Let sit at room temperature if you plan on filling the cookies right after you've baked them; otherwise store it in the fridge and take it out 15 minutes prior to using.

2. Make the cookie dough. Using a handheld mixer or standing mixer with a large bowl, cream together the margarine and confectioners' sugar. Scraping the sides of the bowl frequently, beat the mixture until thick and fluffy, about 3 minutes. Beat in the vanilla and lemon zest, then sift in the flour, cornstarch, baking powder, and salt. Mix until you have a soft, crumbly mixture, 2 to 3 minutes. Beat in the nondairy milk and rum, scraping the sides of bowl frequently, to form a soft but not overly sticky dough.

3. Divide the dough into two pieces and place between sheets of waxed paper. Chill for

30 minutes. While the dough is chilling, place the grated coconut or almonds in small, heavy skillet over medium-low heat. Stir constantly and toast until the coconut is lightly golden, 3 to 4 minutes, and quickly transfer to a plate to prevent the coconut from overbrowning.

4. When ready to bake the cookies, preheat the oven to 325ºF and line a baking sheet with parchment paper. Lightly flour a large piece of waxed paper, take out half of the dough, and pat into a circle. Top with another sheet of waxed paper and roll out the dough to 1/4 to 3/8 inch thick (should be thicker than typical sugar cookies) and cut with a 2-inch-diameter round cookie cutter (one with a decorative edge is particularly nice here). Remove the excess dough and, if necessary, use a thin spatula to carefully lift the cookies onto the prepared baking sheet. You could also shape the cookies by scooping 2 teaspoons of dough, rolling in a ball and placing between sheets of waxed paper. Use a measuring cup to flatten into a circle about 1/4 inch thick. This is a lazy way to do it; your circles won't be shaped as nicely, so the sandwiches may look a little freeform.

5. Bake for 12 to 14 minutes; do not let the cookies become overly browned on the edges. Allow the cookies to cool on the baking sheet for 2 minutes before transferring to wire cooling racks.

6. The cookies can be slightly warm when filling. To assemble an *alfajor*, spread a gener-

ous layer of Thick Dulce de Leche Filling (about a rounded teaspoon) on the underside of one cookie, spreading to the edges. Top with another cookie (the bottom sides of the cookies should face so the pretty sides of the cookie are showing). Press down gently so a little of the filling is visible around the circumference of the cookie. Roll the edges in toasted *coconut*, if desired. Continue with the rest of the cookies and *dulce*. Store in a tightly covered container in a cool place.

THICK DULCE DE LECHE FILLING

1/4 cup brown rice syrup
1/3 cup light brown sugar
1/4 cup soy creamer or rich
  soy milk
2 tablespoons tapioca flour
1 tablespoon nonhydrogenated
  vegan margarine
1 1/2 teaspoons vanilla extract

1. In a measuring cup, whisk together the soy creamer and tapioca flour and pour into a small saucepan. Add the brown rice syrup and brown sugar to the pan and whisk over medium heat until smooth. Bring the mixture to a boil and continue to stir until it becomes very thick, then lower the heat as much as possible and simmer the sauce for 10 minutes, stirring occasionally. The mixture should resemble a thick, caramel-like spread.

2. Stir in the margarine and whisk until smooth. Remove from the heat and stir in the vanilla. Let the sauce cool for 15 minutes before filling the *alfajores*. Store any unused *dulce* in a tightly covered container in the fridge.

Variations

Chocolate-drizzled Alfajores: Melt 1 cup of vegan chocolate chips in a double boiler or a microwave, according to the package directions. Add 1 tablespoon of nonhydrogenated margarine to the softened chips and stir until smooth. Arrange the assembled sandwich cookies on a large sheet of waxed paper. Either load the melted chocolate into a pastry bag with a small round tip or dip a fork into the melted chocolate. Drizzle the chocolate over the tops of the cookies or try dipping a cookie halfway into the chocolate. Let the cookies stand for an hour to allow the chocolate to set, or pop them into the fridge to speed up the process.

Guayaba Alfajores: Gently warm ½ cup of guava paste in a microwave, in a microwave-safe bowl, for 30 to 40 seconds on 60 percent power, until softened. Use a spoon to stir the paste until smooth and spread between the cookies. For extra fun, use both Thick Dulce de Leche (page 242) and guava paste between the cookies, for a one-two punch of buttery sweet and tropical fruity flavor.

VANILLA-COCONUT FLAN

- **Makes 6 servings, just over ½ cup per serving**
- **Gluten Free**

An eggless, milk-free tribute to everyone's favorite Spanish jiggly, caramel-covered custard. It sweetly finishes any Latin meal from a hearty elaborate *posole* stew to a humble empanada, or enjoy on its own with cup of strong *café*.

Because it's vegan, there's no need to turn on the oven or steam anything, but you'll need to focus when making the hard candy caramel that will become the caramel syrup after the flan has set.

Tip: The simplest molds to shape your flan are individual ½- to 1-cup classic ceramic ramekins, or small glass or Pyrex bowls—this size makes it easier when it's time to release the flans from their molds. I have a set of ½-cup Pyrex "condiment" bowls that make perfectly portioned single-serving *flancitos*, plus they have handy lids that make storing flan just too easy. You can also divide it into two larger molds, or if you're overly ambitious you can try a large, round, shallow tin for one big flan.

Tip: Agar flakes are an easier ingredient to find. But if you can find agar powder, this is the way to go for a truly smooth flan, as the occasional rogue agar flake may not melt.

Warning: My preferred method of making caramel is in a microwave, which produces excellent results in mere minutes; the stovetop stuff takes much more time and can be a little unreliable. Whichever method you choose, keep in mind that you'll be working with hot molten sugar—do not touch hot caramel with your bare fingers.

Read the instructions carefully and work safely; you'll also have to work quickly since caramel cools fast. Just have your molds nearby and, before you know it, you'll be coating half the glassware in the house with golden caramel goodness just for kicks. You can prepare your caramel-coated containers hours in advance, before making the rest of the flan.

Caramel Coating

1 cup granulated sugar
3 tablespoons water
1 teaspoon lemon or lime juice

Flan

1/2 cup water
2 1/2 teaspoons agar flakes, or
  1 1/4 teaspoons agar powder
2 cups vanilla soy or almond milk
2 tablespoons cornstarch
1 cup regular or lite coconut milk
1/2 cup granulated sugar
2 tablespoons light brown sugar
2 1/2 teaspoons vanilla extract
1 1/2 teaspoons coconut extract

1. First make the caramel coating. Have ready on your work surface four to six individual clean, dry, glass or ceramic serving cups or two 2-cup serving bowls.

2. "Microwave caramel" is the fastest and my method of choice, but you'll have to watch it closely. To do so, pour the sugar into a microwave-safe Pyrex 2- or 4-cup measuring cup. Add the water, stir gently a few times, and microwave on high for 5 to 6 minutes; do not stir again. At about 4 minutes, the sugar will be melted and rapidly bubbling. Soon after that it will start to turn pale golden, then increasingly amber. Once the browning begins, it will continue to do so very rapidly, so keep a watch on the caramel closely after about 5 1/2 minutes or so. Once it has reached a dark amber color, stop the microwave and use oven mitts to remove the cup of hot caramel immediately; if you leave it in any longer it could burn, so pay attention! If some of the sugar has not melted, don't worry and do not try to microwave it again; you'll have enough caramel to work with.

Alternatively, to make caramel on the stovetop: combine the sugar, 1/4 cup of water, and the lemon juice in a small saucepan (preferably one with an indented lip for pouring). Bring to a boil over medium heat, lower the heat slightly, and cook without stirring for 15 to 20 minutes (this takes enough time that you'll wish you had a microwave); cook until the caramel reaches a deep amber color.

3. When your caramel is hot and ready, quickly pour a thin layer onto the bottoms of the ramekins; you won't need much if it's hot. Gently tilt each ramekin with a circular motion so that some of the caramel flows from the bottom onto the sides of the container; it doesn't have to reach more than 1/2 inch up the sides. Set the molds aside and let cool as you prepare the flan custard.

4. In a large saucepan, combine the water and agar and bring to a boil; lower the heat to a simmer and cook for 5 minutes. In a measuring cup or small bowl, whisk together 1/2 cup of the soy milk and the cornstarch and set aside. After most of agar appears to have to melted (some stubborn flakes may remain, that's why powdered agar is better), stir in the remaining soy milk, coconut milk, granulated sugar, and brown sugar. Increase the heat and bring the mixture to a boil, stirring occasionally, then lower the heat again. Whisk the other soy milk mixture once more and stir rapidly into simmering coconut milk mixture. Cook and stir constantly until the mixture has thickened slightly and the cornstarch is completely cooked (taste the mixture; it should be smooth, not chalky), 6 to 8 minutes. Stir in the vanilla and coconut extract and remove from the heat.

5. Pour into the caramel-lined molds, leaving a minimum of 1/2 inch from the top of the molds. Let cool for 10 minutes, then move the flans into the refrigerator to chill and complete firming for 4 hours or overnight.

6. To serve the chilled flan: Gently run a butter knife a few times along the sides of each flan. Invert the ramekin onto a serving plate, give it couple sharp taps, and it should slide onto the plate. Most of the caramel will have dissolved to form syrupy sauce coating the custard. If your flan still refuses to be evicted, set the flan in a shallow bowl of hot water (not enough to cover, just reach up the sides of the mold) and after a minute or so try again. Some of the caramel will remain in the molds; to remove the caramel, just fill the molds with warm water and let sit for a few hours to dissolve the sugar. Serve the flan within two to three days of preparing.

CAFÉ CON LECHE FLAN

- **Makes 6 servings, just over 1/2 cup per serving**

Flan is very good but it's even better when pretending to be smooth, creamy Latin-style coffee. A touch of espresso transforms the vanilla flan into an exquisite dessert that both coffee fans and custard fans can agree on. It's perhaps my favorite dessert in this chapter (but don't tell the churros that!).

Tip: Look for Italian instant espresso powder in the coffee section of gourmet stores or Italian markets. It brings massive bold coffee flavor to this flan. If instant coffee is all you can find, just use a little bit more.

Caramel Coating

1 cup granulated sugar

3 tablespoons water

1 teaspoon lemon or lime juice

Flan

1/2 cup water

2 1/2 teaspoons agar flakes

2 cups vanilla soy or almond milk

2 tablespoons arrowroot powder or cornstarch

1 cup regular or lite coconut milk

1/2 cup granulated sugar

2 tablespoons brown sugar

2 tablespoons instant espresso powder or instant coffee

2 teaspoons vanilla extract

1. First make the caramel coating. Have ready four to six individual clean, dry glass or ceramic serving cups or two larger 2-cup serving bowls.

2. "Microwave caramel" is the fastest and my method of choice, but you'll have to watch it closely. To do so, pour the sugar into a microwave-safe Pyrex 2- or 4-cup measuring cup. Add the water, stir gently a few times, and microwave on high for 5 to 6 minutes; do not stir again. At about 4 minutes, the sugar will be melted and rapidly bubbling. Soon after that it will start to turn pale golden, then increasingly amber. Once the browning begins, it will continue to do so very rapidly, so keep a watch on the caramel closely after about 5 1/2 minutes or

so. Once it has reached a dark amber color, stop the microwave and use oven mitts to remove the cup of hot caramel immediately; if you leave it in any longer it could burn, so pay attention! If some of the sugar has not melted, don't worry and do not try to microwave it again; you'll have enough caramel to work with. Alternatively, to make caramel on the stovetop: combine the sugar, 1/4 cup of water, and the lemon juice in a small saucepan (preferably one with an indented lip for pouring). Bring to a boil over medium heat, lower the heat slightly, and cook without stirring for 15 to 20 minutes (this takes enough time that you'll wish you had a microwave); cook until the caramel reaches a deep amber color.

3. When your caramel is very hot and ready, quickly pour a thin layer onto the bottoms of the ramekins; you won't need much if it's hot. Gently tilt each ramekin with a circular motion so that some of the caramel flows from the bottom onto the sides of the container; it doesn't have to reach more than 1/2 inch up the sides. Set the molds aside and let cool as you prepare the flan custard.

4. In a large saucepan, combine the water and agar and bring to a boil; lower the heat to a simmer and cook for 5 minutes. In a measuring cup or small bowl, whisk together 1/2 cup of the soy milk and the cornstarch and set aside. After most of agar appears to have to melted (some stubborn flakes may remain, that's why powdered agar is better), stir in the remaining soy milk, coconut milk, granulated sugar, brown sugar, and espresso powder. Increase the heat and bring the mixture to a boil, stirring occasionally, then lower the heat again. Whisk the other soy milk mixture once more and stir rapidly into simmering coconut milk mixture. Cook and stir constantly until the mixture has thickened slightly and the cornstarch is completely cooked (taste the mixture; it should be smooth, not chalky), 6 to 8 minutes. Stir in the vanilla and remove from the heat.

5. Pour into the caramel-lined molds, leaving a minimum of $1/2$ inch from the top of the molds. Let cool for 10 minutes, then move the flans into the refrigerator to chill and complete firming for 4 hours or overnight.

6. To serve the chilled flan: Gently run a butter knife a few times along the sides of each flan. Invert the ramekin onto a serving plate, give it couple sharp taps, and it should slide onto the plate. Most of the caramel will have dissolved to form syrupy sauce coating the custard. If your flan still refuses to be evicted, set the flan in a shallow bowl of hot water (not enough to cover, just reach up the sides of the mold) and after a minute or so try again. Some of the caramel will remain in the molds; to remove the caramel, just fill the molds with warm water and let sit for a few hours to dissolve the sugar. Serve the flan within two to three days of preparing.

● ● ●

APPENDIX A

MUCHOS MENUS
MEALS, MENUS, AND PLATOS TÍPICOS

*L*et this section serve as inspiration for your next friendly weekend dinner, lavish entertaining spread, or not-just-your-average weeknight meal. Or organize a potluck with each guest bringing along an entrée, dessert, or a selection of salsas.

TRADITIONAL MEALS, PLATOS TÍPICOS

A huge plate overflowing with rice, beans, and other hearty fare is typical of many Latin cuisines, so there's little wonder why they are often referred to as *platos típicos*. The whole thing is really a sum of its parts; although it's easy to enjoy fried plantains or beans on their own, they really form something special when served together. These are suggestions for assembling your own more or less authentic *plato típico*. Although you may find yourself serving Brazilian Rice with Colombian Red Beans and a side of Mexican-seasoned Chile-Lime-Beer Marinated Veggies, to heck with tradition and up with new ways to serve your own delightful Latin vegan ensembles.

Presentation and assembly of your *plato típico* is something to always be considered. Choose a big dinner plate; oval or rectangular shapes with high edges are convenient for holding lots of food and containing saucy beans or salsas. Each component could gently overlap, with the main elements such as beans, rice, or protein in the center and sides such as plantains or avocado neatly framing the plate. Each element should be identifiable and alluring instead of heaped in one big pile . . . a little bit of thought put into this is worth it! You've spent all this time making each morsel of food, so take pride in presenting it.

* * *

LARGE DINNERS, ENOUGH FOR 4 TO 6 PEOPLE

Use these menus when you want to cook to impress. Or, make up your own Latin-themed holiday just to have an excuse to cook up a storm.

The Buena Vegan Social Club
   Mojitos
   Cuban Black Bean Soup
   White Rice or Arroz con Coco
   Zesty Orange Mojo Baked Tofu
   Yuca with Cuban Garlic-Lime-Mojo
      Sauce
   Café con Leche Flan
   Cuban-style Coffee

Venezuelan Voyage, Pabaellón Criollo
   Venezuelan-style Black Beans (Caraotas)
   Fried Sweet Plantains, sliced in half and
      into lengthwise strips
   Latin Shredded Seitan, Venezuelan
      variation
   Basic white rice
   Creamy Avocado-Tomato Salsa
      (Venezuelan Guasacaca)
   Small Venezuelan-style *arepas*—sliced and
      spread with margarine and vegan cheese
   Real Brown Sugar Limeade

Colombian Colors, Bandeja Paisa
   Colombian-style Red Beans, made with
      cargamanto or bola roja beans
   Basic white rice
   Fried Sweet Plantains; slice each ripe
      plantain in half lengthwise and fry
      (see page 115)

Quarter or half of a ripe avocado, seeded
      and peeled and placed to the side
   Latin Shredded Seitan, basic recipe,
      or Latin Baked Tofu
   Small side of Tofu Chicharrones
   Small Colombian-style *arepas* or
      Colombian Arepas with Corn and
      Vegan Cheese
   Real Brown Sugar Limeade

Buenos Aires Potluck
   Creamy Corn-Crusted Tempeh Pot Pie, in
      particular baked in individual servings
   Tomato Salad with Sweet Crisp Onions
   Dulce de Batata served with
      store-bought vegan vanilla ice cream
   Argentinean or Chilean Red Wine

Brazilian Feijoada Feasting
   Portobello Feijoada
   Savory Orange Rice, Brazilian Style, or
      plain variation
   Brazilian Braised Shredded Kale
   Peeled whole oranges, sliced in half and
      sliced again into thin wedges
   Fresh Papaya-Lime Sorbet topped with
      Crème de Cassis liquor, or
      Sweet Corn Ice Cream

Peruvian "Surf and Turf"
   Mixed Mushroom Ceviche (the "surf")
   Peruvian Seitan and Potato Skewers (the
      "turf")
   Quinoa-Corn-Peanut Salad with Ají
      Amarillo Dressing
   Dulce de Batata with store-bought
      vegan vanilla or chocolate ice cream

Picnic à la Argentina

Sandwiches made with the following:

Seitan Chorizo (regular recipe), prepared, chilled, sliced in half, and lightly pan-fried in a little olive oil until hot and edges are crisped

Chimichurri Sauce with Smoked Paprika

Toasted crusty French rolls

Thin onion and tomato slices to garnish the sandwiches

Leafy green salad with any dressing

Buttery Cookies with Thick Dulce de Leche Filling

Dry red Argentinian wine

Sofrito So Good

Avocados stuffed with black beans, corn, and jicama

Pan-fried Tempeh with Sofrito

Yellow Rice with Garlic

Chayote-Carrot Salad

Sweet Corn Ice Cream with Un-Dulce de Leche

Tapas with a Side of Tropical Island Breeze

Bite-Size Green Plantain Sandwiches

Mini Potatoes Stuffed with Mushrooms and Olives

Salsa Golf

Crunchy Fried Yuca, sliced into fingers before frying

Any tropical fruit *batidos*

Mojitos or margaritas

Latin Caribbean Buffet

Mofongo

Red Beans with Dominican-style sazón

Basic white rice

Habanero-Melon-Papaya Salsa

Latin Shredded Seitan, either original, Ropa Vieja, or Picadillo style

Classic Cabbage salad with tomatoes

Fresh Mango and Guava Bread Pudín

Batidos or Sangria

Sensational Central American Buffet

Hearty Warm Yuca and Cabbage Salad

Costa Rican Refried Rice and Beans

Latin Baked Tofu or Baked Tofu in Sofrito

Fried Sweet Plantains, Crispy Fried Green Plantains

Slices of ripe avocado

Coconut Tres Leches Cake

An All- (South) American BBQ

So Good, So Green Dipping Sauce

Pickled Red Onions

Peruvian Seitan and Potato Skewers

Yellow Chile Grilled Tempeh

Grilled corn on the cob with olive oil and sea salt (follow basic procedures on page 64)

Peruvian Red Chile–Corn Salad with Limas and Cherry Tomatoes

Un-Dulce de Leche served on store-bought vegan vanilla ice cream and fresh berries

Barbecue Vegano Mexicano

Mexican Side-Street Corn

Tempeh Asado served with plenty of Chocolate-Chile Mole Sauce

Drunken Beans with Seitan Chorizo

Cilantro-Lime Rice

Caesar salad with Creamy Ancho Chile Dressing

Fresh Papaya-Lime Sorbet and lightly
  grilled pineapple
Micheladas or Horchata

Enchilada Grand Slam Holiday Spread
  "Any Noche" Romaine and Fruit Salad
  Potato-Chickpea Enchiladas with
    Green Tomatillo Sauce
  Refried pinto beans
  Cilantro-Lime Rice
  Vanilla-Coconut Flan
  Sangria

Vegan la Raza Tamale Party
(perfecto for Cinco de Mayo!)
  Red Chile–Seitan Tamales
  Black Bean–Sweet Potato Tamales
  Classic Roasted Tomatillo Salsa
  Fresh Tomato Salsa
  Guacamole served with tortilla chips and
    crudité of jicama sprinkled with lime
    juice, ancho chile powder, and salt
  Pineapple-Raisin Sweet Tamales and
    store-bought vegan vanilla or coconut
    ice cream
  Horchata or Micheladas

SMALLER DINNERS SERVING
2 TO 3 PEOPLE
  Chimichurri Baked Tofu
  Savory Orange Rice, Brazilian Style
  Swiss Chard with Raisins and Capers

  Black-Eyed–Butternut Tostadas
  Mango-Jicama Chopped Salad
  Cilantro-Lime Rice

Tempeh Asado
Pan-Grilled Vegetables in
  Chile-Lime Beer
Amaranth Polenta with Roasted Chiles

Creamy Potato Peanut Stew
Pickled Red Onions
Basic white rice
Steamed plain greens, such as kale or
  Swiss chard

Spicy Tortilla Casserole with Roasted
  Poblanos
Spinach-Avocado-Chile Salad
Refried black beans

Pupusas, any filling
Salvadorian Marinated Slaw
Simple Latin Tomato Sauce
Diced avocado

Tropical Pumpkin Soup
Tempeh Asado with Spinach–Brazil Nut–
  Gazpacho Salad
Crepes with Un-Dulce de Leche and
  Sweet Plantains (really about getting
  to dessert but, hey, it's all about the
  crepes)

TWO-RECIPE MEALS FOR
WEEKNIGHT COOKING
For cooking on a Tuesday night and unwind-
ing for a while after work in your kitchen
with two friendly recipes. Recommended for
those whole enjoy two- or more burner cooking or something hearty served with a salad.

Or pair it up with such basics as tortillas, *arepas*, or any rice.

Peruvian Potatoes with
Spicy "Cheezy" Sauce
Green salad with chickpeas, tossed with
Fresh Gazpacho Salsa Dressing

Venezuelan-style Black Beans served
with white rice
Mango-Jicama Chopped Salad

Costa Rican Refried Rice and Beans
Fruity Chile Slaw

Seitan Saltado (Peruvian Seitan and
Potato Stir-fry)
Pan-grilled Vegetables in
Chile-Lime Beer

Quick Red Posole with Beans
Homemade Soft Corn Tortillas

Quinoa–Oyster Mushroom Risotto
Braised Brazilian Shredded Kale

Arroz con Seitan
Black Bean–Corn Salsa Salad

Rice with Pigeon Peas (especially the
deluxe version)
Sweet and Nutty Roasted Stuffed
Plantains

Yellow Chile Grilled Tempeh
Calabacitas

BREAKFAST (DESAYÚNO)

Many of my recipe testers asked for Latin-style breakfast recipes. My usual response is that people in Latin countries often eat for breakfast smaller portions of foods popular eaten for later meals. Tamales, *arepas*, rice and beans, and fried plantains make natural go-to items for a solid start to any day. These foods may take too much time to prepare when juggling getting showered, dressed, and out the door, but they can be made the night before or on Sunday nights for a week of hearty breakfast fare. If sprawling weekend brunches are your thing, then make a complete spread with fried plantains, a selection of salsas, and a light salad.

- Gallo pinto (simplified variation) is a favorite protein- and fiber-packed breakfast of mine, especially when made with brown rice (see page 93 for suggested preparation).
- Stuff a homemade or store-bought wheat tortilla with leftover rice, any bean or refried bean, a few slices of Latin Baked Tofu, a dollop of your favorite salsa, shredded green cabbage, and/or salsa. Fold it all up and you have a different (and somewhat more authentic, if you ask me) kind of "breakfast" burrito.
- Taquitos with Chorizo and Potatoes (page 168) are a nice brunchy item and can be assembled the night before. Keep chilled in a tightly covered container and fry as directed for an additional 3 to 4 minutes, to make sure the centers get hot.

- *Llapingachos*—the Ecuadorian mashed potato pancake—is a filling and tasty breakfast and a fine choice for fans of hash browns or home fries (see page 57). The *salsa de maní* (peanut sauce) is of course amazing, but you can simplify things by serving with a slice of avocado or a few spoonfuls of gently warmed tomato salsa.
- Black Bean–Sweet Potato Tamales (page 189) or Farmers' Market Tamales (page 194), resteamed until hot in the center, unpeeled, and grilled on a lightly oiled cast-iron pan until the edges are crisped
- Corn tortillas (homemade or store-bought), lightly grilled until soft, topped with refried beans and a slice of avocado and/or a dab of salsa
- Sweet Coconut Corn Pudding (page 235), gently warmed in the microwave, using 60 percent heat, or gently heated on a stovetop in a shallow pan of warm water until the center of pudding is warm.
- Simply Arroz con Leche (page 234) made with brown rice. Be sure to double the total liquid amount and cook twice as long. Reduce the sugar by up to one-third and enrich with more fruit or a sprinkle of toasted chopped almonds, if desired.
- Any baked empanada is a meal-on-the-run that's there for you even on your busiest weekday mornings. Of course, you can't make them that morning before work, but if you have a batch ready in your freezer or fridge, they can be heated right then or brought to work and heated in a microwave. Pair your favorite empanada with a small crisp apple as a refreshing follow-up, for a satisfying meal that will keep you going strong well into lunch.
- Fried Sweet Plantains (page 115) are a decadent breakfast treat. Sweet and Nutty Roasted Stuffed Plantains (page 117) don't require frying and are delectable.
- Fried corn-crusted empanadas are perfectly good breakfast fare, too . . . they can be quite rich, so I like to think of them as a savory alternative to doughnuts. Reheat in the oven for optimal crispness or make them from scratch on the weekend for an indulgent brunch with Creamy Avocado-Tomato Salsa (page 39) or Green Onion Salsa (page 44).
- Speaking of doughnuts, Churros (page 223) are the ultimate sweet breakfast or brunch treat with Latin hot chocolate. Plan about 45 minutes to whip up fresh warm churros and chocolate. They are complete as is, but are particularly delightful paired with fresh strawberries or ripe sweet melon.

APPENDIX B

QUICK-START SHOPPING LIST
SHOPPING? ¡EXCELLENTÉ!

*J*f you're like me, exploring a newly discovered ethnic market is almost as fun as taking an exotic vacation. And finding a new hot sauce or seldom-seen tropical fruit is definitely more fun than packing.

To get to your shopping fun faster or easier, the following are a few suggested sites for buying hard-to-find items online. Or, if you prefer to do your shopping in person, I've put together a few shopping lists. Simply photocopy these lists and keep handy in your bag (or give it to your mom if she's the type that likes to buy random things for you . . . instead of paisley curtains, a 5-pound bag of masa harina, please) and next time you're visiting your local Latin neighborhood you'll have a go-to list for those specialty items that may not be so close to home. Don't let another weekend go by without pasilla peppers or *ají amarillo* paste! Stock up on your favorite ingredients now even if you don't intend to make things right that very moment.

If you're technologically minded, I've prepared downloadable PDF cards you can clip and tuck into your wallet. Join my update list at veganlatina.com and you'll be the first to know what else I dream up to make eating Latin vegan effortless, and receive tips on shopping for Latin stuff in your area.

SHOPPING USING
EL INTERNET

Chances are you know how to buy something online. Purchasing unusual nonperishable ethnic food items is a great way to exercise your online shopping muscle, besides being the only option for many foodies living in remote locations across the globe. Here are a few good places to seek out both Latin products and specialty vegan-centric food items.

Latin American Products

Some sites specialize in products from a specific region or country (Mexican- and Spanish-only sites are particularly well stocked) and others feature a more pan-Latin approach. Either way, shelf-stable favorites such as dried chiles and exotic beans are found effortlessly online.

amigofoods.com—A fun site that's indeed like shopping with an *amigo*, offering a little bit of something from most every *país*. Get your Costa Rican Salsa Lizano, Brazilian toasted manioc flour (*farinha de mandioca*), Cuban coffee, and Peruvian *ají* pastes all in one shopping trip and without ever having to put your pants on. A win-win on all counts.

ecuadorianfooddelivery.com—Not just for Ecuador anymore! An impressive array of Latin foods and frozen stuff from everywhere, with an emphasis on organic fruit *dulces* and gluten-free items.

latinmerchant.com—A cute site with a nice selection of dried chiles, herbs, spices, and those gorgeous dried chile *ristras*, the perfect piece of Mexican flare for your *cocina*.

Vegan Products

Online shopping is ideal for stocking up on those long-lasting essentials such as nutritional yeast and vital wheat gluten flour.

Foodfight.com—The rock 'n' roll all-vegan grocery store in Portland that loves to deliver fresh and tasty vegan essentials to your door. Great selection of vegan cheeses, faux meats, and sweets.

cosmosveganshoppe.com—Big selection of dairy alternatives and fake meaty things, too.

Bobsredmill.com—Bob's there for you when it comes to fine flours and grains. Check out their excellent garbanzo bean and vital wheat gluten flours. They also make a very nice Mexican-style masa harina.

• • •

SHOPPING LISTS, BY ME FOR YOU

You don't need to buy everything at once on this list, just build your pantry slowly based on what appeals to you. Unless indicated, I recommend purchasing one package/jar/bottle/unit at a time if you're not cooking up an entire village fiesta.

This list is not conclusive by any means. You may have to make several shopping trips and not have just one place to buy all of your vegan ingredients. Or maybe you have an excellent grocery store that services a Latin community and regularly stocks plantains and masa harina in addition to all of the "regular" nonethnic stuff. I've just organized this list to reflect the Pantry chapter. Hope this helps!

Latin American Stuff

Dried Chiles
- [ ] For moles and sauces, earthy sweet flavors, and mild-to-medium heat, dark reddish-brown: ancho, pasilla, morada
- [ ] Hot and bright sharp flavors, red: costeño, piquín, chile de arbol
- [ ] South American chiles (ají): mild to medium: amarillo, panca, mirasol; hot to very hot: rocoto

Dried Beans
- [ ] Black, pinto
- [ ] White
- [ ] Cargamanto
- [ ] Central American/Salvadorian red
- [ ] Bola roja
- [ ] Canary
- [ ] Garbanzo
- [ ] Pigeon peas

Spices
- [ ] Achiote, a.k.a. annatto seeds
- [ ] Aniseeds or star anise
- [ ] Bay leaves
- [ ] Cinnamon sticks and ground cinnamon
- [ ] Cloves
- [ ] Cumin, ground
- [ ] Epazote, dried
- [ ] Mexican oregano, dried
- [ ] Oregano, dried

Grains and Flours
- [ ] Mexican masa harina
- [ ] Masa harina for tamales
- [ ] Masarepa, a.k.a. Harina PAN (Colombian/Venezuelan harina) for arepas
- [ ] Long-grain white or brown rice
- [ ] Quinoa, white, red, or black
- [ ] Amaranth (for polenta or soup)
- [ ] Toasted manioc flour for farofa (Brazilian specialty item)

Prepared Jarred/Canned Items
- [ ] Peruvian ají paste (crema): amarillo, panca, and rocoto
- [ ] Assorted hot sauces, Mexican: Tapatío, Yucatán, Valentina ; Ecuadorean: La Cholla ; and so on

- [ ] Costa Rican Salsa Lizano
- [ ] Canned black, pinto, kidney, and garbanzo beans
- [ ] Canned Latin specialty beans (see dried list) such as bola roja, cargamanto, and pigeon peas
- [ ] Achiote paste
- [ ] Coconut milk and cream of coconut
- [ ] Guava paste (canned or in a plastic container)
- [ ] Pickled jalapeños
- [ ] Pickled nopales (cactus paddles)
- [ ] Olives: green pimiento-stuffed, black kalamata
- [ ] Capers or alcaparrado (mixed olives, capers, and pimientos)
- [ ] Chipotles in adobo sauce

Fresh Produce

- [ ] Cilantro
- [ ] Other Latin herbs such as culantro, yerba buena, papalo, and epazote
- [ ] Yuca (cassava, manioc) root
- [ ] Other Latin root veggies: yautia, ñame, etc.
- [ ] Green onions
- [ ] Garlic
- [ ] Onions: yellow, red, Spanish, sweet/Vidalia
- [ ] Leeks
- [ ] Plantains, green or ripe
- [ ] Fresh chiles: Anaheim, jalapeño, serrano, poblano, chilaques, and so on
- [ ] Bell peppers, green and red
- [ ] Avocado (buy 2 to 3 days prior to using)
- [ ] Potato, waxy yellow, red, and purple

- [ ] Papaya
- [ ] Limes, lemons, oranges
- [ ] Tomatillos
- [ ] Ripe red tomatoes
- [ ] Calabaza (Latin pumpkin)
- [ ] Fresh nopales, spines removed (cactus paddles)

Frozen

- [ ] Tropical fruit purees: guava, passion fruit (maracujá), soursop (guanábana), pineapple
- [ ] Frozen pigeon peas
- [ ] Frozen fava beans
- [ ] Vegan empanada dough rounds (read ingredients carefully . . . lard may lurk here!)
- [ ] Frozen peeled yuca chunks
- [ ] Choclo corn kernels
- [ ] Frozen whole ají amarillo, rocoto
- [ ] Frozen banana leaves

Miscellaneous

- [ ] Beer (most Mexican beer is vegan)
- [ ] Vegan dry white wine and red wine for cooking
- [ ] Dried corn husks
- [ ] Panela brown sugar, any cone or cake shape
- [ ] Latin chocolate for drinking (Ibarra, Sol, Luker, etc.)
- [ ] Corn or flour (read labels to check for lard) tortillas
- [ ] Cotton kitchen twine for tamales (cheaper in Latin markets!)
- [ ] Parchment paper for wrapping tamales (ditto)

Vegan Ingredients

- [ ] Vegetable broth or bouillon (avoid very "green" cabbagy-tasting brands)
- [ ] "Chicken"-flavored vegetable broth, cubes, or concentrated pastes
- [ ] Vital wheat gluten flour
- [ ] Tofu, Chinese (firm) for savory, Japanese silken (soft) for desserts or crema
- [ ] Soy sauce; use lighter Chinese-style sauce over strong tamari or shoyu varieties

- [ ] Nutritional yeast flakes
- [ ] Vegetarian Worcestershire sauce
- [ ] Tempeh
- [ ] Vegan mayonnaise
- [ ] Nonhydrogenated shortening and margarine

General Ingredients

Most any supermarket should have these groceries in stock.

- [ ] Tomato paste
- [ ] Canned diced tomatoes, preferably organic
- [ ] Canned crushed tomatoes or plain tomato sauce
- [ ] Red wine vinegar, white wine vinegar
- [ ] Olive oil, and vegetable oil for frying and baking

- [ ] Almonds, peanuts
- [ ] Pine nuts
- [ ] Raisins
- [ ] Fresh produce: corn, kale, radishes, green or red cabbage, lettuce, summer squash (zucchini, yellow squash), garlic, Italian parsley, carrot, eggplant, and so on

APPENDIX C

COOKING TERMS AND TECHNIQUES

If you're a newbie cook, browse through the following terms so that you know what to expect . . . especially if it's news that mincing not only applies to words but also garlic!

BASIC COOKING TERMS

Chop: A loose term for taking your knife to innocent vegetables and other items. I use *chop* to indicate that shape or size isn't necessarily important, typically because the chopped items will eventually be pureed, mashed, or otherwise not served in their current state. As a general rule, keep chopped pieces less than 1½ inches across.

Deglaze: Start throwing around this term when you want to really impress your friends with what a master chef you've become. Deglazing happens when a relatively small amount of liquid is added to sauté items in a hot pan once most of the juices have cooked off. Simmering with a little broth or wine lifts of the caramelized bits from the bottom of the pan, dissolves them, and distributes their lovely, improved flavors back into your food.

Not to mention it handily removes the gunk from the pan, making your eventual cleaning job all the easier.

Deep-fry: A *tostone's* best friend. Deep-frying involves a lot more oil than any other form of cooking, at least 2½ inches deep in a thick, heavy pot heated until very hot (around 350°F) but not smoking. Deep-fried foods should be able to float freely in the oil to achieve the proper texture and cooking. I use inexpensive vegetable oil blends, or oils specially designed for high heat, such as high-heat canola or peanut oil. I also like to keep a supply of brown paper bags to use for draining fried stuff; I tear them into single sheets, crumple them up so that they have nooks and crannies to facilitate the oils' draining down, and layer them two or three sheets thick, next to the pot. A long-handled wire mesh skimmer is perfect for retrieving fried items; a pair of long-handled tongs is the next best thing.

Dice, large, small, and in between: Dicing is just a slightly more strategic form of chopping: here, you're chopping foods into square shapes. When I refer to just "dice," I intend for the food to be chopped into squares roughly ½ inch in diameter. Large dice is about 1 inch, and small dice is about ⅜ inch or smaller. Don't feel that you need to break out the ruler (or a sweat!). You can follow the size of your own fingers if you'd prefer: about the size of your thumb knuckle for large dice, a little smaller than your thumb fingernail for regular (just "dice") dice, and your pinkie nail (or smaller) for small dice.

Fold: A purposeful way of mixing together ingredients. Rather than mixing around and around, move your spoon or spatula from underneath, scooping forward and eventually moving to the top. Do it a few times and you'll see it really is a little like folding stuff together. This method is effective when you want to make sure small ingredients are incorporated evenly and quickly into a thicker mixture, such as raisins into a cake batter.

Knead: A method of folding and flipping any dough onto a work surface to help develop and enhance its texture. The simplest way is to lift one end of the dough, fold it on top of the other end, and press down and out firmly with the heel of your palm. Smoosh the dough outward as far as you like, flip it over if it sounds like fun, repeat, and there you have it, you're kneading.

Mince: A slightly more fussy form of dicing that takes a little practice to get the hang of, but is well worth it for pretty sprinkles of cilantro or the even distribution of garlic or other good things into food. With a sharp chef's knife dice your item as small as you can, scrape all the bits toward you into a pile, and quickly chop finely again. It's best to use a chef's knife to achieve the proper rocking motion with a curved blade that makes mincing fly by. When in doubt watch any chefy kind of television show (there's a zillion out there) and at some point someone will do some mincing.

Pan-fry: Frying in a skillet with just enough oil to coat the entire bottom of the pan with about ¼ to ⅛ inch oil, or even a little less. This enables the fried items to get a crisp exterior without floating in oil. Essential for perfectly caramelized sweet plantains or "cheating" at deep-frying such items as *taquitos* (page 168).

Puree: Use a food processor, blender, or immersion blender to chop food until it becomes a thick, smooth mixture. Transforms tofu from a wiggly white block to a miracle ingredient and ordinary vegetable soup into a silky-smooth wonder. Be sure to invest in a decent food processor or immersion blender (page 25).

Sauté: A classy word for frying in a skillet, sautéing involves also occasionally stirring, flipping, and moving things around in the hot pan so that they are evenly heated and cooked.

Simmer: A gentle, slow boil with very little bubbling (and therefore small bubbles). Typically involves lowering the heat on the stovetop burner to the lowest setting possible so that *something* is still happening, only in the slowest possible way. Good for reducing sauces or cooking delicate items a low temperature to prevent over cooking.

Reduce: Another five-dollar chef word, *reduce* involves simmering a volume of liquid so that it, well, reduces in volume over a period of time via evaporation. This helps concentrate the flavors and possibly thicken the texture of your liquid. Consult the recipe regarding how much you should reduce something to, but typically this is about one-third of half of the original whatever-you're-making.

Whisk: What cookbook would be without the mention of whisking? Sometimes done with an actual whisk, this is just a rapid form of mixing involving short, circular strokes with the intention of getting everything in a liquid to mix evenly and quickly. A fork makes an excellent stand-in for a whisk and is just the right size for mixing up a little cup of dressing.

A few cooking techniques and methods are used extensively in Latin cooking:

Long sauté of onions, garlic, peppers, and other aromatic veggies: At its most basic, this creates a hearty foundation of flavor for the rest of the elements of the dish to build upon. In its most refined form, it's *adobo* or *sofrito*, a thick concoction of slowly fried onion, peppers, herbs, spices, and other veggies with a generous helping of oil. Either way, this long, gentle sauté enables the sugars in the vegetables to caramelize and transform raw ingredients into a concoction that's rich in savory umami (the recently discovered "other" taste, perhaps best described as "savory," in addition to salty, sweet, bitter, and sour) flavors that provide depth and character to Latin cuisine.

Steaming, in particular rice and corn masa products: Steaming is an ancient method of cooking tamales and produces the moist and tender texture that makes them so desirable.

Tamale steaming differs from run-of-the-mill vegetable steaming mainly in that it (1) requires a much larger pot than you typically would steam a head of broccoli or a portion of carrots in, and (2) goes on for much longer, usually for an hour or slightly more. The most important part about steaming tamales is that you make sure there is always water in the bottom level of the pot so that it never dries out—no water in the pot can result in burning or scorching all of your hard work.

Just make sure to occasionally check the water level of anything that requires steaming for longer than 25 minutes and replenish with more warm water. A good way to keep an eye on whether there's enough water is to check and see if the pot steams if the lid is lifted, or if you can hear the water boiling and hissing in the pot. Or just use your nose . . . if you smell something burning remove the pot immediately from the burner or you may already have singed tamales!

Steaming rice on the stovetop is the most basic way to make Latin rice, though I do prefer to bake rice when cooking a big portion (2 or more cups of raw rice) or if it includes lots of ingredients such as beans or pumpkin, as those will increase the cooking time and possibly not cook thoroughly on a stovetop. Latin-style rice should be firm but never crunchy, fluffy and moist but never sticky. I find that some rice cookers tend to produce rice that's on the sticky side (and rice cookers in general require a little bit of voodoo and good luck to get it right sometimes) but if you're a rice-cooker champion, then go right ahead.

Deep-frying: This is a cooking method thoroughly embraced by many Latin cultures. The occasional treat of crispy fried yuca, tender crisp empanadas, and of course crunchy *tostones* make all that oil and a mess of paper towels worth it. To ensure that less oil is absorbed by your deep fried treats, always preheat the oil over medium-high heat for at least 6 minutes. When a tiny piece of dough/boiled yuca/plantain rapidly sizzles on contact with the oil, the oil is ready. Some cooks insist on using a deep-fry thermometer to confirm a fry-ready ideal temperature of 350°F, but I find the dough test to be just as valid. And of course, never drop water into hot oil, as it will splatter in a scary way . . . so no drinking and frying! If you do a lot of frying, you may want to invest in a frying screen that can be placed over the pan to catch any rebellious flying drops of hot oil.

Boiling: Everybody boils food, and Latin cuisine is no exception. Boiling is usually the first stage in preparing starchy root vegetables for consumption or for lightly blanching vegetables such as chayote. Use a large pot with a tight-fitting lid, fill the pot halfway or a little more, and heat over high heat. Cover the pot to hasten the boiling and remove the cover once the water is rolling.

Grilling: Either on a proper grill or on the heated dry surface of a pan, grilling is not just for protein foods but also for starchy items such as tortillas and *arepas*. In their respective countries, a *comal* or a *budare* (page 27), a griddlelike item, is used for cooking, but a well-seasoned cast-iron griddle or skillet does exactly the same job. I prefer cast iron for these foods as it readily accepts high heat and distributes it perfectly, not to mention a well-seasoned cast-iron surface is naturally nonstick. Your *comal*, *budare*, or cast-iron skillet should be preheated for at least 5 minutes or more, and is ready to use when a drop of water flicked onto its surface sizzles and pops immediately.

Removing corn from the cob: In many parts of South America, corn kernels are not so much cut off of the cob as they are grated off; a regular box grater works just fine for this. Just firmly grab one side of a corn cob and grate on a large-hole grater side, taking care not to grate off any of the hard cob (or your knuckles), and turn the cob to a new side when you've grated everything there is.

If you need whole intact kernels, I highly recommend getting a corn zipper (page 26), which is a nifty little tool that quickly removes one row of corn kernels at a time. I know that doesn't sound fast, but once you get the hang of it, it really is fast, plus it's fun to say you're unzipping corn. Life without a corn zipper is possible if you possess a very sharp paring or chef's knife and a large, wide bowl. Firmly grasp the narrow end of the ear of corn, balance the other end on the bottom of the bowl, and carefully and gently run your knife down the ear, again making sure to cut exactly where the kernel joins the cob and no lower, or you'll end up with tough undesirable bits of cob in your corn.

Roasting bell and chile peppers: Roasting transforms mild-mannered peppers into juicy, succulent dainties with alluring smoky flavor and sweetness, and concentrates all the deep flavors of these fruits.

The best way to roast just one or two peppers is directly on a gas stovetop. Place a whole, uncut pepper directly on top of a burner turned to a high flame. Roast until the skin starts to blacken, pop, and sizzle. Use metal tongs to rotate the pepper frequently so that all of the sides just a chance to sear. Quickly place the pepper in a sturdy container (I use a heavy pot or tortilla warmer) and cover tightly (or place into paper bag and tightly roll the top shut) and let cool for 10 minutes. This cooling also allows the steam to work its way out of the pepper and help loosen the skin from the pepper's surface.

When the pepper is cool enough to touch, gently peel off as much of the outside, flaking skin as possible and discard. Slice, remove the core of large peppers (not necessary for small, thin chiles such as serranos), and scrape off the seeds, if desired (retaining the seeds will make the dish hotter). If possible, try to catch any of the roasted pepper juices to use in the food, as it's loaded with flavor. Don't wash the charred skin; you'll be also washing away a lot of the flavorful juices you worked so hard to cook.

If you're roasting small chiles (such as jalapeños or serranos) that might slip through the burner grills, place a metal heat diffuser (see page 26) on top of the burner, heat over high heat for a few minutes, and place the chiles on the diffuser to roast. Turn with tongs to blister all sides of the chiles.

Roasting a bunch of peppers? Preheat the oven to 400°F and place the whole, unsliced chiles on a large, rimmed baking sheet lined with parchment paper. Roast for 15 to 25 minutes, or until the chiles are blackened and collapsed. Let cool, and peel and seed as directed above.

APPENDIX D

METRIC CONVERSION CHART

- The recipes in this book have not been tested with metric measurements, so some variations might occur.
- Remember that the weight of dry ingredients varies according to the volume or density factor: 1 cup of flour weighs far less than 1 cup of sugar, and 1 tablespoon doesn't necessarily hold 3 teaspoons.

General Formulas for Metric Conversion

Ounces to grams	→ ounces × 28.35 = grams
Grams to ounces	→ grams × 0.035 = ounces
Pounds to grams	→ pounds × 453.5 = grams
Pounds to kilograms	→ pounds × 0.45 = kilograms
Cups to liters	→ cups × 0.24 = liters
Fahrenheit to Celsius	→ (°F − 32) × 5 ÷ 9 = °C
Celsius to Fahrenheit	→ (°C × 9) ÷ 5 + 32 = °F

Linear Measurements

1/2 inch	=	1 1/2 cm
1 inch	=	2 1/2 cm
6 inches	=	15 cm
8 inches	=	20 cm
10 inches	=	25 cm
12 inches	=	30 cm
20 inches	=	50 cm

Volume (Dry) Measurements

1/4 teaspoon = 1 milliliter
1/2 teaspoon = 2 milliliters
3/4 teaspoon = 4 milliliters
1 teaspoon = 5 milliliters
1 tablespoon = 15 milliliters
1/4 cup = 59 milliliters
1/3 cup = 79 milliliters
1/2 cup = 118 milliliters
2/3 cup = 158 milliliters
3/4 cup = 177 milliliters
1 cup = 225 milliliters
4 cups or 1 quart = 1 liter
1/2 gallon = 2 liters
1 gallon = 4 liters

Volume (Liquid) Measurements

1 teaspoon = 1/6 fluid ounce = 5 milliliters
1 tablespoon = 1/2 fluid ounce = 15 milliliters
2 tablespoons = 1 fluid ounce = 30 milliliters
1/4 cup = 2 fluid ounces = 60 milliliters
1/3 cup = 2 2/3 fluid ounces = 79 milliliters
1/2 cup = 4 fluid ounces = 118 milliliters
1 cup or 1/2 pint = 8 fluid ounces = 250 milliliters
2 cups or 1 pint = 16 fluid ounces = 500 milliliters
4 cups or 1 quart = 32 fluid ounces = 1,000 milliliters
1 gallon = 4 liters

Oven Temperature Equivalents, Fahrenheit (F) and Celsius (C)

100°F = 38°C
200°F = 95°C
250°F = 120°C
300°F = 150°C
350°F = 180°C
400°F = 205°C
450°F = 230°C

Weight (Mass) Measurements

1 ounce = 30 grams
2 ounces = 55 grams
3 ounces = 85 grams
4 ounces = 1/4 pound = 125 grams
8 ounces = 1/2 pound = 240 grams
12 ounces = 3/4 pound = 375 grams
16 ounces = 1 pound = 454 grams

ACKNOWLEDGMENTS

First things first, endless thanks to a long-distance family of home cooks that made sure these recipes could be made by anyone anywhere. From East Coast to West Coast, all points in between, and even as far as the U.K. and Germany, these gorgeous, brilliant, and supremely tasteful testers donated their kitchens and stomachs in the name of making better recipes.

Ana "wannabeavegan" Cruz
Kittee Berns
Melisser Elliott
Andrea "Andi" Espinoza
Jenny Howard (kitchenspoon)
Carla Kelly (Queen V supertester, 130+ recipes tested!)
Teressa Jackson
Erica Johnson
Lisa L.
Kim "Veg-in-Training" and Fred Lahn "Phat Freddie"
Megan McClellan
Monique Martin
Tami Noyes
Thalia C. Palmer

Lisa Pitman (I'm talking to you!)
Laura Poe
Constanze Reichardt
Chantal Reid
Rob and Barbi
Dayna Rozental
Luciana Rushing
Amanda "Esme" Sacco
Leigh Saluzzi
Katy "ají paste fiend" Schwalbe
Stacy Swartz-Thomas
Anne-Kristin Thordin
Jennifer Turnbull-Henn
Cindy Uribe
Sarah "sandybadlands" Willson
Abby Wohl
Liz Wyman
Bahar "bazu" Zaker

Just when it couldn't get even more exciting the follow people deserve tamales and hugs for helping make *Viva Vegan!* a reality. I can't thank you enough, but this is a start:

John Stavropoulos for the shopping, cleaning, hugs, and life management stuff done while I was busy losing my mind. I love you even when you buy parsley instead of cilantro.

My Stavropoulos and Vournas family: Eleni, Christopher, Kiki, Chris, Kathy, Tina, and Cleo the dog for driving me around (not Cleo, she's too young to drive), and allowing me take over their house, basement, fridge, and kitchen for extreme food photography.

My Papá and Mom for answering all those questions about food and stuff en español any time I called. Someday I'll give you your cookbooks back.

Isa Moskowitz for all things Post Punk Kitchen, theppk.com, and getting the whole vegan world-domination thing in motion.

My Queens crew of Jimb, Evelyn, Erica, Frank, Keren, JZN, Paula, Herzy, Abby, John C. (many thanks for the last minute camera!), Eppy (and his slice of Brooklyn), and by extension nerd.nyc.

And to everyone who sparked their imaginations to help us name this book . . . Vegan La Raza!

I would also like to thank:

Katie, Erica, Renee, Lindsey, and Georgia at Da Capo.

Angie Gaul, photographer warrior woman extraordinaire.

Miha, Mark, Paige, and Nikki for the cover shoot, and Ira and Rocco the dog for their lovely digs and kitchen.

Marc Gerald at the Agency Group.

• • •

INDEX

achiote (annatto)
  about, 21
  Annatto-Infused Oil (Aciete de Achiote), 31–32
  Sofrito con Cilantro and Achiote (variation), 33
Aciete de Achiote (Annatto-Infused Oil), 31–32
Agavelicious Horchata (variation), 214
Agave–Orange Flower "Honey," Sopaipillas with, 226–227
Agua de Papelón (Real Brown Sugar Limeade), 214–215
alfajores
  Alfajores (Buttery Cookies with Thick Dulce de Leche Filling), 241–242
  Chocolate-drizzled Alfajores (variation), 243
  Guayaba Alfajores (variation), 243
almonds
  Buttery Cookies with Thick Dulce de Leche Filling (Alfajores), 241–242
  Chocolate-Chile Mole Sauce (an Oaxacan wannabe), 51–53
  Creamy Horchata, 213–214
  Fruity Chile Slaw, 72
Amaranth Polenta with Roasted Chiles, 128–129

Ancho Chile Dressing, Creamy, 70–71
Ancho Chile–Tempeh Asado (variation), 110–111
Annatto-Infused Oil (Aciete de Achiote), 31–32
Anticuchos, Seitan (Peruvian Seitan and Potato Skewers), 104–106
"Any Noche" Romaine and Fruit Salad with Candied Chile Peanuts, 73–75
appetizers. *See* bocadillos, snacks, appetizers
apples
  "Any Noche" Romaine and Fruit Salad with Candied Chile Peanuts, 73–75
  Shredded Carrot-Jicama Salad, 72–73
arepas
  Arepas Stuffed with Oyster Mushrooms and Pimiento Peppers, 180–181
  Arepas (Venezuelan- and Colombian-style "Tortillas"), 177–179
  Arepas with Sexy Avocado-Tempeh Filling (Avocado Pepiada Arepa), 181–182
  Colombian Arepa con Chicharron (variation), 180

Colombian Grilled Arepas with Corn and Vegan Cheese, 179–180
  Traditional Petits Pois Arepas (variation), 182
Arroz con Coco (Savory Coconut Rice), 97
Arroz con Gandules (Rice with Pigeon Peas), 140–142
Arroz con Leche de Coco (variation), 235
Arroz con Leche with Saffron (variation), 235
Arroz con Seitan, 145–147
asparagus, in Pan-Grilled Vegetables in Chile-Lime Beer, 124
avocados
  about, 20–21
  Arepas with Sexy Avocado-Tempeh Filling (Avocado Pepiada Arepa), 181–182
  Bite-Size Green Plantain Sandwiches (Patacones), 65–66
  Black-Eyed–Butternut Tostadas, 173–174
  Creamy Avocado-Tomato Salsa (Venezuelan Guasacaca), 39–40
  Creamy Potato Soup with Avocado (Locro), 149–150

avocados *(continued)*
  Eggplant Torta Sandwich,
    55–57
  Spinach-Avocado-Chile
    Salad, 72
  The Only Guacamole Recipe
    I Ever Make, 48–49
  Tostones with Avocado and
    Palm Ceviche, 61

Baked Tofu with Salsa de Mani
    (variation), 103
Banana Smoothie, Truly Tropical
    (variation), 216
basic recipes. *See also* doughs
  Annatto-Infused Oil (Aciete
    de Achiote), 31–32
  Basic Beans from Scratch,
    83–85
  Basic Onion-Pepper Sofrito,
    32–33
  Chorizo Seitan Sausages,
    36–37
  Classic Stovetop Long-Grain
    White or Brown Rice,
    94–95
  homemade tortilla chips, 174
  Home-style Refried Beans,
    86–87
  Steamed Red Seitan, 34–35
  Steamed White Seitan,
    35–36
batidos
  Merengada (variation), 216
  Tropical Fruit Shake (Batido),
    215–216
  Truly Tropical Banana
    Smoothie (variation), 216
beans
  about, 12, 13, 22, 85
  Basic Beans from Scratch,
    83–85
  Bean and Tofu Chicharrones,
    164
  Beans, Rice, and Sweet
    Plantain Empanadas,
    210–212

Black Bean–Corn Salsa
    Salad, 72
Black Bean Soup Habanero
    (variation), 152
Black Bean–Sweet Potato
    Tamales, 189–191
Black-Eyed–Butternut Tostadas,
    173–174
burrito fillings, 170–171
Chocolate Mole Veggie
    Tamales, 193–194
Colombian-style Red Beans, 90
cooking pots for, 88
corn empanada fillings, 207
Costa Rican Refried Rice and
    Beans (Gallo Pinto), 92–93
Creamy Corn-Crusted Tempeh
    Pot Pie (variation), 145
Creamy Potato Peanut Stew
    (variation), 140
Cuban Black Bean Soup,
    150–152
Drunken Beans with Seitan
    Chorizo, 91–92
Eggplant Torta Sandwich,
    55–56, 55–57
Farmer's Market Tamales,
    194–196
Green Posole Seitan Stew with
    Chard and White Beans,
    137–138
Hearty Pumpkin and Cranberry
    Bean Stew (Porotos
    Granados), 152–154
Hearty Warm Yuca and
    Cabbage Salad, 78–79
Home-style Refried Beans,
    86–87
Onion-Flavored Beans
    (bean-cooking tip), 85–86
pupusa fillings, 164
Pupusas Stuffed with Black
    Beans and Plantains,
    162–165
Peruvian Red Chile–Corn
    Salad with Limas and Cherry
    Tomatoes, 80–81

Portobello Feijoada (Brazilian
    Black Bean Stew with
    Portobello Mushrooms),
    147–148
Potato-Chickpea Enchiladas
    with Green Tomatillo Sauce,
    133–135
Quick Red Posole with Beans,
    136–137
Quinoa-Corn "Chowder" with
    Limas and Ají, 156–157
Red Beans with
    Dominican-style Sazón,
    87–88
Rice with Pigeon Peas (Arroz
    con Gandules), 140–142
Sancocho (Vegetable, Roots,
    and Plantain Soup), 154–155
Spinach–Brazil Nut–Gazpacho
    Salad, 72
taco toppings, 176
Venezuelan-style Black Beans
    (Caraotas), 89
beer
  about, 9
  Arroz con Seitan, 145–147
  Chipotle, Seitan, and Potato
    Tacos, 174–177
  Drunken Beans with Seitan
    Chorizo, 91–92
  Michelada (Spicy, Salty,
    Ice-Cold Beer), 220–221
  Pan-Grilled Vegetables in
    Chile-Lime Beer, 124
beets, in "Any Noche" Romaine
    and Fruit Salad with
    Candied Chile Peanuts,
    73–75
bell peppers
  about, 19
  Arroz con Seitan, 145–147
  Basic Onion-Pepper Sofrito,
    32–33
  Costa Rican Refried Rice and
    Beans (Gallo Pinto), 92–93
  Creamy Potato Peanut Stew
    (Guatita), 138–140

Cuban Black Bean Soup,
150–152
Red Beans with Dominican-
style Sazón, 87–88
beverages. *See* drinks
Bite-Size Green Plantain
Sandwiches (Patacones),
65–66
black beans
Beans, Rice, and Sweet
Plantain Empanadas,
210–212
Black Bean–Corn Salsa
Salad, 72
Black Bean Soup Habanero
(variation), 152
Black Bean–Sweet Potato
Tamales, 189–191
Costa Rican Refried Rice and
Beans (Gallo Pinto), 92–93
Cuban Black Bean Soup,
150–152
Eggplant Torta Sandwich,
55–56
Home-style Refried Beans,
86–87
Pupusas Stuffed with Black
Beans and Plantains,
162–165
Portobello Feijoada (Brazilian
Black Bean Stew with
Portobello Mushrooms),
147–148
Quick Red Posole with Beans,
136–137
Spinach–Brazil Nut–Gazpacho
Salad, 72
Venezuelan-style Black Beans
(Caraotas), 89
Black-Eyed–Butternut Tostadas,
173–174
bocadillos, snacks, appetizers
Bite-Size Green Plantain
Sandwiches (Patacones),
65–66
Calabacita Torta
(variation), 57

Cubano Vegano Sandwich,
66–67
Eggplant Torta Sandwich, 55–57
Mashed Potato Pancakes with
Peanut Sauce
(Llapingachos), 57–58
Mexican Side-Street Corn,
63–64
Mixed Mushroom Ceviche,
59–60
Stuffed Mini Potatoes with
Mushrooms and Olives
(Papas Rellenas), 62–63
Tostones with Avocado and
Palm Ceviche, 61
Bolivian Salteñas (Sweet and
Spicy Seitan-Potato
Empanadas), 204–206
Braised Brazilian Shredded Kale,
121–122
brandy, in Sangria, 219
Brazilian Shredded Kale, Braised,
121–122
Brazilian Style Savory Orange
Rice, 98
Brazilian-style White Rice
(variation), 98
Brazil Nut–Spinach–Gazpacho
Salad, 72
burritos, 170–171
Butternut–Black-Eyed Tostadas,
173–174
Buttery Cookies with Thick Dulce
de Leche Filling (Alfajores),
241–242

cabbage
Classic Cabbage Salad, 71–72
Fruity Chile Slaw, 72
Hearty Warm Yuca and
Cabbage Salad, 78–79
Salvadorian Marinated Slaw
(Curdito), 79–80
Cachapas (Savory Fresh Corn
Pancakes), 182–184
Caesar Mexicano Salad,
Chipotle, 73

Café con Leche, 217–218
Café con Leche Flan, 245–247
Cake, Chocolate Orange Spice,
with Dulce de Batata,
238–239
Cake, Coconut Tres Leches,
230–232
Calabacitas (Mixed Squash
Sauté), 122–123
Calabacita Torta (variation), 57
calabaza pumpkin. *See* pumpkin
Candied Chile Peanuts, "Any
Noche" Romaine and Fruit
Salad with, 73–75
capers
Arroz con Seitan, 145–147
Chayote and Potato Salad with
Capers and Peas, 75–76
Farmer's Market Tamales,
194–196
Puerto Rican "Picadillo" Style
Seitan (variation), 108
Rice with Pigeon Peas
(variation), 141
Swiss Chard with Raisins and
Capers, 123
Caraotas (Venezuelan-style
Black Beans), 89
Carrot-Jicama Salad, Shredded,
72–73
Cashew Crema, 51
cazuelas. See stews and casseroles
Ceviche, Mixed Mushroom,
59–60
Ceviche, Tostones with Avocado
and Palm, 61
chard
Green Posole Seitan Stew with
Chard and White Beans,
137–138
Potato-Chard Soup with
Sizzling Chorizo (variation),
160
Swiss Chard with Raisins and
Capers, 123
Chayote and Potato Salad with
Capers and Peas, 75–76

cheese. *See* vegan cheese

"Cheezy" Sauce, Peruvian Potatoes with Spicy, 125–126

Chia, Whole Wheat Flour Tortillas with, 166–168

chicharrones
- Bean and Tofu Chicharrones, 164
- Colombian Arepa con Chicharron (variation), 180
- Tofu Chicharrones, 101–102

chickpeas
- Creamy Corn-Crusted Tempeh Pot Pie (variation), 145
- Creamy Potato Peanut Stew (variation), 140
- Hearty Warm Yuca and Cabbage Salad, 78–79
- Potato-Chickpea Enchiladas with Green Tomatillo Sauce, 133–135
- Sancocho (Vegetable, Roots, and Plantain Soup), 154–155

Chile-Braised Seitan, Mexican (variation), 107

Chile-Lime Beer, Pan-Grilled Vegetables in, 124

chiles, 15–18, 22

Chile Sauce, Red, 45–46

Chile-Seitan Tamales, Red, 191–192

Chilena, Ensalada (Tomato Salad with Sweet Crisp Onions), 76–77

Chimichurri Baked Tofu, 100–101

Chimichurri Sauce with Smoked Paprika, 42

chipotles
- Chipotle, Seitan, and Potato Tacos, 174–177
- Chipotle Adobo Seitan (variation), 108
- Chipotle Caesar Mexicano Salad, 73
- Chipotle Chorizo (variation), 37

Chipotle in Adobo Salad Dressing (variation), 71

Sweet Potato–Chipotle Bisque, 155–156

Choclo, Pastel de (Creamy Corn-Crusted Tempeh Pot Pie), 144–145

choclo corn, to prepare (tip), 59

chocolate
- Chocolate-Chile Mole Sauce (an Oaxacan wannabe), 51–53
- Chocolate-drizzled Alfajores (variation), 243
- Chocolate Mole Veggie Tamales, 193–194
- Chocolate Orange Spice Cake with Dulce de Batata, 238–239
- Chocolate para Churros, 225–226
- Real Hot Chocolate and Variations, 216–217

chorizo
- Chipotle Chorizo (variation), 37
- Chorizo Seitan Sausages, 36–37
- Chorizo-Spinach Sopes, 171–173
- Drunken Beans with Seitan Chorizo, 91–92
- Hot Ají Chorizo (variation), 37
- *pupusa* fillings, 164
- Potato-Kale Soup with Sizzling Chorizo, 159–160
- Rice with Pigeon Peas (variation), 141–142
- Taquitos with Chorizo and Potatoes, 168–169
- to serve, 38

Churros, 223–225

Churros, Chocolate para, 225–226

Cilantro and Achiote, Sofrito con (variation), 33

Cilantro-Citrus Vinaigrette, 69–70

Cilantro-Lime Rice, 95–96

Classic Cabbage Salad, 71–72

Classic Roasted Tomatillo Salsa, 47–48

Classic Stovetop Long-Grain White or Brown Rice, 94–95

coconut
- Arroz con Coco (Savory Coconut Rice), 97
- Arroz con Leche de Coco (variation), 235
- Buttery Cookies with Thick Dulce de Leche Filling (Alfajores), 241–242
- Coconut-Pineapple Tamales (variation), 197
- Coconut Tres Leches Cake, 230–232
- Dulce de Batata (variation), 237

coconut milk
- about, 12
- Arroz con Coco (Savory Coconut Rice), 97
- Arroz con Leche de Coco (variation), 235
- Café con Leche Flan, 245–247
- Coconut Tres Leches Cake, 230–232
- richer hot chocolate (variation), 217
- Sweet Coconut Corn Pudding (Majarete), 235–236
- Sweet Corn Ice Cream, 240
- Vanilla-Coconut Flan, 243–245

coffee
- Café con Leche, 217–218
- Café con Leche Flan, 245–247
- Cuban-Style Coffee, 217–218

Colombian- and Venezuelan-style "Tortillas" (Arepas), 177–179

Colombian Grilled Arepas with Corn and Vegan Cheese, 179–180

Colombian-style Red Beans, 90

condiments. *See* salsas and condiments

cookies
Buttery Cookies with Thick
Dulce de Leche Filling
(Alfajores), 241–242
Chocolate-drizzled Alfajores
(variation), 243
Guayaba Alfajores
(variation), 243
corn
Black Bean–Corn Salsa
Salad, 72
Calabacitas (Mixed Squash
Sauté), 122–123
Colombian Grilled Arepas with
Corn and Vegan Cheese,
179–180
Creamy Corn-Crusted Tempeh
Pot Pie (Pastel de Choclo),
144–145
Creamy Corn-Filled Empanadas
(Empanadas Humitas),
201–202
Farmer's Market Tamales,
194–196
Mexican Side-Street Corn,
63–64
Peruvian Red Chile–Corn
Salad with Limas and Cherry
Tomatoes, 80–81
Porotos Granados (Hearty
Pumpkin and Cranberry
Bean Stew), 152–154
Quinoa-Corn "Chowder" with
Limas and Ají, 156–157
Quinoa Salad with Spinach,
Olives, and Roasted
Peanuts, 82
roasted, 64
Sancocho (Vegetable, Roots,
and Plantain Soup), 154–155
Savory Fresh Corn Pancakes
(Cachapas), 182–184
Sweet Coconut Corn Pudding
(Majarete), 235–236
Sweet Corn Ice Cream, 240
corn-crusted empanada
fillings, 207

Corn-Crusted Pumpkin-Potato
Empanadas, 207–210
Corn Tortillas, Homemade Soft,
165–166
Costa Rican Refried Rice and
Beans (Gallo Pinto),
92–93
Cranberry Bean Stew, Hearty
Pumpkin and (Porotos
Granados), 152–154
Creamy Ancho Chile Dressing,
70–71
Creamy Avocado-Tomato Salsa
(Venezuelan Guasacaca),
39–40
Creamy Corn-Crusted Tempeh
Pot Pie (Pastel de Choclo),
144–145
Creamy Corn-Filled Empanadas
(Empanadas Humitas),
201–202
Creamy Horchata, 213–214
Creamy Potato Peanut Stew
(Guatita), 138–140
Creamy Potato Soup with
Avocado (Locro), 149–150
Crema, Cashew, 51
Crema, Pine Nut, 45
Crepes à la Mode (variation), 226
Crepes with Un-Dulce de Leche
and Sweet Plantains,
228–230
Crispy Fried Green Plantains
(Tostones), 118–120
Crunchy Fried Yuca (Yuca Frita),
126–127
Cuban Black Bean Soup,
150–152
Cuban Garlic-Lime-Mojo Sauce,
Yuca with, 127–128
Cubano Vegano Sandwich,
66–67
Cuban "Ropa Vieja" Style Seitan
(variation), 107
Cuban-Style Coffee, 217–218
Curdito (Salvadorian Marinated
Slaw), 79–80

desserts
Arroz con Leche de Coco
(variation), 235
Arroz con Leche with Saffron
(variation), 235
Buttery Cookies with Thick
Dulce de Leche Filling
(Alfajores), 241–242
Café con Leche Flan, 245–247
Chocolate-drizzled Alfajores
(variation), 243
Chocolate Orange Spice Cake
with Dulce de Batata,
238–239
Chocolate para Churros,
225–226
Churros, 223–225
Coconut-Pineapple Tamales
(variation), 197
Coconut Tres Leches Cake,
230–232
Crepes à la Mode
(variation), 230
Crepes with Un-Dulce de
Leche and Sweet Plantains,
228–230
Dulce de Batata (Sweet Potato
Sweet Mash), 236–237
Fresh Mango and Guava Bread
Pudín, 232–234
Fresh Papaya-Lime Sorbet, 239
Guayaba Alfajores
(variation), 243
Pineapple-Raisin Sweet
Tamales, 196–197
Simply Arroz con Leche,
234–235
Sopaipillas with Orange
Flower–Agave "Honey,"
226–227
Sweet Coconut Corn Pudding
(Majarete), 235–236
Sweet Corn Ice Cream, 240
Thick Dulce de Leche
Filling, 242
Un-Dulce de Leche, 227–228
Vanilla-Coconut Flan, 243–245

Dominican-style Sazón, Red Beans with, 87–88
doughs
Arepas (Venezuelan- and Colombian-style "Tortillas"), 177–179
for corn-crusted empanadas, 208
for Pupusas Stuffed with Black Beans and Plantains, 162–165
frozen empanada dough, 200
Homemade Soft Corn Tortillas, 165–166
Savory Vegan Masa Dough, 188–189
Wheat Empanada Dough, 199–201
Whole Wheat Flour Tortillas with Chia, 166–168
Dried Chile Salsa (variation), 50
dried herbs and spices, 21
drinks
Café con Leche, 217–218
Creamy Horchata, 213–214
Cuban-Style Coffee, 217–218
Merengada (variation), 216
Michelada (Spicy, Salty, Ice-Cold Beer), 220–221
Mojito, 220
Real Brown Sugar Limeade (Agua de Papelón), 214–215
Real Hot Chocolate and Variations, 216–217
Sangria, 219
Simple Syrup for, 218
Toddy Caliente (variation), 217
Tropical Fruit Shake (Batido), 215–216
Drunken Beans with Seitan Chorizo, 91–92
Dulce de Batata (Sweet Potato Sweet Mash), 236–237
Dulce de Batata, Chocolate Orange Spice Cake with, 238–239

dulce de leche. See also un-dulce de leche
Buttery Cookies with Thick Dulce de Leche Filling (Alfajores), 241–242

Eggplant Torta Sandwich, 55–57
empanadas
Beans, Rice, and Sweet Plantain Empanadas, 210–212
corn-crusted empanada fillings, 207
Corn-Crusted Pumpkin-Potato Empanadas, 207–210
Creamy Corn-Filled Empanadas (Empanadas Humitas), 201–202
frozen empanada dough, 200
Richer Wheat Dough (variation), 201
Shredded Seitan and Mushroom Empanadas with Raisins and Olives, 202–204
Shredded Seitan Empanadas (variation), 212
Sweet and Spicy Seitan-Potato Empanadas (Bolivian Salteñas), 204–206
Wheat Empanada Dough, 199–201
enchilada fillings from leftovers, 135
Enchiladas, Potato-Chickpea, with Green Tomatillo Sauce, 133–135
ensaladas. See salads

Farmer's Market Tamales, 194–196
fava beans
about, 12, 22
Hearty Warm Yuca and Cabbage Salad, 78–79
Sancocho (Vegetable, Roots, and Plantain Soup), 154–155
Flan, Café con Leche, 245–247
Flan, Vanilla-Coconut, 243–245
flautas (taquito variation), 169

Flour Tortillas with Chia, Whole Wheat, 166–168
Fresh Gazpacho Salsa Dressing, 70
Fresh Mango and Guava Bread Pudín, 232–234
Fresh Papaya-Lime Sorbet, 239
Fresh Tomato Salsa with Roasted Chiles, 50
Fried Sweet Plantains, 115–117
fruits. See also specific types
"Any Noche" Romaine and Fruit Salad with Candied Chile Peanuts, 73–75
frozen purees, 22
Sangria, 219
Tropical Fruit Shake (Batido), 215–216
Fruity Chile Slaw, 72

Gallo Pinto (Costa Rican Refried Rice and Beans), 92–93
gandules (pigeon peas)
frozen, 12, 22
Rice with Pigeon Peas (Arroz con Gandules), 140–142
Garlic, Yellow Rice with, 96–97
Garlic-Lime-Mojo Sauce, Cuban, Yuca with, 127–128
Gazpacho Salsa Dressing, Fresh, 70
Gazpacho–Spinach–Brazil Nut Salad, 72
Golf, Spicy Salsa, 53
Green Ají Sauce (So Good, So Green Dipping Sauce), 43–44
green beans, in Farmer's Market Tamales, 194–196
Green Onion Salsa, 44–45
Green Posole Seitan Stew with Chard and White Beans, 137–138
greens
Braised Brazilian Shredded Kale, 121–122
Green Posole Seitan Stew with Chard and White Beans, 137–138

INDEX

Potato-Kale Soup with Sizzling Chorizo, 159–160

Swiss Chard with Raisins and Capers, 123

Green Tomatillo Sauce, 40–41

groceries. *See* pantry items

Guacamole Recipe I Ever Make, The Only, 48–49

Guasacaca, Venezuelan (Creamy Avocado-Tomato Salsa), 39–40

Guatita (Creamy Potato Peanut Stew), 138–140

guava paste
  Fresh Mango and Guava Bread Pudín, 232–234
  Guayaba Alfajores (variation), 243

Habanero-Melon-Papaya Salsa, 53–54

hearts of palm
  Spinach–Brazil Nut–Gazpacho Salad, 72
  Tostones with Avocado and Palm Ceviche, 61

Hearty Pumpkin and Cranberry Bean Stew (Porotos Granados), 152–154

Hearty Warm Yuca and Cabbage Salad, 78–79

herbs and spices, 21

Homemade Soft Corn Tortillas, 165–166

homemade tortilla chips, 174

Home-style Refried Beans, 86–87

hominy
  Green Posole Seitan Stew with Chard and White Beans, 137–138
  Quick Red Posole with Beans, 136–137

Horchata, Agavelicious (variation), 214

Horchata, Creamy, 213–214

Hot Ají Chorizo (variation), 37

Hot Chocolate, Real, and Variations, 216–217

Huancaína Verde, Salsa a la (variation), 126

Humitas, Empanadas (Creamy Corn-Filled Empanadas), 201–202

Ice Cream, Sweet Corn, 240

ingredients. *See* pantry items

jicama
  "Any Noche" Romaine and Fruit Salad with Candied Chile Peanuts, 73–75
  Arepas with Sexy Avocado-Tempeh Filling (Avocado Pepiada Arepa), 181–182
  Mango-Jicama Chopped Salad, 77–78
  Shredded Carrot-Jicama Salad, 72–73

Kale, Braised Brazilian Shredded, 121–122

Kale-Potato Soup with Sizzling Chorizo, 159–160

kitchen tools and equipment, 23–27

Latin Baked Tofu, 103

Latin Shredded Seitan, 106–108

lima beans
  Peruvian Red Chile–Corn Salad with Limas and Cherry Tomatoes, 80–81
  Quinoa-Corn "Chowder" with Limas and Ají, 156–157
  Sancocho (Vegetable, Roots, and Plantain Soup), 154–155

Limeade, Real Brown Sugar (Agua de Papelón), 214–215

Lime-Papaya Sorbet, Fresh, 239

Llapingachos (Mashed Potato Pancakes with Peanut Sauce), 57–58

Locro (Creamy Potato Soup with Avocado), 149–150

Majarete (Sweet Coconut Corn Pudding), 235–236

mangoes
  Arroz con Coco (Savory Coconut Rice), 97
  Fresh Mango and Guava Bread Pudín, 232–234
  Mango-Jicama Chopped Salad, 77–78
  to slice, 233

Mani, Salsa de, (Peanut Sauce), 41–42

Mani, Salsa de, Baked Tofu with (variation), 103

masa, about, 13–15, 186. *See also* doughs

Mashed Potato Pancakes with Peanut Sauce (Llapingachos), 57–58

"Mechada" Style Seitan, Venezuelan (variation), 107

Melon-Papaya-Habanero Salsa, 53–54

Merengada (*batido* variation), 216

Mexican Chile-Braised Seitan (variation), 107

Mexican Side-Street Corn, 63–64

Michelada (Spicy, Salty, Ice-Cold Beer), 220–221

mint
  Mojito, 220
  Salsa a la Huancaína Verde (variation), 126

Mixed Mushroom Ceviche, 59–60

Mixed Squash Sauté (Calabacitas), 122–123

Mofongo, 120–121

Mojito, 220

mojo
  Mojo Oven-Roasted Seitan, 104
  Mojo Sauce with Tostones (variation), 128
  Yuca with Cuban Garlic-Lime-Mojo Sauce, 127–128
  Zesty Orange Mojo Baked Tofu, 102

mole
  Chocolate-Chile Mole Sauce
    (an Oaxacan wannabe),
    51–53
  Chocolate Mole Veggie
    Tamales, 193–194
  Tempeh Asado with Oaxacan-
    style Mole (variation), 111
mushrooms
  Arepas Stuffed with Oyster
    Mushrooms and Pimiento
    Peppers, 180–181
  Mixed Mushroom Ceviche,
    59–60
  Portobello Feijoada (Brazilian
    Black Bean Stew with
    Portobello Mushrooms),
    147–148
  Quinoa–Oyster Mushroom
    Risotto (Quinotto), 130–131
  Shredded Seitan and
    Mushroom Empanadas with
    Raisins and Olives, 202–204
  Stuffed Mini Potatoes with
    Mushrooms and Olives
    (Papas Rellenas), 62–63

ñame, in Sancocho (Vegetable,
    Roots, and Plantain Soup),
    154–155
navy beans
  Green Posole Seitan Stew with
    Chard and White Beans,
    137–138
  Hearty Pumpkin and Cranberry
    Bean Stew (Porotos
    Granados), 152–154
  Sancocho (Vegetable, Roots,
    and Plantain Soup), 154–155
nondairy milks, 10
nopales
  about, 125
  Pan-Grilled Vegetables in
    Chile-Lime Beer
    (variation), 124
nutritional yeast
  about, 11

Chorizo Seitan Sausages,
    36–37
Mashed Potato Pancakes
    with Peanut Sauce
    (Llapingachos), 57–58
Mexican Side-Street Corn
    (variation), 64
Peruvian Potatoes with Spicy
    "Cheezy" Sauce, 125–126
Steamed Red Seitan, 34–35
Steamed White Seitan, 35–36
nuts
  "Any Noche" Romaine and
    Fruit Salad with Candied
    Chile Peanuts, 73–75
  Buttery Cookies with Thick
    Dulce de Leche Filling
    (Alfajores), 241–242
  Cashew Crema, 51
  Chocolate-Chile Mole Sauce
    (an Oaxacan wannabe),
    51–53
  Creamy Horchata, 213–214
  Fruity Chile Slaw, 72
  Pine Nut Crema, 45
  Quinoa Salad with Spinach,
    Olives, and Roasted
    Peanuts, 82
  Spinach–Brazil Nut–Gazpacho
    Salad, 72
  Stuffed Mini Potatoes with
    Mushrooms and Olives
    (Papas Rellenas), 62–63
  Sweet and Nutty Roasted
    Stuffed Plantains, 117–118

Oil, Annatto-Infused (Aciete de
    Achiote), 31–32
okra, in Pan-Grilled Vegetables in
    Chile-Lime Beer, 124
olives
  Arroz con Seitan, 145–147
  Creamy Corn-Crusted Tempeh
    Pot Pie (Pastel de Choclo),
    144–145
  Peruvian Potatoes with Spicy
    "Cheezy" Sauce, 125–126

Puerto Rican "Picadillo" Style
    Seitan (variation), 108
Quinoa Salad with Spinach,
    Olives, and Roasted
    Peanuts, 82
Rice with Pigeon Peas
    (variation), 141
Shredded Seitan and
    Mushroom Empanadas with
    Raisins and Olives, 202–204
Stuffed Mini Potatoes with
    Mushrooms and Olives
    (Papas Rellenas), 62–63
Sweet and Spicy Seitan-Potato
    Empanadas (Bolivian
    Salteñas), 204–206
onions
  Basic Onion-Pepper Sofrito,
    32–33
  Green Onion Salsa, 44–45
  Onion-Flavored Beans (bean-
    cooking tip), 85–86
  Pickled Red Onions, 45
  Tomato Salad with Sweet Crisp
    Onions (Ensalada Chilena),
    76–77
Orange Flower–Agave "Honey,"
    Sopaipillas with, 226–227
oranges
  "Any Noche" Romaine and
    Fruit Salad with Candied
    Chile Peanuts, 73–75
  Fruity Chile Slaw, 72
  Mojo Oven-Roasted Seitan, 104
  Sangria, 219
  Savory Orange Rice, Brazilian
    Style, 98
  Zesty Orange Mojo Baked
    Tofu, 102

Pancakes, Mashed Potato, with
    Peanut Sauce
    (Llapingachos), 57–58
Pancakes, Savory Fresh Corn
    (Cachapas), 182–184
panela
  about, 12–13

Real Brown Sugar Limeade (Agua de Papelón), 214–215

Sweet and Nutty Roasted Stuffed Plantains, 117–118

Pan-fried Tempeh with Sofrito, 112–113

Pan-Grilled Vegetables in Chile-Lime Beer, 124

pantry items
basic staples, 7–10
dried herbs and spices, 21
Latin produce, 17–22
Latin staples, 12–17, 186
vegan staples, 10–12

Papas Rellenas (Stuffed Mini Potatoes with Mushrooms and Olives), 62–63

Papaya-Lime Sorbet, Fresh, 239

Papaya-Melon-Habanero Salsa, 53–54

Papelón, Agua de (Real Brown Sugar Limeade), 214–215

pupusas
fillings, 164
Pupusas Stuffed with Black Beans and Plantains, 162–165

Pastel de Choclo (Creamy Corn-Crusted Tempeh Pot Pie), 144–145

Patacones (Bite-Size Green Plantain Sandwiches), 65–66

peanut butter
Baked Tofu with Salsa de Mani (variation), 103
Creamy Potato Peanut Stew (Guatita), 138–140
Peanut Sauce (Salsa de Mani), 41–42

Peanuts, "Any Noche" Romaine and Fruit Salad with Candied Chile, 73–75

Peanuts, Roasted, Quinoa Salad with Spinach, Olives, and, 82

peas
Arroz con Seitan, 145–147

Chayote and Potato Salad with Capers and Peas, 75–76

Chocolate Mole Veggie Tamales, 193–194

Farmer's Market Tamales, 194–196

Sweet and Spicy Seitan-Potato Empanadas (Bolivian Salteñas), 204–206

Traditional Petits Pois Arepas (variation), 182

pecans, in Chocolate-Chile Mole Sauce (an Oaxacan wannabe), 51–53

pepitas
Green Posole Seitan Stew with Chard and White Beans, 137–138
Spicy Tortilla Casserole with Roasted Poblanos, 142–144

peppers. See also bell peppers
chiles, 15–18, 22
sweet, 19

Peruvian Potatoes with Spicy "Cheezy" Sauce, 125–126

Peruvian Red Chile–Corn Salad with Limas and Cherry Tomatoes, 80–81

Peruvian Seitan and Potato Skewers (Seitan Anticuchos), 104–106

Peruvian Seitan and Potato Stir-Fry (Seitan Saltado), 108–110

"Picadillo" Style Seitan, Puerto Rican (variation), 108

Pickled Red Onions, 45

pickles, in Cubano Vegano Sandwich, 66–67

pigeon peas (gandules)
frozen, 12, 22
Rice with Pigeon Peas (Arroz con Gandules), 140–142

Pimiento Peppers, Arepas Stuffed with Oyster Mushrooms and, 180–181

pimientos, in Rice with Pigeon Peas (variation), 141

pineapple
"Any Noche" Romaine and Fruit Salad with Candied Chile Peanuts, 73–75
Arroz con Coco (Savory Coconut Rice), 97
Coconut-Pineapple Tamales (variation), 197
Pineapple-Raisin Sweet Tamales, 196–197

Pine Nut Crema, 45

pink beans
Costa Rican Refried Rice and Beans (Gallo Pinto), 92–93
Home-style Refried Beans, 86–87

pinto beans
Chocolate Mole Veggie Tamales, 193–194
Drunken Beans with Seitan Chorizo, 91–92
Eggplant Torta Sandwich, 55–56
Home-style Refried Beans, 86–87
Quick Red Posole with Beans, 136–137

Pizza Pupusa, 164

plantains
about, 18
Beans, Rice, and Sweet Plantain Empanadas, 210–212
Bite-Size Green Plantain Sandwiches (Patacones), 65–66
Chocolate-Chile Mole Sauce (an Oaxacan wannabe), 51–53
Colombian-style Red Beans, 90
Crepes with Un-Dulce de Leche and Sweet Plantains, 228–230
Crispy Fried Green Plantains (Tostones), 118–120

plantains (*continued*)
Fried Sweet Plantains, 115–117
Mofongo, 120–121
Pupusas Stuffed with Black Beans and Plantains, 162–165
roasted, 118
Sancocho (Vegetable, Roots, and Plantain Soup), 154–155
Sweet and Nutty Roasted Stuffed Plantains, 117–118
to ripen, 116
Tostones with Avocado and Palm Ceviche, 61
Poblanos, Spicy Tortilla Casserole with Roasted, 142–144
Polenta, Amaranth, with Roasted Chiles, 128–129
pomegranate, in "Any Noche" Romaine and Fruit Salad with Candied Chile Peanuts (variation), 74
Porotos Granados (Hearty Pumpkin and Cranberry Bean Stew), 152–154
Portobello Feijoada (Brazilian Black Bean Stew with Portobello Mushrooms), 147–148
Posole, Quick Red, with Beans, 136–137
Posole Seitan Stew, Green, with Chard and White Beans, 137–138
potatoes
Chayote and Potato Salad with Capers and Peas, 75–76
Chipotle, Seitan, and Potato Tacos, 174–177
Chocolate Mole Veggie Tamales, 193–194
Corn-Crusted Pumpkin-Potato Empanadas, 207–210
Creamy Potato Peanut Stew (Guatita), 138–140
Creamy Potato Soup with Avocado (Locro), 149–150

Mashed Potato Pancakes with Peanut Sauce (Llapingachos), 57–58
Pastel de Choclo (Creamy Corn-Crusted Tempeh Pot Pie), 144–145
Peruvian Potatoes with Spicy "Cheezy" Sauce, 125–126
Peruvian Seitan and Potato Skewers (Seitan Anticuchos), 104–106
Potato-Chickpea Enchiladas with Green Tomatillo Sauce, 133–135
Potato-Kale Soup with Sizzling Chorizo, 159–160
Quinoa-Corn "Chowder" with Limas and Ají, 156–157
Seitan Saltado (Peruvian Seitan and Potato Stir-Fry), 108–110
Spicy Tortilla Casserole with Roasted Poblanos, 142–144
Stuffed Mini Potatoes with Mushrooms and Olives (Papas Rellenas), 62–63
Sweet and Spicy Seitan-Potato Empanadas (Bolivian Salteñas), 204–206
Sweet Potato–Chipotle Bisque, 155–156
Taquitos with Chorizo and Potatoes, 168–169
Tropical Pumpkin Soup, 158–159
Pot Pie, Creamy Corn-Crusted Tempeh (Pastel de Choclo), 144–145
puddings
Café con Leche Flan, 245–247
Fresh Mango and Guava Bread Pudín, 232–234
Simply Arroz con Leche, 234–235
Sweet Coconut Corn Pudding (Majarete), 235–236
Vanilla-Coconut Flan, 243–245

Puerto Rican "Picadillo" Style Seitan (variation), 108
pumpkin
Calabacitas (Mixed Squash Sauté), 122–123
Chocolate Mole Veggie Tamales, 193–194
Corn-Crusted Pumpkin-Potato Empanadas, 207–210
Hearty Pumpkin and Cranberry Bean Stew (Porotos Granados), 152–154
Rice with Pigeon Peas (variation), 141–142
Sancocho (Vegetable, Roots, and Plantain Soup), 154–155
Tropical Pumpkin Soup, 158–159
pumpkin seeds
Green Posole Seitan Stew with Chard and White Beans, 137–138
Spicy Tortilla Casserole with Roasted Poblanos, 142–144

Quick Red Posole with Beans, 136–137
Quinoa-Corn "Chowder" with Limas and Ají, 156–157
Quinoa–Oyster Mushroom Risotto (Quinotto), 130–131
Quinoa Salad with Spinach, Olives, and Roasted Peanuts, 82

raisins
Arroz con Coco (Savory Coconut Rice), 97
Chocolate-Chile Mole Sauce (an Oaxacan wannabe), 51–53
Fresh Mango and Guava Bread Pudín, 232–234
Pastel de Choclo (Creamy Corn-Crusted Tempeh Pot Pie), 144–145

Pineapple-Raisin Sweet
Tamales, 196–197
Shredded Seitan and
Mushroom Empanadas with
Raisins and Olives, 202–204
Simply Arroz con Leche,
234–235
Stuffed Mini Potatoes with
Mushrooms and Olives
(Papas Rellenas), 62–63
Sweet and Spicy Seitan-Potato
Empanadas (Bolivian
Salteñas), 204–206
Swiss Chard with Raisins and
Capers, 123
Real Brown Sugar Limeade (Agua
de Papelón), 214–215
Real Hot Chocolate and
Variations, 216–217
red beans
Colombian-style Red Beans, 90
Costa Rican Refried Rice and
Beans (Gallo Pinto), 92–93
Red Beans with Dominican-
style Sazón, 87–88
Red Chile Enchiladas
(variation), 135
Red Chile Sauce, 45–46
Red Chile–Seitan Tamales,
191–192
Red Onions, Pickled, 45
Red Seitan, Steamed, 34–35
Refried Beans, Home-style, 86–87
Refried Rice and Beans, Costa
Rican (Gallo Pinto), 92–93
rice
about, 8
Arroz con Coco (Savory
Coconut Rice), 97
Arroz con Leche de Coco
(variation), 235
Arroz con Leche with Saffron
(variation), 235
Arroz con Seitan, 145–147
Beans, Rice, and Sweet
Plantain Empanadas,
210–212

Brazilian-style White Rice
(variation), 98
brown rice, to substitute for
white rice, 95
Cilantro-Lime Rice, 95–96
Classic Stovetop Long-Grain
White or Brown Rice, 94–95
Costa Rican Refried Rice and
Beans (Gallo Pinto), 92–93
Creamy Horchata, 213–214
for burritos, 170–171
Rice with Pigeon Peas (Arroz
con Gandules), 140–142
Savory Orange Rice, Brazilian
Style, 98
Simply Arroz con Leche,
234–235
variations for stovetop rice, 95
Yellow Rice with Garlic, 96–97
Risotto, Quinoa–Oyster
Mushroom (Quinotto),
130–131
Roman beans
Hearty Pumpkin and Cranberry
Bean Stew (Porotos
Granados), 152–154
Red Beans with
Dominican-style Sazón,
87–88
"Ropa Vieja" Style Seitan, Cuban
(variation), 107

salad dressings
Chipotle in Adobo
(variation), 71
Cilantro-Citrus Vinaigrette,
69–70
Creamy Ancho Chile Dressing,
70–71
Fresh Gazpacho Salsa
Dressing, 70
salads
"Any Noche" Romaine and
Fruit Salad with Candied
Chile Peanuts, 73–75
Black Bean–Corn Salsa
Salad, 72

Chayote and Potato Salad with
Capers and Peas, 75–76
Chipotle Caesar Mexicano, 73
Classic Cabbage, 71–72
Fruity Chile Slaw, 72
Hearty Warm Yuca and
Cabbage Salad, 78–79
Mango-Jicama Chopped Salad,
77–78
Peruvian Red Chile–Corn
Salad with Limas and Cherry
Tomatoes, 80–81
Quinoa Salad with Spinach,
Olives, and Roasted
Peanuts, 82
Salvadorian Marinated Slaw
(Curdito), 79–80
Shredded Carrot-Jicama, 72–73
Spinach-Avocado-Chile
Salad, 72
Spinach–Brazil Nut–Gazpacho
Salad, 72
Tomato Salad with Sweet Crisp
Onions (Ensalada Chilena),
76–77
salsas and condiments
Cashew Crema, 51
Chimichurri Sauce with
Smoked Paprika, 42
Chocolate-Chile Mole Sauce
(an Oaxacan wannabe),
51–53
Classic Roasted Tomatillo
Salsa, 47–48
Creamy Avocado-Tomato Salsa
(Venezuelan Guasacaca),
39–40
Dried Chile Salsa
(variation), 50
Fresh Tomato Salsa with
Roasted Chiles, 50
Green Onion Salsa, 44–45
Green Tomatillo Sauce, 40–41
Habanero-Melon-Papaya Salsa,
53–54
Peanut Sauce (Salsa de Mani),
41–42

salsas and condiments *(continued)*
    Pickled Red Onions, 45
    Pine Nut Crema, 45
    Red Chile Sauce, 45–46
    salsa a la Huancaína (yellow cheese sauce), 125–126
    Simple Latin Tomato Sauce, 46–47
    So Good, So Green Dipping Sauce (Green Ají Sauce), 43–44
    Spicy Salsa Golf, 53
    The Only Guacamole Recipe I Ever Make, 48–49
    Winter Salsa (variation), 50
Saltado, Seitan (Peruvian Seitan and Potato Stir-Fry), 108–110
Salteñas, Bolivian (Sweet and Spicy Seitan-Potato Empanadas), 204–206
Salvadorian Marinated Slaw (Curdito), 79–80
Sancocho (Vegetable, Roots, and Plantain Soup), 154–155
sandwiches. *See* bocadillos, snacks, appetizers
Sangria, 219
sauces. *See* salsas and condiments
sausage. *See* chorizo
Savory Coconut Rice (Arroz con Coco), 97
Savory Fresh Corn Pancakes (Cachapas), 182–184
Savory Orange Rice, Brazilian Style, 98
Savory Vegan Masa Dough, 188–189
Sazón, Red Beans with Dominican-Style, 87–88
seitan. *See also* chorizo
    about, 11
    Arroz con Seitan, 145–147
    Bite-Size Green Plantain Sandwiches (Patacones), 65–66

Chipotle, Seitan, and Potato Tacos, 174–177
Chipotle Adobo Seitan (variation), 108
Chocolate Mole Veggie Tamales, 193–194
Creamy Potato Peanut Stew (variation), 140
Cubano Vegano Sandwich, 66–67
Cuban "Ropa Vieja" Style (variation), 107
for burritos, 170–171
Green Posole Seitan Stew with Chard and White Beans, 137–138
Latin Shredded Seitan, 106–108
Mexican Chile-Braised Seitan (variation), 107
Mojo Oven-Roasted Seitan, 104
pupusa fillings, 164
Peruvian Seitan and Potato Skewers (Seitan Anticuchos), 104–106
Portobello Feijoada (substitution tip), 147
Potato-Chickpea Enchiladas with Green Tomatillo Sauce (variation), 135
Puerto Rican "Picadillo" Style Seitan (variation), 108
Red Chile–Seitan Tamales, 191–192
Rice with Pigeon Peas (variation), 141–142
Sancocho (Vegetable, Roots, and Plantain Soup), 154–155
Seitan Saltado (Peruvian Seitan and Potato Stir-Fry), 108–110
Shredded Seitan and Mushroom Empanadas with Raisins and Olives, 202–204
Shredded Seitan Empanadas (variation), 212

Steamed Red Seitan, 34–35
Steamed White Seitan, 35–36
Sweet and Spicy Seitan-Potato Empanadas (Bolivian Salteñas), 204–206
Venezuelan "Mechada" Style (variation), 107
Sexy Avocado-Tempeh Filling, Arepas with (Avocado Pepiada Arepa), 181–182
Shake, Tropical Fruit (Batido), 215–216
Shredded Carrot-Jicama Salad, 72–73
Shredded Seitan and Mushroom Empanadas with Raisins and Olives, 202–204
side dishes
    Amaranth Polenta with Roasted Chiles, 128–129
    Braised Brazilian Shredded Kale, 121–122
    Calabacitas (Mixed Squash Sauté), 122–123
    Crispy Fried Green Plantains (Tostones), 118–120
    Crunchy Fried Yuca (Yuca Frita), 126–127
    Fried Sweet Plantains, 115–117
    Mofongo, 120–121
    Pan-Grilled Vegetables in Chile-Lime Beer, 124
    Peruvian Potatoes with Spicy "Cheezy" Sauce, 125–126
    Quinoa–Oyster Mushroom Risotto (Quinotto), 130–131
    Sweet and Nutty Roasted Stuffed Plantains, 117–118
    Swiss Chard with Raisins and Capers, 123
    Yuca with Cuban Garlic-Lime-Mojo Sauce, 127–128
Simple Latin Tomato Sauce, 46–47
Simple Syrup, 218
Simply Arroz con Leche, 234–235

Smoothie, Truly Tropical Banana
(variation), 216
snacks. *See* bocadillos, snacks,
appetizers
sofrito
Basic Onion-Pepper Sofrito,
32–33
Cuban Black Bean Soup
(shortcut tip), 150
Pan-fried Tempeh with Sofrito,
112–113
Sofrito con Ají (variation), 33
Sofrito con Cilantro and
Achiote (variation), 33
Sofrito con Tomate
(variation), 33
Tofu in Sofrito (variation), 103
So Good, So Green Dipping Sauce
(Green Ají Sauce), 43–44
Sopaipillas with Orange
Flower–Agave "Honey,"
226–227
Sopes, Chorizo-Spinach, 171–173
Sorbet, Fresh Papaya-Lime, 239
soups. *See also* stews and casseroles
Black Bean Soup Habanero
(variation), 152
Creamy Potato Soup with
Avocado (Locro), 149–150
Cuban Black Bean Soup,
150–152
Potato-Kale Soup with Sizzling
Chorizo, 159–160
Quinoa-Corn "Chowder" with
Limas and Ají, 156–157
Sancocho (Vegetable, Roots,
and Plantain Soup), 154–155
Sweet Potato–Chipotle Bisque,
155–156
Tropical Pumpkin Soup,
158–159
Soy Curls, in Creamy Potato
Peanut Stew (Guatita),
138–140
Spicy, Salty, Ice-Cold Beer
(Michelada), 220–221
Spicy Salsa Golf, 53

Spicy Tortilla Casserole with
Roasted Poblanos, 142–144
spinach
Chorizo-Spinach Sopes,
171–173
Quinoa Salad with Spinach,
Olives, and Roasted
Peanuts, 82
Spinach-Avocado-Chile
Salad, 72
Spinach–Brazil Nut–Gazpacho
Salad, 72
Spinach with Raisins and
Capers (variation), 123
squash, summer
Calabacitas (Mixed Squash
Sauté), 122–123
Calabacita Torta (variation), 57
Chayote and Potato Salad with
Capers and Peas, 75–76
Farmer's Market Tamales,
194–196
Pan-Grilled Vegetables in
Chile-Lime Beer, 124
pupusa fillings, 164
squash, winter
Black-Eyed–Butternut Tostadas,
173–174
Calabacitas (Mixed Squash
Sauté), 122–123
Chocolate Mole Veggie
Tamales, 193–194
Corn-Crusted Pumpkin-Potato
Empanadas, 207–210
Farmer's Market Tamales,
194–196
Hearty Pumpkin and Cranberry
Bean Stew (Porotos
Granados), 152–154
pupusa fillings, 164
Rice with Pigeon Peas
(variation), 141–142
Sancocho (Vegetable, Roots,
and Plantain Soup), 154–155
Tropical Pumpkin Soup,
158–159
Steamed Red Seitan, 34–35

Steamed White Seitan, 35–36
stews and casseroles
Creamy Corn-Crusted Tempeh
Pot Pie (Pastel de Choclo),
144–145
Creamy Potato Peanut Stew
(Guatita), 138–140
Green Posole Seitan Stew with
Chard and White Beans,
137–138
Hearty Pumpkin and Cranberry
Bean Stew (Porotos
Granados), 152–154
Portobello Feijoada (Brazilian
Black Bean Stew with
Portobello Mushrooms),
147–148
Potato-Chickpea Enchiladas
with Green Tomatillo Sauce,
133–135
Quick Red Posole with Beans,
136–137
Red Chile Enchiladas
(variation), 135
Rice with Pigeon Peas (Arroz
con Gandules), 140–142
Spicy Tortilla Casserole with
Roasted Poblanos, 142–144
Stovetop Long-Grain White or
Brown Rice, Classic, 94–95
strawberries, in "Any Noche"
Romaine and Fruit Salad
with Candied Chile Peanuts,
73–75
Stuffed Mini Potatoes with
Mushrooms and Olives
(Papas Rellenas), 62–63
summer squash. *See* squash,
summer
Sweet and Nutty Roasted Stuffed
Plantains, 117–118
Sweet and Spicy Seitan-Potato
Empanadas (Bolivian
Salteñas), 204–206
Sweet Coconut Corn Pudding
(Majarete), 235–236
Sweet Corn Ice Cream, 240

Sweet Plantains, Fried, 115–117
sweet potatoes
    Black Bean–Sweet Potato
        Tamales, 189–191
    Chipotle, Seitan, and Potato
        Tacos, 174–177
    Dulce de Batata (Sweet Potato
        Sweet Mash), 236–237
    Mixed Mushroom Ceviche,
        59–60
    Sweet Potato–Chipotle Bisque,
        155–156
Sweet Tamales, Pineapple-Raisin,
    196–197
Swiss Chard with Raisins and
    Capers, 123

Tacos, Chipotle, Seitan, and
    Potato, 174–177
taco toppings, 176
tamales
    Black Bean–Sweet Potato
        Tamales, 189–191
    Chocolate Mole Veggie
        Tamales, 193–194
    Coconut-Pineapple Tamales
        (variation), 197
    Farmer's Market Tamales,
        194–196
    Pineapple-Raisin Sweet
        Tamales, 196–197
    Red Chile–Seitan Tamales,
        191–192
    Savory Vegan Masa Dough for,
        188–189
    tips, 185–188, 193
tapas. See bocadillos, snacks,
    appetizers
Taquitos with Chorizo and
    Potatoes, 168–169
tempeh
    about, 11
    Ancho Chile–Tempeh Asado
        (variation), 111
    Arepas with Sexy Avocado-
        Tempeh Filling (Avocado
        Pepiada Arepa), 181–182

Creamy Corn-Crusted Tempeh
    Pot Pie (Pastel de Choclo),
    144–145
for burritos, 170–171
Pan-fried Tempeh with Sofrito,
    112–113
Tempeh Asado, 110–111
Tempeh Asado with
    Oaxacan-style Mole
    (variation), 111
to steam (tip), 110
Yellow Chile Grilled Tempeh
    (with Ají Amarillo),
    111–112
textured vegetable protein. See
    TVP
The Only Guacamole Recipe
    I Ever Make, 48–49
Thick Dulce de Leche Filling, 242
Toddy Caliente (variation), 217
tofu
    about, 10–11
    Baked Tofu with Salsa de Mani
        (variation), 103
    Bean and Tofu Chicharrones,
        164
    Chimichurri Baked Tofu,
        100–101
    Coconut Tres Leches Cake,
        230–232
    for burritos, 170–171
    Hearty Warm Yuca and
        Cabbage Salad, 78–79
    Latin Baked Tofu, 103
    Mofongo, 120–121
    Pine Nut Crema, 45
    Rice with Pigeon Peas
        (variation), 141–142
    Sweet Corn Ice Cream, 240
    Tofu Chicharrones, 101–102
    Tofu in Sofrito (variation), 103
    to press, 100
    Zesty Orange Mojo Baked
        Tofu, 102
tomatillos
    Classic Roasted Tomatillo
        Salsa, 47–48

Green Posole Seitan Stew with
    Chard and White Beans,
    137–138
Green Tomatillo Sauce,
    40–41
Potato-Chickpea Enchiladas
    with Green Tomatillo Sauce,
    133–135
tomatoes
    Creamy Avocado-Tomato Salsa
        (Venezuelan Guasacaca),
        39–40
    Fresh Gazpacho Salsa
        Dressing, 70
    Fresh Tomato Salsa with
        Roasted Chiles, 50
    Peruvian Red Chile–Corn
        Salad with Limas and Cherry
        Tomatoes, 80–81
    Simple Latin Tomato Sauce,
        46–47
    Sofrito con Tomate
        (variation), 33
    Tomato Salad with Sweet Crisp
        Onions (Ensalada Chilena),
        76–77
Torta, Calabacita (variation), 57
Torta Sandwich, Eggplant,
    55–57
Tortilla Casserole with Roasted
    Poblanos, Spicy, 142–144
tortilla chips, homemade, 174
Tortillas, Homemade Soft Corn,
    165–166
"Tortillas," Venezuelan- and
    Colombian-style (Arepas),
    177–179
Tortillas with Chia, Whole
    Wheat Flour, 166–168
Tostadas, Black-Eyed–Butternut,
    173–174
tostones
    Bite-Size Green Plantain
        Sandwiches (Patacones),
        65–66
    Crispy Fried Green Plantains
        (Tostones), 118–120

Mojo Sauce with Tostones (variation), 128

to crush, 119

Tostones with Avocado and Palm Ceviche, 61

Tres Leches Cake, Coconut, 230–232

Tropical Fruit Shake (Batido), 215–216

Tropical Pumpkin Soup, 158–159

Truly Tropical Banana Smoothie (variation), 216

TVP
about, 11–12
Creamy Potato Peanut Stew (Guatita), 138–140
Green Posole TVP Stew with Chard and White Beans (variation), 138
Portobello Feijoada (Brazilian Black Bean Stew with Portobello Mushrooms), 147–148
Sancocho (Vegetable, Roots, and Plantain Soup), 154–155

un-*dulce de leche*
Crepes with Un-Dulce de Leche and Sweet Plantains, 228–230
Un-Dulce de Leche, 227–228

Vanilla-Coconut Flan, 243–245

vegan cheese
Bite-Size Green Plantain Sandwiches (variation), 66
Colombian Grilled Arepas with Corn and Vegan Cheese, 179–180

Cubano Vegano Sandwich, 66–67

Mashed Potato Pancakes with Peanut Sauce (tip), 57–58

pupusa fillings, 164

Pupusas Stuffed with Black Beans and Plantains, 162–165

Savory Fresh Corn Pancakes (Cachapas), 182–184

Sweet and Nutty Roasted Stuffed Plantains, 117–118

Taquitos with Chorizo and Potatoes (variation), 169

vegan ham, in Cubano Vegano Sandwich, 66–67

vegetables. *See also specific types*
Pan-Grilled Vegetables in Chile-Lime Beer, 124
Vegetable, Roots, and Plantain Soup (Sancocho), 154–155
Veggie Suprema Pupusas, 164

Venezuelan- and Colombian-style "Tortillas" (Arepas), 177–179

Venezuelan Guasacaca (Creamy Avocado-Tomato Salsa), 39–40

Venezuelan "Mechada" Style Seitan (variation), 107

Venezuelan-style Black Beans (Caraotas), 89

vital wheat gluten
about, 11
Chorizo Seitan Sausages, 36–37
Steamed Red Seitan, 34–35
Steamed White Seitan, 35–36

walnuts
Stuffed Mini Potatoes with Mushrooms and Olives (Papas Rellenas), 62–63

Sweet and Nutty Roasted Stuffed Plantains, 117–118

Wheat Empanada Dough, 199–201

white beans
Green Posole Seitan Stew with Chard and White Beans, 137–138
Hearty Pumpkin and Cranberry Bean Stew (Porotos Granados), 152–154

White Seitan, Steamed, 35–36

Whole Wheat Flour Tortillas with Chia, 166–168

wine, in Sangria, 219

Winter Salsa (variation), 50

winter squash. *See* squash, winter

Yellow Chile Grilled Tempeh (with Ají Amarillo), 111–112

Yellow Rice with Garlic, 96–97

yuca
about, 18–19
Crunchy Fried Yuca (Yuca Frita), 126–127
Hearty Warm Yuca and Cabbage Salad, 78–79
Pastel de Choclo (Creamy Corn-Crusted Tempeh Pot Pie), 144–145
Sancocho (Vegetable, Roots, and Plantain Soup), 154–155
Yuca with Cuban Garlic-Lime-Mojo Sauce, 127–128

Zesty Orange Mojo Baked Tofu, 102

zucchini. *See* squash, summer